Qualitative Research in Nursing and Healthcare

Qualitative Research in Nursing and Healthcare

Immy Holloway

Faculty of Health and Social Sciences,
Bournemouth University, Poole, United Kingdom

Kathleen Galvin

School of Sport and Health Sciences,
University of Brighton, Brighton, United Kingdom

FIFTH EDITION

WILEY Blackwell

This edition first published 2024

Edition History
Blackwell Publishing Ltd. (1e, 1996 and 2e, 2002); Immy Holloway and Stephanie Wheeler (3e, 2010);
John Wiley & Sons, Ltd. (4e, 2017)

Registered Offices
John Wiley & Sons, Inc., 111 River Street, Hoboken, NJ 07030, USA
John Wiley & Sons Ltd, The Atrium, Southern Gate, Chichester, West Sussex, PO19 8SQ, UK

For details of our global editorial offices, customer services, and more information about Wiley products
visit us at www.wiley.com.

Wiley also publishes its books in a variety of electronic formats and by print-on-demand. Some content that
appears in standard print versions of this book may not be available in other formats.

Library of Congress Cataloguing-in-Publication Data applied for:
Paperback ISBN: 9781119630609

Cover Design: Wiley
Cover Image: © MirageC/M/omentGetty Images

Set in 9.5/13 MeridienLTStd by Straive, Pondicherry, India

Printed and bound by CPI Group (UK) Ltd, Croydon, CR0 4YY
C9781119630609_280324

Contents

Part Four: Data Analysis and Completion

16 Data Analysis: Strategies and Procedures, 281

Preface

The readership of this book will be those who intend to carry out qualitative research in clinical, academic or educational settings, specifically in the healthcare arena. It aims to introduce third-year undergraduates to qualitative research and to assist postgraduate students in their study of qualitative approaches before they move on to more sophisticated and specialised texts.

This fifth edition of the book is an update of earlier versions. Approaches in qualitative research are constantly evolving, and this is shown in the new edition. The fundamental principles of qualitative research, of course, stay the same, reflecting the firm epistemological ground on which this research approach stands; hence, there are not many drastic changes; the formula of writing and extending individual approaches with integrating updated examples from healthcare research has been retained.

Immy Holloway and Kathleen Galvin

About the Authors

Immy Holloway is Professor Emerita at Bournemouth University in the Faculty of Health and Social Sciences. She has extensively taught, supervised, researched and examined qualitative research and is the co-founder of the Centre for Qualitative Research at Bournemouth, she is still one of its members. Her activities include supervising and teaching postgraduate students in the area of nursing and healthcare. Her special interest lies in developing understanding and skills of students in using a variety of approaches to qualitative research. She has written several books in the field of qualitative inquiry and also published book chapters and articles in this area.

Kathleen Galvin is Professor of Nursing Practice at School of Sport and Health Sciences at the University of Brighton. She has also held positions of Associate Dean (Research, Scholarship and Enterprise) in the Faculty of Health and Social Care at the University of Hull and Deputy Dean, Research and Enterprise at the Bournemouth University and has been an active member of the Centre for Qualitative Research. She too has a portfolio of published articles, books and book chapters in the area of qualitative research and has supervised numerous postgraduate and PhD theses. She is particularly interested in the application of methodologies which can help the public to engage in a more embodied way with qualitative research findings, and in making use of the humanities and the arts in developing qualitative research for the purposes of new deep understanding of well-being and its absence.

Acknowledgement

We would like to thank the many postgraduate students we have worked with over the years for the engaging conversations we have enjoyed together. Without these discussions we could not have developed the book in varied directions. Thank you for the many ways in which you have helped us.

Part One

Introduction to Qualitative Research: Starting Out

Chapter 1

The Essentials of Qualitative Research

What is qualitative research?

Qualitative research is a form of social inquiry that focuses on the way people make sense of their experiences and the world in which they live. A number of different approaches exist within the wider framework of this type of research, and many of these share the same aim – to understand, describe and interpret social phenomena as perceived by individuals, groups and cultures. Researchers use qualitative approaches to explore the behaviour, feelings and experiences of people and what lies at the core of their lives. For example, ethnographers focus on culture and customs; grounded theorists investigate social processes and interaction, while phenomenologists consider and illuminate a phenomenon and describe the 'lifeworld' or *Lebenswelt*. Qualitative approaches are useful in the exploration of change or conflict. The basis of qualitative research lies in the interpretive approach to social reality and in the description of the lived experience of human beings.

KEY POINT

Qualitative research is exploratory, discovery orientated and evolving.

The characteristics of qualitative research

Different types of qualitative research share common features and use similar procedures though differences in data collection and analysis do exist.

The following elements are part of most qualitative approaches:

- The data have primacy; the theoretical framework is not predetermined but derive directly from the data.
- Qualitative research is context-bound, and researchers should be context sensitive.

Qualitative Research in Nursing and Healthcare, Fifth Edition.
Immy Holloway and Kathleen Galvin.
© 2024 John Wiley & Sons Ltd. Published 2024 by John Wiley & Sons Ltd.

- Researchers immerse themselves in the natural setting of the people whose situations, behaviours and thoughts they wish to explore.
- Qualitative researchers focus on the 'emic' perspective, the 'inside view' of the people involved in the research and their perceptions, meanings and interpretations.
- Qualitative researchers use 'thick description': they describe, analyse and interpret but also go beyond the reports, descriptions and constructions of the participants.
- The relationship between the researcher and the researched is close and based on a position of immersion in the field and equality as human beings.
- Reflexivity in the research makes explicit the stance of the researcher.

The primacy of data

Researchers usually approach people with the aim of finding out about their concerns; they go to the participants to collect the rich and in-depth data that can then become the basis for theorising. The interaction between the researcher and the participants leads to an understanding of experiences and the generation of concepts. The data themselves have primacy, they generate new theoretical ideas and they help modify already existing theories or uncover the essence of phenomena. It means that the research design cannot be predefined before the start of the research. In other types of research, assumptions and ideas lead to hypotheses which are tested (though this is not true for all quantitative research); sampling frames are imposed; in qualitative research, however, the data have priority. The theoretical framework of the research project is not predetermined but based on the incoming data. Although the researchers do have knowledge of some of the theories involved, the incoming data might confirm or contradict existing assumptions and theory.

This approach to social science is, initially at least, inductive. Researchers move from the specific to the general, from the data to theory or analytic description. They do not impose ideas or follow-up assumptions but give accounts of reality as seen by the participants. Researchers must be open-minded, though they cannot help having some 'hunches' about what they may find, especially if they are familiar with the setting and some of the literature on the topic.

While some qualitative inquiry is concerned with the generation of theory such as grounded theory, many researchers do not achieve this; others, such as phenomenologists, focus on a particular phenomenon to delineate, illuminate and describe it. All approaches provide descriptions or interpretation of participants' experiences – and the phenomenon to be studied, but researchers go to a more abstract and theoretical level in the written work, especially when they carry out postgraduate research. Qualitative inquiry is not static but developmental and dynamic in character; the focus is on process as well as outcomes. We recommend looking at general texts such as Aurini *et al.* (2021), Denzin and Lincoln (2023), Mason (2018) and Leavy (2020).

KEY POINT

In qualitative research the data have priority: researchers are led by the data.

Contextualisation

Researchers must be sensitive to the context of the research and therefore immerse themselves in the setting and situation. Both personal and social contexts of all the participants are important. When people enter a setting, they do not come as a 'tabula rasa'; for instance, in a clinical setting, patients and researchers might have particular religious or cultural beliefs, or personal perspectives on blood or pain, and that would affect their behaviour.

The context of participants' lives or work affects their behaviour, and therefore researchers have to realise that the participants are grounded in their history and temporality. Researchers take into account the total context of people's lives – including their own – and the broader political and social framework of the culture in which it takes place. Group or organizational affiliation might also influence the inquiry. The conditions in which researchers gather the data, the locality, time and history are all involved. Events and actions are studied as they occur in everyday 'real-life settings' and environments. It is important to respect the context and culture in which the study takes place. If researchers understand the context, they can locate the actions and perceptions of individuals and grasp the meanings that they communicate. The interest in context and contextualisation goes beyond that which influences the research; it also affects its outcomes and applications in the clinical situation. An example of contextualisation would be the effects of culture in a specific hospital on the actions and language of health professionals and researchers.

Immersion in the setting

Qualitative researchers use the strategies of observing, questioning and listening, immersing themselves in the 'real' world of the participants. Observing, listening to stories of participants and asking questions will lead to rich data. Involvement in the setting also assists in focusing on the interactions between people and the way they construct or change rules and situations. Qualitative inquiry can trace progress and development over time, as perceived by the participants.

For the understanding of participants' experiences, it is necessary to become familiar with their world which consists not only of physical space but also of culture, views and attitudes. Immersion might mean attending meetings with or about informants, becoming familiar with other similar situations, reading documents or observing interaction in the setting. This can even start before the formal data collection phase.

When professionals do research, they are often part of the setting they investigate and know it intimately. This might mean that they could miss important issues or considerations. To be able to better examine the world of the participant, researchers must not take this world for granted but should question their own assumptions and act like strangers to the setting or as 'naïve' observers. They 'make the familiar strange' (Delamont and Atkinson, 1995). This 'defamiliarisation' has its origin in the performative arts but cannot be taken too far, as the researcher is still involved with the participants and their world.

Most qualitative inquiry investigates patterns of interaction, seeks knowledge about a group or a culture or explores the lifeworld of individuals. In clinical, social care or educational settings, this may be interaction between professionals and clients or relatives, or interaction with colleagues. It also means listening to people and attempting to see the world from their point of view. The research can be a macro or micro study – for instance, it may take place in a hospital ward, a classroom, a residential home, a reception area or indeed the community. Immersion in the culture of a hospital or hospital ward, for instance, does not just mean getting to know the physical environment but also the particular ideologies, values and ways of thinking of its members. Researchers need sensitivity to describe or interpret what they observe and hear. Human beings are influenced by their experiences; therefore, qualitative methods encompass processes and changes over time in the culture or subculture under study.

The 'emic' perspective

Qualitative approaches are linked to the subjective nature of social reality; they provide insights from the perspective of participants, enabling researchers to see events as their informants do; they explore 'the insiders' view'. Anthropologists and linguists call this the *emic perspective* (Harris, 1976). The term was initially coined by the linguist Pike in 1954. It means that researchers attempt to examine the experiences, feelings and perceptions of the people they study, rather than immediately imposing a framework of their own that might distort the ideas of the participants. They 'uncover' the meaning people give to their experiences and the way in which they interpret them, although meanings should not be reduced to purely subjective accounts of the participants as researchers search for patterns in process and interaction or the invariant constituents of the phenomenon or phenomena they study. The term has gained wider use in qualitative research.

Qualitative research is based on the premise that individuals are best placed to describe situations and feelings in their own words. Of course, these meanings may be unclear or ambiguous and they are not fixed; the social world is not frozen in a particular moment or situation but dynamic and changing. By observing people and listening to their accounts, researchers seek to understand the process by which participants make sense of their own behaviour and the rules that govern their actions. Taking into account their informants' intentions and motives, researchers gain access to their social reality. Of course, the reports individuals give are *their* explanations of an event or action, but as the researcher wishes to find people's own definition of reality, these reports are valid data. Researchers cannot always rely on the participants' accounts but are able to take their words and actions as reflections of underlying meanings. The qualitative approach requires 'empathetic understanding', that is the investigators must try to examine the situations, events and actions from the participants' – the social actors' – point of view and not impose their own perspective. The meanings of participants are interpreted or a phenomenon identified and described. Researchers have access to the participants' world through experience and observation. This type of research is thought to empower participants, because they do not merely react to the questions of the researchers but have a voice and guide the study. For this reason, the people studied are generally called *participants* or *informants* rather than subjects. It is necessary that the relationship between researcher and informant is one of trust; this close relationship and the researcher's in-depth knowledge of the informant's situation make deceit unlikely (though not impossible).

Of course, researchers theorise or infer from observed behaviour or participants' words. The researcher's view, the analytical and more abstract interpretation and description, is the *etic perspective* – the outsider's view (Harris, 1976). Researchers move back and forth between the emic perspective of the participants and their own etic view, and the process of research is iterative. The two terms 'emic' and 'etic' show the difference between 'lay language' and 'academic language'. It must be kept in mind, however, that the emic view cannot be simply translated into an etic perspective but demands analysis and reflection from the researcher.

Thick description

Immersion in the setting will help researchers use *thick description* (Geertz, 1973; first used by the philosopher Gilbert Ryle). It involves detailed portrayals of the participants' experiences, going beyond a report of surface phenomena to their interpretations, uncovering feelings and the meanings of their actions. This also means that researchers create and produce another layer constructed from that of the participants. Thick description develops from the data and context.

The task involves describing the location and the people within it, giving visual pictures of settings, events and situations as well as individuals' accounts of their perceptions and ideas in context.

The description of the situation or discussion should be thorough; this means that writers describe everything in vivid detail. Indeed Denzin (1989: 83) defines thick description as 'deep, dense, detailed accounts of problematic experiences ... It presents detail, context, emotion and the webs of social relationship that join persons to one another'. Thick description is not merely factual but also includes theoretical and analytic description. Thick description describes human behaviour in context.

Thick description helps readers of a research study to develop an active role in the research because the researchers share their knowledge of the participants' perspective with the readers of the study. Through clear description of the culture, the context and the process of the research, the reader can follow the path of the researcher and share some understanding of the phenomenon or the culture under study. Thick description not only shows readers of the story what they themselves would experience were they in the same situation as the participants, but it also generates theoretical and abstract ideas which the researcher has developed.

Ponterotto (2006) develops the concept of 'thick description', traces its evolution and stresses the importance of context. He states that the discussion of a qualitative research report 'successfully merges the participants' lived experiences with the interpretations of these experiences ...' (p. 547).

The research relationship

In order to gain access to the true thoughts and feelings of the participants, researchers adopt a non-judgemental stance towards the thoughts and words of the participants. The relationship should be built on mutual trust. This is particularly important in interviews and observations. The listener becomes the learner in this situation, while the informant is the teacher who is also encouraged to be reflective. Rapport does not automatically imply an intimate relationship or deep friendship (Spradley, 1979), but it does lead to negotiation and sharing of ideas, although each relationship is unique in the context of time and place. Rapport and trust make the research more interesting for the participants because they feel free to ask questions. Negotiation is not a once and for all event but a continuous process, indeed Boulton (2007: 2191) speaks of social science relationships as 'more enduring, negotiated and equal'. In qualitative inquiry, the participants have more power because they can guide the researcher to issues that are of concern for them. Miller and Boulton (2007: 2200) state that the relationship between participants is one of continuously shifting boundaries between the professional and the personal.

The researcher should answer questions about the nature of the project as honestly and openly as possible without creating bias in the study.

Insider/outsider research

Closely connected to this topic is the issue of insider/outsider perspectives. The insider perspective is one when the researcher is part of the specific subculture that he or she is studying; a health visitor might study the role of other health visitors, a clinical psychologist the perception of others in the profession and a surgeon the experience of other surgeons. Suzy Hansford (2019), a psychotherapist, for instance, explored the use of language and communication between counsellors and their clients. Researchers' own experience becomes a resource and source of knowledge. This position has both advantages and disadvantages. On the one hand, it can give greater insights as the group is already known to the researcher and some of its obvious rules and roles are familiar and need not be explained by the participants, who might disclose more to a colleague. On the other hand, the researchers might have preconceptions and close their minds to the meanings of others in their subculture and are not able to take the necessary distance from the research which might prevent the generation of new knowledge. Blythe *et al.* (2013) describe some of the issues in the insider perspective. They declare the main challenges as assumed understanding, ensuring analytic objectivity and the problem of managing the participants' expectations. Jenny Roddis, while working as an administrator, carried out outsider research of people with thrombophilia and diabetes. (An article was published in 2019.)

Even as an insider, the researcher might take the stance of a 'person from Mars' to fully explore the ideas of the participants and not take the way they would make sense of the situation as a given. In any case, many insider researchers differ from participants in some characteristics such as age, gender, ethnic group or belief. Thus, the researcher's position is always located on a continuum between an outsider and an insider.

Reflexivity

Reflexivity is critical reflection on what has been thought and done in a qualitative research project. It locates the researcher in the research project. Finlay (2002: 531) names reflexivity as the process 'where researchers engage in explicit, self-aware analysis of their own role'. It is a conscious attempt by researchers to acknowledge their own involvement in the study – a form of self-monitoring in relation to the research that is being carried out. It also includes awareness of the interaction between the researcher, the participants and the research itself and it takes into account how the process of the research affects findings and eventual outcomes.

According to Etherington (2004) 'critical subjectivity' means adopting a critical stance to oneself as researcher. Personal response and thoughts about the research and research participants are taken into account, and researchers are aware and take stock of their own social location and how this affects the study. Indeed, Etherington (2017) speaks of different layers of personal experience. Bott (2010) stresses the importance for researchers to 'constantly locating and relocating themselves in their work' (p. 160). This is of major importance in health research where researchers often have been socialised into professional ways of thinking. Although they do not take centre stage in the research, they have a significant place in its process during collection and interpretation of data as well as in the relationship they have with participants and with the readers of their research. The researchers' own standpoint and values shape the research, and this needs to be made explicit in qualitative inquiry. Researchers should be aware of and uncover their own preconceptions and assumptions while attempting to understand the effect they have on the data and be conscious of both structural and subjective elements in their research. The researcher is part of the research but also the conditions and problems which are encountered and the context in which it occurs; all these become a focus for reflexivity. In other words, reflexivity is a critical reflection not only on the researcher's place in the inquiry but also on the epistemological process of producing knowledge. Thus, the concept of reflexivity is concerned with the awareness of socially located and constituted knowledge.

The concept of reflexivity fits into a wider discussion on ontology and epistemology (Berger, 2015). It examines the role of the self in the generation and construction of knowledge. The researchers need to examine their own location in the research, their assumptions and presuppositions – especially when carrying out insider research. Reflexivity assists in acting ethically and sensitively, without bias. Palaganas *et al.* (2017) call reflexivity an 'elusive concept'. It is not a magical cure-all (Day, 2012), nor is it easy to achieve. It takes place on a personal level as it is not only to do with the researchers' background and their feelings and how to cope with them.

Dangers are inherent in reflexivity even on the simplest level: the researchers might take self-reference too far, and some qualitative writers are prone to this (in popular language it is often called navel gazing) by constantly focusing on their own feelings rather than those of 'the other'. The voice of the participants and the illumination of the phenomenon under study should have priority. Nevertheless, *the researcher is the main research instrument*; they decide what constitutes data and where the focus should be located; researchers analyse the data and determine how to illuminate the phenomenon under study. They also write the research report and choose what to include and exclude. The term 'researcher as main tool' in qualitative inquiry, however, has been criticised by writers: it suggests objectification and distances researchers from the participants.

The place of theory in qualitative research

What place has theory in qualitative research? Theory is a framework or set of statements about concepts that are related to each other and useful for understanding the phenomena under study. Morgan (2018) explains theory as 'links between a set of key concepts'. Novice researchers sometimes believe that they do not need theories in the beginning of their research because qualitative inquiry is inductive, that is, it goes from the specific and unique cases to the general and hence develops theory or theories. Indeed, many qualitative approaches explicitly develop theory, such as grounded theory, and theorising prior to the study is not encouraged. However, the inductive nature and the lack of a hypothesis in the beginning of research do not mean that no existing theories are needed or used in the research. For instance, a colleague might research ethnic differences in professional education. Data from interviews have primacy. This means that the theories of culture, ethnicity and social interaction are part of the framework of the research, regardless of the data obtained and the theory developed. To give an example: in chronic illness, theories of identity or gender might be important. Existing theory illuminates the findings (Reeves *et al.*, 2008) and might even be modified through these. Researchers also need some knowledge about the related literature on major theoretical concepts which could be important for the research. Health researchers often present atheoretical studies. For practical purposes in an empirical context these are useful and acceptable, but not enough in an academic project.

Creswell and Creswell (2018) ascribe a place to theory and calls it a general 'orientating lens' through which the research can be seen. It helps researchers to formulate the research question and – eventually – locate their own research inside or outside an existing framework. In addition to the theories already mentioned, there are many pre-existing social theories, such as feminist theory, critical theory, symbolic interactionism and so on, and any of these might explain the standpoint of the researcher. Too much theory in the beginning of the research, however, might generate preconceptions and assumptions rather than leaving the researchers with an open mind and freedom to develop their own theoretical ideas.

The use of qualitative research in healthcare

Qualitative researchers adopt a person-centred and holistic perspective. The approach helps develop an understanding of human experiences, which is important for health professionals who focus on caring, communication and interaction. Through this perspective, nurses and other health researchers gain knowledge and insight about human beings – be they patients, colleagues or other professionals. They generate in-depth accounts that present a lively picture of the participants' reality. The focus is on human beings within their social and cultural context, not just on specific clinical conditions or professional and educational tasks. Qualitative health research is in tune with the nature of the phenomena examined; emotions, perceptions and actions are qualitative experiences.

The essence of work in the field of healthcare contains elements of commitment and patience, understanding and trust, give and take, flexibility and openness (Paterson and Zderad, 1988). These traits mirror those of qualitative inquiry. Indeed, flexibility and openness are as essential in qualitative study as they are in the tasks of the health worker. In the clinical arena too, health professionals often have to backtrack as they do in research, return to the situation and try something new, because the situation is constantly evolving.

Health professionals, in particular midwives and nurses, have long recognised that individuals are human beings and not just body parts (or 'diagnostic cases', a phrase Leininger used in 1985) of qualitative health research, and therefore the inquiry must focus on the whole. The researcher, taking a holistic view, observes people in their natural environment, and the researcher–participant relationship is also based on trust and openness. Both professional caring and qualitative research depend on this and knowledge of the social context. The settings in which individuals live or stay for a time, the social support they have and the people with whom they interact have a powerful effect on their lives as well as on health and illness.

In-built ethical issues exist in both caring and qualitative research. Health researchers are ethically bound to act in the interest of clients or participants in the setting and to empower them to make autonomous decisions. This does not mean that conventional forms of inquiry have no ethical basis; however, the closer relationships forged in qualitative research require even more focus on ethical values and empathy with the participants.

In their assessment, health professionals use inductive thinking but also make deductions before coming to conclusions, piecing together the full picture of the patient's or client's condition from specific observations and individual pieces of information. Listening carefully and asking relevant questions without being judgemental enable them to gain insights into problems and a deeper understanding of the people with whom they interact. Qualitative research, too, proceeds from collecting specific data to more general conclusions.

There are many uses and applications of qualitative inquiry for health researchers and reasons why it is helpful in clinical or educational settings. In the social and political arena, it can reveal the perspectives of the policymakers in health services and organisations as well as examine strategies for development. More importantly, however, qualitative research can explore the cultural, social and uniquely personal aspects of living with illness, pain and disability. While studying how people make sense of their experience and suffering, nurses and other health researchers also gain their perspectives on care and treatment and are able to evaluate management and self-management of illness and health from both the professional and client perspectives. In professional education too, qualitative inquiry can be a useful tool to study the thoughts and ideas of both teachers and students.

In uncovering motivations, values and expectations, health researchers translate the findings of research to clinical practice. Kuper *et al.* (2008) argue that this research helps health professionals in the understanding of clinical issues; for instance, reasons for adhering to or abandoning medical commendations can be elicited.

There are many more cases where qualitative inquiry can be of use. Sandelowski (2004: 1368) summarises the topics and utilisation of qualitative research which can be helpful to examine the following:

- The social constructions of illness, prevention, treatment and risk
- Experiencing and managing the effects of disease and its treatment
- Decision-making around the areas of birth, dying and potential technological interventions
- Factors affecting the quality of care either positively or negatively, linked to access to care, promotion of good health and prevention of disease and the reduction of inequalities

Indeed, she suggests that other researchers too now use some of the language which started in qualitative inquiry. Evidence-based practice, which is meant to include the best evidence on which to develop patient care, has generally meant the evaluation and utilisation of evidence from the field of randomised controlled trials. However, it has recently been recognised that qualitative research too can contribute to the evidence base (Newman *et al.*, 2006) and indeed add to practical knowledge which is valued highly because of its applicability to the clinical setting. Sandelowski confirms the recent return to emphasis on the 'primacy of the practical' over pure knowledge, and the latter could be translated into utilisation in professional practice.

> **KEY POINT**
>
> Qualitative research is about 'meaning, not measurement'.

Choosing an approach for health research

Adopting approaches because researchers find them easy or interesting is not an appropriate way of doing research. Methodology and procedures depend on the following:

- The nature and type of the research question or problem
- The epistemological stance of the researcher

- The capabilities and knowledge of the researcher
- Skills and training of the researcher
- The resources available for the research project

Researchers do have to think of the practicalities of the research such as their own competence and interest, the scope and time of the research and available funds and resources, all factors that influence the undertaking of a project. A qualitative methodology is generally applied in healthcare settings when the focus is on 'what it is like,' 'what goes on', perceptions, experience and thoughts, change and conflict.

Researchers do have a variety of choices on the approach to adopt. Holloway and Todrew (2003: 355) advise health researchers to consider carefully the research question, including the phenomenon to be studied, and the type of knowledge which they seek. Once they have chosen their approach, they need to study it with care and get to know it in detail, even though they might eventually diverge from some of its more rigid elements.

If researchers wish to study a specific phenomenon or the lifeworld of the participants, they might take a *phenomenological approach*, usually through interviewing participants. For instance, a researcher might interview new fathers or mothers about the phenomenon of becoming a parent.

A *grounded theory* method would generate theory directly from the data; although it can be used in any field of qualitative health research, it often focuses on interaction and has interviewing and/or participant observation as its main data collection procedures; a researcher might observe the interaction between hospital consultants and patients or doctors and nurses. After observation, the researcher might interview the people who were observed about these interactions.

In *narrative analysis*, for instance, the researcher will ask for a first-hand account of insiders who are asked for their experiences; for instance, they might narrate the story about living with multiple sclerosis or chronic pain. *Ethnographers* study the culture or subculture of a particular group in which they have an interest. The culture of midwifery teachers or that of orthopaedic nursing might be explored through observation and interviews. Of course, the preceding are not the only approaches, but each has a distinct focus and theoretical base or framework. These are some examples that could be or have been investigated.

References

Aurini, J., Heath, M. and Howells, S. (2022) *The How to of Qualitative Research*, Sage, London.

Berger, R. (2015) Now I see it, now I don't: researcher's position and reflexivity in qualitative research. *Qualitative Research*, **15** (2), 219–234.

Blythe, S., Wilkes, L., Jackson, D. and Halcomb, E. (2013) The challenges of being an insider in storytelling research. *Nurse Researcher*, **21** (1), 8–13.

Bott, E. (2010) Favourites and others: reflexivity and the shaping of subjectivities and data in qualitative research. *Qualitative Research*, **10** (2), 968–975.

Boulton, M. (2007) Informed consent in a changing environment. *Social Science and Medicine*, **65** (11), 2187–2198.

Creswell, J.W. and Creswell J.D. (2018) *Research Design: Qualitative, Quantitative and Mixed Methods Approaches*, 5th edn, Sage, Los Angeles, CA.

Day, S. (2012) A reflexive lens: exploring dilemmas of qualitative methodology through the concept of reflexivity. *Qualitative Sociology Review*, **8** (1), 60–85.

Delamont, S. and Atkinson, P. (1995) *Fighting Familiarity: Essays on Education and Ethnography*, Hampton Press, Cresskill, NJ.

Denzin, N.K. (1989) *Interpretive Interactionism*, Sage, Newbury Park, CA.

Denzin, N.K. and Lincoln, Y.S. (2023) *The Sage Handbook of Qualitative Research*, 6th edn, Kindle Edition Sage, Thousand Oaks, CA.

Etherington, K. (2004) *Becoming a Reflexive Researcher: Using Our Selves in Research*, Jessica Kingley, London.

Etherington, K. (2017) Personal experience and critical reflexivity in counselling and psychotherapy research. *Counselling and Psychotherapy Research*, **17** (2), 85–94.

Finlay, L. (2002) Outing the researcher: the provenance, process and practice of reflection. *Qualitative Health Research*, **12** (4), 531–545.

Geertz, C. (1973) *The Interpretation of Cultures*, Basic Books, New York, NY.

Hansford, S. (2019) Seeing new landscapes, or having new eyes; How does the meaning we make from language impact on the therapeutic relationship in counselling and psychotherapy? Unpublished thesis, Leeds University PhD thesis, University of Leeds.

Harris, M. (1976) History and significance of the emic/etic distinction. *Annual Review of Anthropology*, **5**, 329–350.

Holloway, I. and Todrew, L. (2003) The status of method: flexibility, consistency and coherence. *Qualitative Research*, **3** (3), 345–357.

Kuper, A., Reeves, S. and Levinson, W. (2008) An introduction to reading and appraising qualitative research. *British Medical Journal*, **337**, a288.

Leavy, P. (ed.) (2020) *The Oxford Handbook of Qualitative Research*, OUP, Oxford.

Leininger, M. (1985) *Qualitative Research Methods in Nursing*, Grune & Stratton, Orlando, FL.

Mason, J. (2018) *Qualitative Researching*, Sage, London.

Miller, T. and Boulton, M. (2007) Changing constructions of informed consent: qualitative research and complex social worlds. *Social Science and Medicine*, **65** (11), 2199–2211.

Morgan, D.L. (2018) Themes, theories and models. *Qualitative Health Research*, **28** (3), 339–345.

Newman, M., Thompson, C. and Roberts, A.P. (2006) Helping practitioners to understand the contribution of qualitative research to evidence-based practice, *Human Behaviour*, Summer Institute of Linguistics, Glendale, CA.

Palaganas, E.C., Sanchez, M.C., Molintas, M.P. and Caricativo, R.D. (2017). Reflexivity in qualitative research: a journey of learning. *The Qualitative Report*, **22** (2), 426–438. Available at http://nsuworks.nova.edu/tqr/vol22/iss2/5.

Paterson, J.G. and Zderad, L.T. (1988) *Humanistic Nursing*. New edn. National League for Nursing, New York, NY.

Ponterotto, J.G. (2006) Brief note on the origins, evolution and meaning of the qualitative research concept 'thick description'. *The Qualitative Report*, **11** (3), 538–549. Available at http://www.nova.edu/ssss/QR/QR11-3/ponterotto.pdf.

Reeves, S., Albert, M., Kuper, A. and Hodges, B.D. (2008) Why use theories in qualitative research? *British Medical Journal*, **33** (7), 94.

Roddis, J.K., Holloway, I., Galvin, K. and Bond, C. (2019) Acquiring knowledge prior to diagnosis. *Patient Experience Journal*, **6** (1), 10–18.

Sandelowski, M. (2004) Using qualitative research. *Qualitative Health Research*, **14** (10), 1366–1386.

Spradley, J.P. (1979) *The Ethnographic Interview*, Harcourt Brace Johanovich College Publishers, Fort Worth, TX.

Further Reading

Finlay, F. (2017) Championing 'reflexivities'. *Qualitative Psychology*, **4** (2), 120–125.

Gair, S. (2012) Feeling their stories: contemplating empathy, insider/outsider positioning, and enriching qualitative research. *Qualitative Health Research*, **23** (1), 124–143.

Hammarberg, K., Kirkman, M. and de Lacey, S. (2016) Qualitative methods: when to use them and how to judge them. *Human Reproduction*, **31** (3), 498–501.

Holloway, I. and Biley, F. (2011) Being a qualitative researcher. *Qualitative Health Research*, **21** (7), 968–975.

Chapter 2

The Paradigm Debate: The Place of Qualitative Research

Most experienced qualitative health researchers are acquainted with the common arguments surrounding the paradigm debate. The qualitative research field has evolved and is complex to such an extent that many methodologists now dismiss the unhelpful term about the 'paradigm wars' from the 1980s. Understanding the nature of qualitative evidence and the epistemological issues underpinning this debate is however vital. For novice qualitative researchers, it is useful to rehearse at least some of these arguments and give an (admittedly simple) overview of the issues, as was offered in previous editions.

Theoretical frameworks and ontological position

Social inquiry can be approached in several different ways, and researchers will have to select between varieties of approaches. Whilst often making a choice on practical grounds, they must also understand the theoretical and philosophical ideas on which the research is based.

Approaches to social inquiry consist not only of the procedures of sampling, data collection and analysis, but they are rooted in particular ideas about the world and the nature of knowledge which sometimes reflect conflicting and competing views about social reality. Some of these positions towards the social world are concerned with the very nature of reality and existence (*ontology*) (for a helpful explanation, see Ormston *et al.* (2014)). From this, basic assumptions about knowledge arise: *epistemology* is the theory of knowledge and is concerned with the question of what counts as valid knowledge. *Methodology* refers to the principles and ideas on which researchers base their procedures and strategies (*methods*). To assist in understanding the background to the interpretive/descriptive approach to research, the following section will describe epistemological and methodological ideas about the rise and development of qualitative research. (See the very accessible discussion in the book by Willis (2007), chapters 1 and 2 in particular.)

Qualitative Research in Nursing and Healthcare, Fifth Edition.
Immy Holloway and Kathleen Galvin.
© 2024 John Wiley & Sons Ltd. Published 2024 by John Wiley & Sons Ltd.

Conflict and tension between different schools of social science have been in existence for a long time. Several sets of assumptions underlie social research; in their most basic form, they describe the dichotomy between quantitative and qualitative research or positivism and interpretivism. In the early days of positivism, the focus was on the methods of natural science that became a model for the social sciences such as psychology and sociology. Interpretivists stressed that human beings differ from the material world and the distinction between humans and matter should be reflected in the methods of investigation. Much social research developed from these ideas. Qualitative research was critical of the natural science model and a reaction against its tenets. Researchers held a 'separatist' position and believed the world views of qualitative and quantitative researchers to be incompatible. Many researchers, particularly those who advocate mixed methods research, would now disagree (see chapter on mixed methods).

Social scientists continue to raise the paradigm debate, but have for a long time stressed that simplistic polarisation between positivist and qualitative inquiry will not do. For example, Atkinson (1995), in particular, criticised the use of the concept of the term *paradigm* and the 'paradigm mentality'. Health researchers, too, historically accused their professions of unwarranted 'paradigmatic thinking' and emphasised that it restricts rather than extends knowledge (see Thorne *et al.*, 1999). Nevertheless, qualitative researchers are still defensive of their methodology and tend to develop arguments against other approaches. Indeed, they occasionally do that of which they accuse quantitative researchers and sometimes seem to be absolutist in their statements and uncritical of their own approach.

The natural science model: positivism, objectivism and value neutrality

From the nineteenth century onwards, the traditional and favoured approaches to social and behavioural research were quantitative. Quantitative research has its root in the positivist and early natural science model that has influenced social science throughout the nineteenth and the first half of the twentieth century. The description that follows here is core to the debate.

Positivism was an approach to science based on a belief in universal laws and attempts to present an objective picture of the world. Positivists followed the natural science approach by testing theories and hypotheses. The methods of natural – in particular physical – science stem from the seventeenth, eighteenth and nineteenth centuries. Comte (1798–1857), the French philosopher who created the terms 'positivism' and 'sociology', suggested that the emerging social sciences must proceed in the same way as natural science by adopting natural science research methods.

One of the traits of this type of research is the quest for objectivity and distance between researcher and those studied so that biases can be avoided. Investigators searched for patterns and regularities and believed that universal laws and rules, or law-like generalities, exist for human action. Behaviour could be predicted, so they believed, on the basis of these laws. Researchers thought that findings would and should be generalisable to all similar situations and settings. Even today many researchers think that numerical measurement, statistical analysis and the search for cause and effect lie at the heart of much research, and of course, that is so. Not many researchers now feel, however, that detachment and objectivity are possible, and that only numerical measurement results in objective knowledge. In the positivist approach, researchers control the theoretical framework, sampling frames and the structure of the research. This type of research seeks causal relationships and focuses on prediction and control.

Popper (1959) claimed falsifiability as the main criterion of science. The researcher formulates a hypothesis – an expected outcome – and tests it. Scientists refute or falsify hypotheses. When a deviant case is found, the hypothesis is falsified. Knowledge is always provisional because new incoming data may contradict it. (There has been criticism of Popper's ideas but the debate cannot be developed here. It is discussed in philosophy of science texts.)

The positivist approach develops from a theoretical perspective, and a hypothesis is often, although not always, established before the research begins. The model of science adopted is hypothetico-deductive; it moves from the general to the specific, and its main aim is to test theory. The danger of this approach is that researchers sometimes treat perceptions of the social world as objective or absolute and neglect everyday subjective interpretations and the context of the research.

Nineteenth-century positivists believed that scientific knowledge can be proven and is discovered by rigorous methods of observation and experiments, and derived through the senses. However, this is a simplistic view of science and there has been a major change. Even natural scientists – for instance biologists and physicists – do not necessarily agree on what science is and adopt a variety of different scientific approaches and use inductive methods as well as deduction. Social scientists, too, use a number of approaches and differ in their understandings about the nature of science. Scientific knowledge is difficult to prove.

The search for objectivity may be futile for all scientists. They can strive for it, but their own biases and experiences intrude. Science, whether natural or social science, cannot be 'value free', that is, it cannot be fully objective as the values and background of the researchers affect the research.

The paradigm debate

In the 1960s, the traditional view of science was criticised for its aims and methods by both natural and social scientists. The new and different evolutionary stance taken within disciplines such as biology and psychology had gone beyond the simplistic positivist approach.

The thinking of Kuhn (1962, 1970) has had great impact on the paradigm debate. 'Normal science', with its community of scholars, he asserts, proceeds through a series of crises that hinder its development. Earlier methods of science are questioned and new ways adopted; certain theoretical and philosophical pre-suppositions are replaced by another set of assumptions taking precedence over the model from the past. Eventually, one scientific view of the world is replaced by another. Although Kuhn wrote about the physical sciences and was a natural scientist, later writers have used his work to draw analogies with the shift in the ideas of social science. Kuhn's (1962: 162) definition of paradigm is an 'entire constellation of beliefs, values, techniques, and so on, shared by the members of a given community'.

Thus, a paradigm consists of theoretical ideas and technical procedures that a group of scientists adopt and which are rooted in a particular world view with its own language and terminology. Kuhn's ideas have been extensively criticised (Fuller, 2000), but the critique cannot be developed here.

Qualitative social researchers often claim that a 'paradigm shift' in social science has occurred – in the same way in which Kuhn discussed it – that a whole world view is linked to the new paradigm. They attack the positivist stance for its emphasis on social reality as being 'out there', separate from the individual, and maintain that an objective reality, independent of the people they study, is difficult to grasp.

Quantitative research, in all its variations, is useful and valuable, but it is sometimes seen as limited by qualitative researchers, because it neglects the participants' perspectives within the context of their lives. Lather (2004) reminds researchers, that the shift to qualitative approaches in the 1970s was partly due to the difficulties of measurement and the 'limits of causal models'. (Although she speaks of education in particular, her ideas can also be applied to health research.)

The controlled conditions of traditional approaches sometimes limit practical applications. This type of research does not always or easily answer complex questions about the nature of the human condition. Researchers using these approaches are not inherently concerned about human interaction or feelings, thoughts and perceptions of people in their research but with facts, measurable behaviour and cause and effect; of course both types of research are necessary.

KEY POINT

Qualitative and quantitative methodologies in research are of equal importance, but researchers ask different questions on selection of suitable methods coherent to each approach and therefore generate different kinds of answers.

It must not be forgotten that natural scientists, too, have criticised the often mechanistic natural science view of the world which in the view of many researchers, including many natural scientists, is at least to some extent socially constructed and defined. Indeed, one could argue that there has not been a 'scientific revolution' with a new paradigm. Over two decades ago, many, such as Atkinson (1995) and Thorne *et al.* (1999), challenged the notion of paradigm shift and suggested that the debate is an oversimplification of complex issues. This debate remains and permeates many healthcare fields. In addition, public health interventions have raised important questions recently within all these complexities (for example Greenhalgh *et al.*, 2020).

The interpretive/descriptive approach

The interpretive or interpretivist model and descriptive research (descriptive phenomenologists would point to complexity in their approach in relation to the general meaning interpretive) have their roots in philosophy and the human sciences, particularly in history, philosophy and anthropology. The methodology centres on the way in which human beings make sense of their subjective and shared reality and attach meaning to it. Social scientists view people not as individual entities who exist in a vacuum but explore their world within the whole of their life context. Researchers with this world view believe that understanding human experiences is as important as focusing on explanation, prediction and control. The interpretive/descriptive model has a long history, from its roots in the nineteenth century and Dilthey's philosophy, Max Weber's sociology and George Herbert Mead's social psychology.

The interpretivist view can be linked to Weber's *Verstehen* approach. Philosophers and historians such as Dilthey (1833–1911) and Windelband (1848–1915) considered that the social sciences need not imitate the natural sciences; they should instead emphasise empathetic understanding. Understanding in the social sciences is inherently different from explanation in the natural sciences. Weber (1864–1920) was well aware of the two approaches that existed in the nineteenth century. The concept of *Verstehen* – understanding something in its context – has elements of empathy, not in the psychological sense as intuitive and nonconscious feeling, but as reflective reconstruction and interpretation of the action of others. Weber believed that social scientists should be concerned with the interpretive understanding of human beings. He claimed that meaning could be found in the intentions and goals of the individual.

Weber argued that *understanding* in the social sciences is inherently different from *explanation* in the natural sciences, and he differentiates between the nomothetic, rule-governed methods of the latter and idiographic methods that are not related to general laws and rules but to the actions of human beings. This was linked to the *Methodenstreit* – the conflict between methods – which historians and philosophers had discussed in the nineteenth century. Weber believed that numerically measured probability is quantitative only, and he wanted to stress that social science concerns itself with the qualitative. We should treat the people we study, he advised, 'as if they were human beings' and try to gain access to their experiences and perceptions by listening to them and observing them. Weber did not have a direct impact on early qualitative researchers (Platt, 1985), nor did he discuss qualitative inquiry as we now understand it, but he influenced sociologists in particular, and his ideas have helped shape the qualitative perspective. Sociologists developed further the interpretive perspective that initially stemmed from the writings of Mead, Weber, Schütz and others in the early twentieth century; grounded theory as well as some other approaches acknowledge these influences.

Phenomenology as a qualitative research approach is based on philosophy, particularly continental philosophy, in the nineteenth and early twentieth centuries too, starting with Dilthey, but in particular on the ideas of the mathematician and philosopher Husserl (1859–1938) and the philosopher Heidegger (1889–1976) who focused on ontological questions of meaning, being and what is sometimes termed lived experience. The phenomenologically oriented theoretical framework has developed through time and includes the work of other philosophers. In practical terms it has benefited from the work of psychologists and sociologists. Qualitative researchers claim that the experiences of people and other phenomena are essentially context-bound, that is, they cannot be free from time and location or the mind of the human actor. Researchers are urged to grasp the socially constructed nature of the world and realise that values and interests become part of the research process. Complete objectivity and neutrality are impossible to achieve; the values of all participants become an integral part of the research. Researchers are not divorced from the phenomenon under study (Mantzoukas, 2004). This means reflexivity on their part; they must take into account their own position in the setting and situation, as the researcher is the main research tool. Language itself is context-bound and depends on the researchers' and informants' values as well as their social location (see also Chapter 1). Detailed replication or duplication of a piece of research is impossible because the research relationship, history and location of participants differ from study to study.

Qualitative methodology is not completely precise, because human beings do not always act logically or predictably. Indeed, many writers argue that those who cannot bear ambiguity should not attempt this type of research. Investigators using a qualitative lens turn to the human participants for guidance, control and direction throughout the research. Structure and order are, of course, important for the research to be scientific. The social world, however, is not orderly or systematic; therefore, it is all the more important that the researcher proceeds in a well-structured and systematic way.

Focus on postmodernism and social constructionism

In recent years, qualitative researchers have stressed two related influences on qualitative research, those of postmodernism and social constructionism. Postmodernism is not a unitary concept but a set of ideas rooted in philosophy and sociology, and it also permeates recent literature, music and visual arts, and in particular, architecture. Postmodernists are critical of the traditionalist values of society and stress the plurality of beliefs. Questioning the existence of objectivity and neutrality in research, they believe that much depends on the presenter's and audience's stance and location. They suggest that much which people consider as facts is relative and subjective. Research is bound to the local context and is valid only in relation to our own time and community (Cahoone, 2003).

Postmodernism challenges traditional knowledge, and in qualitative research it stresses the multiplicity of perspectives and lack of a unitary view of truth. Postmodernist researchers are anti-foundationalist, which means they believe that there is no absolute and universal knowledge and truth; indeed, knowledge is provisional and uncertain (Willis, 2007) and there are often a variety of alternative explanations for a phenomenon.

Postmodernism and social constructionism (or similarly constructivism) are closely related. Social constructionists argue that the so-called social reality is a product of social processes; it is tied and relative to context, time and culture; human beings construct it themselves (see Charmaz, 2013). It is believed that the participants, the researcher and the reader together construct the research; in this way research is produced by social interaction. Holstein and Gubrium (2008), however, refute in the introduction to their book that constructionism and qualitative research are synonymous, and not all this type of inquiry can be labelled social constructionist.

Critical theory is another basis of some qualitative research approaches such as critical ethnography and critical discourse analysis. The critical approach takes account of power and inequalities in society and has its roots in Marxist and neo-Marxist thought. Proponents are Habermas (b. 1929) and the members of the 'Frankfurt School' (desiring social change after the Second World War) who point to oppressive relationships in society. Researchers who base their inquiry on critical theory take account of these unequal relationships and aim their research at empowerment of those whose voices cannot be heard (Willis, 2007). Critical theorists want to change existing inequalities through their research.

It can be seen that qualitative research in some form can be involved in a variety of different approaches, but it usually includes in-depth ways of exploring the world and perspectives of the participants and the investigation and description of a phenomenon seen from the viewpoint of a group or individuals (Ormston et al., 2014).

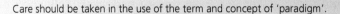

KEY POINT

Care should be taken in the use of the term and concept of 'paradigm'.

Conflicting or complementary perspectives?

Some social scientists believe that qualitative and quantitative approaches are merely different methods of research to be used pragmatically, dependent on the research question (Bryman, 2012). Others decide that they are incompatible and mutually exclusive on the basis of their different epistemologies (Lincoln and Guba, 1985; Leininger, 1992; Denzin and Lincoln, 2018). Researchers sometimes carry out one or the other, depending on their own epistemological stance, or they use both. Silverman (2011) and many others argue that neither school is better or more valid than the other, and that an emphasis on the polarities does not result in a useful debate as both are valid approaches.

Many sociologists, psychologists and health professionals work in the quantitative tradition. In much of health, education and social work, however, the qualitative perspective has been in the ascendant for some decades, in particular in nursing. One might suggest that qualitative research is a coherent way of researching human thought, perception and behaviour (not new or unilinear, but developed to answer different questions from those of traditional approaches).

The positivist and the interpretive/descriptive models of social research have their roots in different assumptions about social reality. While early positivism is based on the belief that reality has existence outside and is independent of individuals, those who adopt new approaches to research claim that *social* reality is constructed and is not independent from the people creating it, although they usually do acknowledge that there is a reality 'out there'. Not only qualitative researchers hold this view, many quantitative researchers also believe this.

Oakley (2000) has claimed that qualitative researchers sometimes use the term 'positivism' as a form of abuse. She criticises this and those researchers who neglect experimental and other forms of quantitative research. She asserts that both qualitative and quantitative approaches have a place. In any case, the terms are not absolute, as numbers are often used in qualitative research, and quantitative inquiry includes elements of quality. Also, research, whether quantitative or qualitative, can be presented in a positivist or non-positivist frame, aim or direction. Crotty (1998: 41) suggests '. . . it is a matter of positivism vs. nonpositivism, not a matter of qualitative vs. quantitative'. Methodological debates often suffer from oversimplification.

Bryman (2012) suggests that qualitative research became popular initially because of dissatisfaction with quantitative research. The latter could not, in the view of many researchers, answer the important questions in which they were interested. In qualitative health research, the 'voices' of patients and clients are heard, and feelings and experiences can be grasped. Although there are distinct differences between the major methodological approaches, many argue against their polarisation. Ercikan and Roth (2006) reiterate the view of these and claim that the dichotomy between qualitative and quantitative research is meaningless: the phenomena under investigation have both qualitative and quantitative features.

Qualitative research is often seen as subjective and quantitative as objective and neutral. In research, however, subjectivity and objectivity are at the end of a continuum – qualitative inquiry is at the more subjective end, while quantitative research has some subjective features but attempts to be more objective. There is neither total objectivity nor complete subjectivity in either approach.

The two approaches should not be seen as dichotomous, although of course they are different.

Final comment

To add to the confusion and ambiguity of the paradigm debate, many researchers see other types of research such as those based on critical theory or mixed methods research as separate 'paradigms'. The term 'paradigm' though over-used, is still seen as a valid concept in methodology (Morgan, 2007). There are many philosophical and epistemological directions which have had an impact on qualitative research; there is no space for all these in this text. Qualitative researchers choose a variety of approaches and procedures to achieve their aims. These include ethnography, grounded theory, phenomenology, narrative research, conversation analysis, discourse analysis and others. Some forms of social inquiry such as action research, ethnography and feminist approaches often use qualitative methods and techniques but sometimes include quantitative strategies.

Regardless of the epistemological stance or perspective of the researchers who carry out this type of inquiry, however, they must at least appreciate some of the important issues which might affect qualitative research. This includes knowledge of the paradigm dialogue and the philosophical and theoretical ideas which have had an influence on qualitative research.

References

Atkinson, P. (1995) Some perils of paradigms. *Qualitative Health Research*, **5** (1), 117–124.
Bryman, A. (2012) *Social Research Methods*, 4th edn, Oxford University Press, Oxford.
Cahoone, L. (ed.) (2003) *From Modernism to Postmodernism: An Anthology*, Blackwell, Malden, MA.
Charmaz, K. (2013) *Constructing Grounded Theory*, 2nd edn, Sage, Thousand Oaks, CA.

Crotty, M. (1998) *The Foundations of Social Research: Meaning and Perspective in the Research Process*, Sage, London.

Denzin, N.K. and Lincoln, Y.S. (eds.) (2018) *SAGE Handbook of Qualitative Research*, 5th edn, Sage, Thousand Oaks, CA.

Ercikan, K. and Roth, W.M. (2006) What good is polarisation between qualitative and quantitative research? *Educational Researcher*, **35** (5), 13–23.

Fuller, S. (2000) *Thomas Kuhn: A Philosophical History for Our Times*, University of Chicago Press, Chicago, IL.

Greenhalgh, T., Schmid, M.B., Czypionka, T. *et al.* (2020) Face masks for the public during the covid-19 crisis. *BMJ*, **369**, m1435. doi:10.1136/bmj.m1435.

Holstein, J.A. and Gubrium, J.F. (eds.) (2008) *Handbook of Constructionist Research*, Guilford Publications, New York, NY.

Kuhn, T.S. (1962) *The Structure of Scientific Revolutions*. Chicago, University of Chicago Press.

Kuhn, T.S. (1970) *The Structure of Scientific Revolutions*, 2nd edn (first edition 1960), University of Chicago Press, Chicago, IL.

Lather, P. (2004) This is your father's paradigm: government intrusion and the case of qualitative research. *Qualitative Inquiry*, **10** (1), 15–34.

Leininger, M. (1992) Current issues, problems, and trends to advance qualitative paradigmatic research methods for the future. *Qualitative Health Research*, **2**, 392–415.

Lincoln, Y.S. and Guba, E.G. (1985) *Naturalistic Inquiry*, Sage, Beverly Hills, CA.

Mantzoukas, S. (2004) Issues of representation within qualitative inquiry. *Qualitative Health Research*, **14** (7), 924–1007.

Morgan, D. (2007) Paradigms lost and pragmatism regained: methodological implications of combining qualitative and quantitative methods. *Journal of Mixed Methods Research*, **1** (1), 48–76.

Oakley, A. (2000) *Experiments in Knowing: Gender and Method in the Social Sciences*, Polity Press, Cambridge.

Ormston, R., Spencer, L., Barnard, M. and Snape, D. (2014) The foundations of qualitative research, in *Qualitative Research Practice* (eds. J. Ritchie, J. Lewis, C. McNaughton Nicholls and R. Ormston), SAGE Publications Ltd., pp. 1–25.

Platt, J. (1985) Weber's Verstehen and the history of qualitative research: the missing link. *British Journal of Sociology*, **36**, 448–466.

Popper, K. (1959) *The Logic of Scientific Discovery*, Routledge & Kegan Paul, London.

Silverman, D. (2011) *Interpreting Qualitative Data*, 5th edn, Sage, London.

Thorne, S.E., Kirkham, S.R. and Henderson, A. (1999) Ideological implications of the paradigm discourse. *Nursing Inquiry*, **4**, 1–2.

Willis, J.W. (2007) *Foundations of Qualitative Research*, Sage, Thousand Oaks, CA.

Further Reading

Maxwell, J.A. (2012) *Qualitative Research Design: An Interactive Approach*, 3rd edn, Sage, Thousand Oaks, CA.

Ravitch, M. and Mittenfelner Carl, N. (2016) *Qualitative Research: Bridging the Theoretical, Conceptual and Methodological*, Sage, Thousand Oaks, CA.

Most textbooks on qualitative research contain chapters on these issues. A very clear article discussing the paradigm debate for a health worker readership is the following: Weaver, K. and Olsen, J. (2006) Understanding paradigms used for nursing research. *Journal of Advanced Nursing*, **53** (4), 459–469.

Chapter 3
Initial Steps in the Research Process

At the start of their journey, researchers engage in a process of selecting the research topic and defining the research question. The overall approach, the research design and the chosen methods should be appropriate to the topic and the research question. Qualitative researchers use a specific terminology and base their work on distinctive principles, often dissimilar from other types of research, and this is reflected in the way they design their project. The initial phase is important as it sets the scene for the progress of the research. The choices at each subsequent stage must be coherent with this early phase. Qualitative inquiry is chosen for a research question where little is known about the specific topic, and where the context is complex and perhaps 'hard to reach' or fraught with sensitive issues. It is important that researchers do not base their work on assumptions or preconceived ideas (see Holloway and Brown, 2012, chapter 2).

Selecting and formulating the research question

The first step in the process is the selection of the research area, topic and question. Although the terms are often used interchangeably, Punch (2016) believes that they are a hierarchy of concepts with different levels of abstraction. The research area is more general than the research question. The research question, which is based on a perceived problem or concern, is about an issue or topic that researchers examine to gain new information. The topic, according to Clancy (2013) (quoted from the book by Layder published the same year) should be 'specific, concrete and empirical'. The research question differs from data collection questions, which are at the lowest level of abstraction. The latter are the steps to gather data in order to answer the research question. The conclusions of any study are intended to answer the research question in relation to its aim. The question should be explicit as well as meaningful and coherent (Mantzoukas, 2008).

An *area* of research may be 'living with … (a chronic condition), or 'experiencing a mental health problem'. A *topic* would be a more specific aspect of the area, for instance, 'old people's experience of chronic pain' or 'living with

Qualitative Research in Nursing and Healthcare, Fifth Edition.
Immy Holloway and Kathleen Galvin.

rheumatoid arthritis and its effect on identity'. The *research question* or *problem* might be phrased: 'How do old people experience and manage pain?' or 'Chronic illness in young manual workers and changes in self-perception'. A *data collection question* is much more specific, such as 'How did you feel when you had that asthma attack?' or 'Tell me how you coped with your pain?' These are *not* research questions but interview questions.

Clancy again quotes Layder (2013) and points to some of the context in which small scale research – which is generally qualitative – is carried out. The environment and interactions with others influence the participant's identity, feelings and thoughts. The setting itself and group affiliation affects behaviour, actions and interactions. Time and power too are important factors that have an impact on all those involved in research.

Nurses and other health researchers often notice problems in their work setting which they feel need investigation so that solutions or remedies for unsatisfactory situations or behaviour may be found. Sometimes the topic emerges from the literature linked to a particular area of professional work where gaps in knowledge can be identified. Nursing/midwifery and other health research studies contribute to existing knowledge and enhance understanding of the area under investigation. Knowledge and understanding of an issue are not always enough, however; health professionals also seek solutions to problems in the clinical setting hence the aim of their qualitative research is sometimes followed by 'in order to …', for instance, 'the aim of this research is to explore the experience of first-time mothers' breastfeeding in order to help them in their endeavour'. Clinical or practical research can indeed be seen as 'actions in response to problems' (a term used by Jacobs (2013)).

Personal observation and experience, as well as discussion with others, guide individuals towards the topic for research though they must be careful not to let their own presuppositions direct the research. Events and interactions often provide an interest or a puzzle and generate the wish to know more. The research question is a statement about what they want to find out and stems directly from a problem experienced in the clinical area or in their personal and professional lives. Holliday (2016) argues that research questions develop during the process of the research; they vary on a continuum from the broader and more general to the very specific, and they might change during the course of the study. This rarely happens in quantitative research. Many health researchers, of course, have a question from the beginning of the study based on their clinical work.

It is important that the problem is related to professional work; for instance, if nurses are working in the field of elderly care, it would be inappropriate (though not wrong) for them to undertake a project with children, however much it might attract their interest (unless they use theoretical sampling – see Chapter 9). A nurse in a ward for confused elderly people who had worried about accidents and falls might explore nurses' perspectives on the care of old people and the problems involved in their care. A midwife who notices the difficulties and barriers that some women experience when they wish to breastfeed might use this as an area of investigation.

Certain criteria should be considered when identifying a research problem:

- The question must be researchable.
- The topic must be relevant and appropriate.
- The work must be feasible within the allocated time span and resources.
- The research should be of interest to the researcher.

The question must be researchable

Health researchers are often confronted with an important ethical or philosophical dilemma that cannot be solved through research. A moral or philosophical question is not researchable; for instance, the question of whether nurses or doctors should become involved in euthanasia is answerable only in philosophical but not in research terms.

Although the research problem need not be a practical one, it must nevertheless result in findings and outcomes. Research could not answer the question whether health professionals 'should' use euthanasia, but the topic of nurses' perceptions of euthanasia would be researchable. 'Do' and 'should' questions are difficult to answer. 'Do new mothers have feelings of inadequacy?' would become 'What are the feelings of new mothers about coping with their babies?' to transform it into a research question. The following are examples of researchable questions and topics.

Example 3.1 Researchable Questions and Topics

Interactions between nurses and elderly people in residential care.
What is it like to experience psychosis?
Mothers' feelings and thoughts on the birth of their first child.
Physiotherapists' communication with patients.
How do people manage their chronic conditions?
Nurses' and doctors' perceptions of their complementary roles.
(These questions would be more specific in the design of a study.)

The topic should be relevant and appropriate

Relevance means that the research is linked to problems or improvements in practice, professional issues, clinical and social settings or the education of health professionals. The question might also be important for people who use services, patients or clients, the health professions or for society in general, and the answer will advance practice, and contribute to new theoretical perspectives in nursing and healthcare knowledge. The results should be applicable to practice, education or management, legitimising existing practices or leading the way towards change.

The work must be feasible

Health professionals are sometimes overambitious, especially if they are new to research. Rather than reflecting on the time the study may take and some of the detailed procedures and the complexity of analysis, they want to start the study straight away, before they have a thorough knowledge of methodology. Learning about methodology should be one of the first steps in research. It is important at each stage to reflect on the methodology and personal resources that will be needed to complete the research, including time.

Time can become a problem in qualitative research because it is eaten up by transcribing, coding and categorising data. A simple, small-scale study using a well-documented research strategy is far less time-consuming than a complex piece of triangulation. It is better to deliver a small-scale, in depth, insightful study well, rather than try to deliver something that is overambitious and may not be completed or achieve any new insights.

The research should be feasible in terms of resources and accessibility of participants, and researchers should identify whose resources will be used. The topic might be inappropriate because of major ethical and access problems which cannot be overcome, such as superiors not giving permission to do the research, or patients' vulnerability. The research should also be feasible in terms of participant numbers or availability. Last but not least, it must be within the researcher's knowledge and capability and the time frame available.

The research should be of interest to the researcher

If the topic is interesting, it can stimulate and motivate rather than generate boredom during the course of the study, and it can be sustained only if the researcher is fully involved. The storyline of the project is not merely controlled by the participants but it reflects the interest of the researcher. Occasionally, we find that a superior or tutor suggests a topic to a novice researcher; it is not often that the latter is as enthusiastic about it as about a topic they chose themselves. If the suggestion cannot be declined, the researchers, however, can make it their own study by changing some of the details or directions.

The selection of the focus takes time, reflection and discussion with others who have knowledge in the field of study. Students in particular should discuss the focus of their work with their tutors and supervisors. All too often, new researchers in qualitative research choose a question that is designed to deal with factual issues and needs a survey rather than a qualitative approach.

Quantitative researchers focus on a very specific area and plan every detail before the start of the study, while qualitative researchers initially formulate the question in more general terms and develop and focus it during the research process. Qualitative researchers generally begin with a broad question and become more specific in the process of the research, responding to what they hear and find in the setting (progressive focusing). The research design is evolutionary rather than strictly pre-defined. This needs flexibility and open-mindedness on the part of researchers.

Example 3.2 Qualitative or Quantitative?

A specialist nurse decides to find out details of charities helping people with thrombophilia in the United Kingdom. She decides to obtain information about accessibility of these services and to find out detailed information about the assistance they provide. This study would not lend itself to qualitative research but a survey would need to be carried out. However, if the researcher wishes to explore the perspectives of these people on the help some specific charities provide, how they accessed help, whether it was useful or not and the barriers to help, a qualitative study with interviews about the topic might be appropriate.

Example 3.3 Qualitative or Quantitative?

A nurse practitioner aims to find out how men feel about and manage the symptoms of prostate cancer and what it means in everyday life. The researcher decides to develop a theory about how different stages in the journey through the condition and a cancer diagnosis influence the perceptions of individuals. The initial findings show that many individuals just want to live 'a normal life' and disregard their symptoms of cancer until they need expert treatment. The researcher could then follow up the idea of 'the wish to lead a normal life' with patients who have other cancers and discover a typology of individuals who have achieved 'normalisation' and those who have not done so.

Practical issues

Beginners, such as undergraduate students, might undertake a simple study suitable to show that they understand the research process and can produce a valid and useful project. We advise novice researchers not to carry out research involving patients except in exceptional circumstances, for instance if they have long nursing experience, special expertise in their field and expert supervision. For inexperienced researchers, it is particularly important to be clear and straightforward. The clearer the question, the clearer and more useful is the outcome of the study.

The research design and choice of approach

The research design needs to be appropriate for the chosen topic and research question. The design of the study depends entirely on the topic to be studied and on developing the research question. There is of course no reason why researchers may not choose to develop a qualitative research project but the method must fit the problem or question. If the researchers are interested in generating theories, they would use a grounded theory approach. If they are examining a culture, subculture or group, they might carry out an ethnographic study. Phenomenological research, as well as narrative inquiry, demands a deeper understanding of individuals and their lifeworld. (See specific approaches in later chapters.)

The literature review

After identifying the research question, investigators review the important literature consisting of the information published and closely related to the area of the project, including both *primary* and *secondary* sources. Primary sources are produced by researchers who developed original work on a subject or researched this topic. For the researcher this means searching for the topic area in research and academic journals and books. Secondary information consists of reports, summaries or references to original work originating from a person other than the researcher. Library catalogues and online data bases are useful locations for research in the general area of the researcher's topic; Hansen (2020) adds government reports and conferences to the list of places for finding relevant literature. The literature reviewed before the start of the inquiry and during the process would include foundational early texts and up-to-date references. The literature search involves searching databases and journals which are of relevance for the topic area. Bold (2012: 34) identifies similar sources, including policy documentation, popular media as well as practice-based and research-based literature that enhance both practical and theoretical understanding.

Researchers review the literature for the following reasons at the beginning:

- To find out what is already known about the subject and acknowledge those who have worked in this area.
- To identify gaps in knowledge.
- To describe how the study contributes to existing knowledge of a topic area.
- To avoid duplicating other people's work.
- To assist in defining the research question.
- To place their research in the context of other studies.
- To show that they have reflected on the research question.

Punch (2016) points out the specific importance of certain aspects:

1 The identification of the literature relevant to the topic.
2 The relationship of the literature to the proposed study.
3 The way the researcher uses the literature in the research.

Through reading reports (articles and books) researchers can identify what knowledge about the subject of their study already exists, the way in which it was generated and the methods that were adopted. They may find a large number of studies on the particular topic and decide to avoid it, not wishing to focus on issues that others have thoroughly examined at an earlier stage. There is little justification for researchers to keep to their original research question if the topic has already been addressed exhaustively and adequately elsewhere. However, the literature sometimes points to problems within the subject area that have not yet been investigated.

Example 3.4 Literature Informs the Knowledge Gap

A physiotherapist might be interested in the experiences of elderly people (over 65 years) about their management of chronic pain. He decides that the focus of this research should be on their interaction with health professionals. However, on searching the literature on this topic, he might find that a large number of studies exist on the perspectives of elderly people with chronic pain, but nobody has investigated the interaction of health professionals with people over 80 years who have chronic pain. The final aim of the project then could be 'to explore the interaction of physiotherapists and elderly people over 80 years with chronic pain'.

A simple description of the literature is not enough. It must be critically reviewed and evaluated, even in the initial literature review; researchers appraise others' work within the context of what they themselves intend to do and where their study fits into the broader understanding of the research area. Aveyard (2019: 14) stresses the importance of 'identifying, critiquing and synthesizing' the appropriate literature.

The use of literature in qualitative research

Although the literature review is not extensive in a qualitative proposal, researchers need to know from the beginning how other writers' work is used in a piece of qualitative research; they also must be aware that the initial literature review is not necessarily exhaustive, its purpose is to make a case for the research question and to delineate the research. The use of literature in qualitative research and the form of the literature review are contentious. However, the key principle is that the researcher should be sensitised by what is already known in the field but this does not preclude an inductive, discovery-oriented approach. Therefore, the literature does not direct the study since researchers initially take an inductive approach. We suggest that qualitative researchers use the heading: 'the initial literature review' and make explicit from the beginning that the review is an ongoing process.

There is a long-standing debate about the place of the literature in qualitative research. We know that in quantitative studies researchers read the literature about a topic area and give a detailed evaluative report in the literature review before they start the fieldwork. In the early days of qualitative investigations, researchers were encouraged to start without a literature review so that they would not be directed in their research, as it was believed that a detailed review would invalidate the qualitative research study; indeed, Glaser (2004 and on YouTube 2010) strongly advises against any type of literature review on the specific topic in the beginning of the study, and advocates instead a wider view which includes the areas around a study rather than specifically addressing the particular topic area. This treatment of the literature has been criticized since. The trawl and search for literature should be carried out, because an answer to the question may already exist in the public domain. In any case, researchers' minds are not a *tabula rasa*, a blank sheet, especially not when they are already experienced professionals. Although it is inappropriate to start with a fully developed theoretical model and an in-depth literature review, it is dangerous to start without any prior ideas of what has already been done in the field. The introductory literature review (or overview) should not be seen to direct the research. However, as Haverkamp and Young (2007) point out, the literature review for a research project is not about the knowledge researchers already possess, but how they make use of what they know while carrying out a study.

Researchers do not start the qualitative study with a rigid framework, hypotheses or fully developed theories for their research. In this type of research, a flexible conceptual framework is necessary, as the study is linked to other research and ideas about the topic. For instance, one of our students researched a specific topic in which gender and class were important aspects. His theoretical position on gender and class were developed from the beginning and formed a framework within which his study proceeded.

As suggested earlier, an overview of the literature often takes place prior to the study, but the literature search and review proceeds throughout. The literature might even become another source for data in the main body of the study, where it is guided by the findings and emerging themes of the researcher. The researchers compare or contrast their own findings with those of other studies and engage in an active debate and dialogue with the literature. This happens throughout the study. Metcalfe (2003) advises researchers that previous authors should be treated as 'experts' or authorities in the field in much the same way that witnesses are called to court to give evidence. The researcher must make a case for calling on the work of these authors and show that they have credibility. Hence, it is not necessary to quote each single piece of research that has ever been done; it suffices if credible experts have been consulted in each major area of the research. Their studies and writing are to confirm or challenge (disconfirm) the findings and the argument that the researcher has established, indeed, they form 'building blocks' for the argument. The publications chosen, however, must demonstrate that the researcher does not show only one single point of view but has presented a balanced choice. Of course, this means that quantitative publications should also be perused.

Often, a category or construct which researchers discover and develop is reflected in other disciplines or areas of knowledge. Ideas about the emerging concepts can then be followed up in the literature. A look at the nursing or health literature does not always suffice; psychological, educational or sociological literature might also be useful.

The literature will become integrated at a later stage. As data collection and analysis proceed at the same time in many qualitative approaches, there is an ongoing process of searching the literature that is linked to the findings in the data. Qualitative researchers have an ongoing dialogue with the literature related to their themes, categories or constructs.

Practicalities

Hart (2018) outlines some ideas for the literature review which would be relevant also for qualitative inquiry:

- The collection of background information.
- A map of the literature related to the topic.
- A search of the relevant sources.
- Build up early bibliographies.
- A critical evaluation of the literature

Other steps to be done could be suggested: Many researchers summarise research studies from the literature and the major concepts involved on cards that they file alphabetically from the beginning of their research. This way they can access the ideas and topic areas more quickly when they want them at a later stage.

Novice researchers often take an uncritical stance to the literature, but it is important to evaluate critically rather than merely describe. If factual claims are made in the introduction or literature review (for instance, 'Recent research has shown …' or 'Midwife researchers suggest …'), they must be substantiated with names and dates; evidence should be given. Sometimes older foundational texts are used; reasons for the inclusion of this work must, however, be given otherwise the review does not seem up-to-date for the reader. Data bases for healthcare, education and allied fields which can be found in academic libraries, online, computerized, or commercial can be accessed, for relevant papers. Key words and phrases are, of course, important. They are generally discussed in the literature section in order of priority.

Writing a research proposal

In an academic situation the term research proposal is used, but in professional settings it is sometimes called the research protocol (see for instance Kaba *et al.*, 2021). Before starting the project, researchers write a proposal – a summary of what they will be examining, why they adopt the particular research focus, and how they will proceed. It also includes information about where and when the research will be carried out. It is useful to add intended outcomes and the potential benefits for patients and service. Researchers also describe the design of the study.

The proposal justifies and clarifies the proposed study for submission to ethics committees, funding agencies, official gatekeepers such as managers and, for student work, to supervisors. The proposal is a detailed plan of action to convince the reader that the researcher knows enough to undertake the project and can show that the completed study will contribute to knowledge in the field. Kaba *et al.* (2021) give 10 clear steps for the development of a research protocol. Most text books give similar advice. Our own *follows*.

Structure of a proposal

The proposal consists of the following main elements:

1 Working title
2 Abstract
3 Introduction
   • Problem statement and rationale of the study (justification; demonstration of importance for the profession and clinical practice).
   • Context and setting.
   • The aim of the research.
4 Brief discussion of the relevant literature
   • A discussion of other researchers' work demonstrating the need for this particular study.
5 Design and methodology
   • Theoretical basis and justification of the methodology (including references on the chosen approach).
   • Delimitations and limitations of the study.
   • Sample selection and sampling procedure.
   • Data collection and analysis.
   • Ethical and entry issues.
   • Bibliography and references.
6 Timetable and costing
7 Potential dissemination

Researchers generally proceed in this order, though reviewers (supervisors, ethics committees or funding bodies) might have their own format for the proposal. There may be change and reformulation at a later stage during the process. Although the research design is not rigid, we advise inexperienced researchers to follow clearly structured, conventional guidelines.

Working title

The working title can be changed as the research evolves, although permission for change might have to be sought from supervisors, research committees or funding bodies. (More detailed discussion of this and some of the following sections in the writing up chapter.)

Abstract of proposal

The abstract in the research proposal is a brief summary of the aim, methods, sample, findings, potential outcomes and usefulness.

Introduction

This section sets the scene for the research and must be clear and precise. Readers can only understand the proposal in context. In the introduction researchers demonstrate quality and feasibility of the study and the reasons for it.

The problem statement and rationale

This briefly describes the research focus, the way in which researchers became aware of the problem, and why they want to find out about it. They describe the context in which it takes place. It is important that the research problem is not trivial but has significance for healthcare. The potential usefulness of the project for the profession and clinical setting might be explained. Researchers can address a new problem that occurred in the setting or adopt a new approach to a familiar problem. They demonstrate the significance of the work by explaining why the research is important, and/or how it could possibly help in improving healthcare practice. Research funded by the National Health Service or related funding agencies must identify potential benefits to the National Health Service.

The rationale gives the reasons for the research that might have emerged through observation of a problem in a particular situation or were stimulated by reading about an event, a crisis or question in the clinical or community setting. At this stage researchers can mention some of the claims and suggestions that other writers make about the topic or area of study. The investigation of the problem should fill a gap in professional knowledge, however small that gap may be. The proposal is a starting point for the writing-up stage; indeed, some sections can be taken over directly into the research report and then extended or modified appropriately.

Context and setting

The context includes the environment and the conditions in which the study takes place as well as the culture of the participants and location. The setting is the physical location of the research, for instance a ward in a hospital, a clinic or the community.

The aim of the research

The aim of the study – a statement of the researcher's intentions and purpose – is made explicit. A statement of the aim is sufficient; objectives might constrict the study by directing it from the outset rather than following the guidance from the ideas of participants. Specific steps to reach the aim will develop as the research proceeds. The overarching purpose of the study reflected in the stated aim is usually concerned with an understanding of participants' feelings, experiences and perceptions as they have developed in the setting and context. Some researchers fail to distinguish the aim from the outcome of the research – the aim is always the specific research aim. For instance, 'the aim of the study is to develop a model of ...' is not a research aim but an outcome of the inquiry. Instead the sentence should read something like 'the aim of the study is to explore ... in order to develop a model ...'.

Creswell and Creswell (2018) advise qualitative researchers to keep the aim non-directional, not to describe cause and effect but to give a general sense of the main idea using terms such as 'discover', 'develop' 'describe' or 'explore'. Generally, the statement of the study's aim should be crisp and not too long, otherwise it becomes unmanageable and unclear.

Example 3.5 Researchable Aims

The aim of this research is to examine the interactions between ward nurses and consultants.

The purpose of my work is to study the emotional impacts on patients of physiotherapy and to describe its emotional outcomes.

I wish to find out how people live with a life-threatening condition and manage it.

As a GP I would like to find out how patients view my interaction with their health professionals in order to improve my own work.

The intent of the present study is to research the perspectives of nursing students on their course.

The aim of this study is to explore general practitioners' thoughts about recent health policies.

This study aims to explore the experiences of midwives in the light of changes in the profession.

The literature

This is sometimes called the 'initial literature review' or 'overview of the literature' in qualitative research as it is not an exhaustive description and evaluation of all the major literature or research studies in the field of the research project. At this stage, the literature in a qualitative account broadly demonstrates the amount and level of knowledge that exists in the area of study. On the basis of an initial scan of relevant studies done by others, the researcher can decide whether to proceed with the work. It is important to mention foundational, classic studies on the subject – those which Hart (2018) calls 'landmark studies' – but also to include the most recent writing.

In a qualitative literature overview, the discussion of the literature tends to be more limited than in other types of research. As the data have primacy, qualitative researchers avoid taking too much direction from the literature, and in consequence they discuss only a few major research studies.

Resources

Researchers specify the use of resources and other costs to demonstrate that the research can be adequately funded. Resourcing and costs are of major importance in proposals for grant-giving bodies and must be detailed. These include clerical costs, paper, computer, letters and mailing as well as the researcher's time.

The research design and methodology

The research design is the overall plan and includes strategies and procedures. Researchers must also show how the conceptual framework will be developed during the research process. As stated before, methodology is concerned with the ideas and principles on which procedures are based. Methods consist of the procedures and strategies rooted in a methodology. Students must identify, describe and justify the methodology they adopt and the strategies and procedures involved. It is, of course, important that the methods fit the research question. It must be remembered that some of the details of a qualitative research project cannot be pre-specified as they arise during the research process.

Limitations of the study

Researchers should list the constraints and limitations of the study, and how they would overcome them. Locke *et al.* (2014) see limitations as weaknesses which constrain the research while delimitations are the boundaries around the research. By stating these, researchers show their careful preparation for the study. For example, one of the limitations of qualitative research that must be acknowledged is the lack of generalisability of findings. When stating the limitations, researchers can sometimes suggest ways to overcome them. It may be explained, for instance, how the lack of generalisability need not be a problem by describing attempts to achieve typicality or specificity, or how theoretical ideas might be generalisable. As to delimitations, the researcher cannot study every individual who might be appropriate for the research at any time or specific place. Hence, some people are included and others excluded. The inclusion and exclusion criteria depend on the time, place and person; for instance, some vulnerable people might be excluded for ethical or practical reasons. The inclusion and exclusion criteria need to be made explicit in every piece of research.

Sample selection and procedure

The access to participants and the initial sample size must be explained as well as other sampling procedures. An explanation of purposive and theoretical sampling is required, depending on the type of study.

Data collection and analysis

This section describes the way in which the data will be collected and analysed. These may include interviews, observations, diaries or other forms of data collection. The specifics of data analysis will also have to be discussed – for instance, constant comparative or thematic data analysis and so on.

Ethical and entry issues

Researchers will give an indication as to how they will deal with these issues, where and how they will recruit their sample, for instance. They will also demonstrate how they will protect the participants from risk and safeguard them from disclosure of identity and lack of confidentiality. A statement about ethics committee approval should also be included. There is further discussion of ethical issues later in this chapter and in Chapter 4.

References

The referencing must be exact, consistent and, in case of research students, compatible with the advice given by the university in which the student is registered. It is advisable to up-date the referencing towards the end of the study so that the latest edition of a book is consulted and referenced. A piece of research for a higher degree should contain the original source of an idea as far as it is known.

Timetable and costing

Reviewers wish to see a timetable for the research to become convinced of its feasibility. Therefore, qualitative researchers submit a projected work schedule for the research even though they cannot always predict exactly how long each step is going to take. Each step is recorded on the time line. This time line can be written or drawn as a diagram. It must be remembered that the analysis of data in qualitative research takes a long time. The literature has to be searched after the identification of major categories and built into the findings and discussion. The write-up is revised until a storyline is clearly discernible. All *this takes time*.

Dissemination

Researchers identify the readership for which they write and explain the usefulness of the study for the particular group they address. They can state how they will disseminate the results of the study, be it through journals, books or other media such as conferences, digital outputs, film and audio files. They might also plan a dissemination or public engagement event.

Example 3.6 Example of Time Frame for a Master's Dissertation

(This could be presented in diagrammatic form.)

June–July
Initial literature review/formulation of research question
Gaining approval from gatekeepers, ethics committees and participants
Writing the pro

September–October
Initial data collection (for instance, interviewing, participant observation)
Start of analysis

October–February
Further data collection and analysis
Literature review related to emerging findings
Final decision on categories and major themes

March–April
Writing up the penultimate draft

May–June
Final draft of study with corrections

Of course, this plan should be flexible depending on time available, ethics and gatekeeper permissions and other factors.

Useful reading about evaluating proposals can be found in Morse (2003). It is a good idea to look at one's own proposal in the light of an evaluation checklist.

Access and entry to the setting

Health researchers, be they experienced professionals or students, must ask permission for entry to the setting and access to the participants. It is usual for all research in health or social care settings to require approval from a research ethics and research governance committee, before gaining any access. Where the research is conducted outside formal organisations or agencies, for example, through local community networks, or informal 'snowball sampling', there is still a requirement to seek ethical approval, usually via a university ethics committee. Gaining access means that researchers can observe the situation, talk to the individuals involved, read the necessary documents and interview potential participants. Formal permission is important in any research and protects both researchers and participants. Access is sought in various ways. Some health professionals put up a notice on a public board in the hospital in which they work; others ask permission from a self-help group, such as a group of carers, to talk to the members and find out whether they wish to participate. There are a number of ways to access potential informants, but voluntary participation must be ensured.

Following the required ethical approval and permissions, there are steps in the process of access and entry:

1 Gaining access to the participants (sometimes with the help of gatekeepers) and asking for permission to carry out the research.
2 Explaining the aim and scope of the research.
3 Thinking of ethical issues, particularly in their sampling decisions.
4 Taking account of organisational or institutional issues.
5 Counteracting the effects of reactivity.

First then, researchers need to make contact with people in the setting who can give permission for access and speak to those whom they wish to observe and interview.

Second, the researcher explains early and clearly the type of project and its scope and aims. The explanation cannot be too detailed, however, as the research might be prejudiced if everything is explained at this early stage, and participants would be guided towards specific issues rather than give their own ideas and perceptions to the researcher. (At the end of interviews and observation, more details of the research must be given.)

Third, sensitive areas for research and vulnerable people must be treated with thoughtfulness and care.

Fourth, the researcher must be aware of the hierarchy in the system and know that conflicts between the interests of those at the top and those at the bottom of the hierarchy may exist. All individual participants involved should, of course, be asked for permission to undertake the study.

Fifth, the researcher might have an effect on the setting. This may not only be threatening to the people involved but could also skew the research. The threat can be diminished if researchers get to know the people in the setting and establish a relationship of trust.

The choice of setting

Researchers search for an appropriate setting. The location where the research takes place must be suitable. For this the researcher has to know the setting intimately. There is, of course, a very important difference between general knowledge of, say, a paediatric oncology setting and researching it on the particular unit in which the professional has previously worked. Some settings are inappropriate or too complex for the particular research question to be answered. There is no point in planning an ambitious study if access to the setting proves impossible or difficult.

It is not advisable that health researchers carry out research in their own settings both for ethical and practical reasons (this is debated in Chapter 3). Qualitative researchers do not always choose a single setting but in an attempt to demonstrate the typicality of their findings, carry out the research in several settings. The answer to the research question needs to contribute to nursing knowledge and the existing literature (Morse, 2003).

Access to gatekeepers

Researchers negotiate with the 'gatekeepers' – the people who have the power to grant or withhold access to the setting. There may be a number of these at different places in the hierarchy of the organisation. Researchers should not ask just the person directly in charge but also others who hold power to start and stop the research. This includes managers, clinicians, consultants, nurses, general practitioners or other personnel, whose patients or clients might be observed or interviewed. For instance, if nurses wish to observe interaction on a ward, they must not only ask the consent of the manager of the NHS Trust and the research ethics committee but also that of the ward manager, the people working on the ward and, most importantly, the patients involved. All gatekeepers have power and control of access, but those at the top of the hierarchy are most powerful and should be asked first because they can restrict access even if everybody else agrees. If they cooperate, the path of the research can be smoothed, and their recommendations might make others more willing to collaborate, though their power might influence participants to take part, and the researcher has to ascertain that participation is entirely voluntary. Wood (2013: 333) warns, that researchers 'may have the figurative door closed to them by organizational gatekeepers or the observed behaviours stage-managed when the outsider is present'.

There can be problems with gatekeepers. They may make demands that the researchers cannot fulfil, trying to guide them in a particular direction or denying access to some individuals. Often their knowledge of research is based on familiarity with randomised controlled trials or surveys; hence, the nature of qualitative research and the aims and objectives of the study must be explained. The topic might have to be negotiated to fit in with the social organisation, physical environment or timetable of the setting. Although researchers cannot start without permission and must take the wishes of the gatekeepers into account, it is important that participants do not see researchers as a tool of management because this would affect the data.

Usually, gatekeepers do not interfere in the research process, though ethics committees can and do. In research carried out with financial and social support from superiors, there is sometimes a danger that gatekeepers have their own expectations and attempt to manipulate the research, intentionally or unintentionally. This can affect the researchers' direction or report of the work, and they might find that they are influenced by these expectations. As gatekeepers are in a position of power, resistance might be difficult. Powerful people within the setting can generate difficulties for the researcher who often has to compromise. Contract arrangements might lead to more constraints on researchers as institutional objectives might take precedence over individual research interest because of the prioritising of resources. Staff time costs.

Researchers are denied access for a variety of reasons:
- The gatekeeper sees the researcher as unsuitable.
- It is feared that an observer might disturb the setting.
- There is suspicion and fear of criticism.
- Sensitive issues are being investigated.
- Potential participants in the research may be embarrassed or fearful.

Powerful gatekeepers might see researchers as unsuitable because of gender, age or lack of trustworthiness. They must be convinced that the researcher is both able to cope with the study and trustworthy. Friends and acquaintances who are already involved in the chosen location can sometimes persuade those in power of the ability and trustworthiness of the researcher. If researchers are very young, the gatekeepers might feel that they lack credibility; some female researchers suggest that they have problems with male colleagues in positions of power.

Managers might deny access if they feel that the setting will be disturbed by the presence of researchers. A ward climate might change because everybody feels that the researchers are watching every task and movement that occurs; therefore, it is important that observers and interviewers immerse themselves in the setting until they become part of it and do not create an 'observer effect'.

Researchers ask potential participants for permission to interview or observe, stating clearly the right of refusal or withdrawal and assuring confidentiality. When the main steps have been taken, the research can begin, always taking into account appropriate timing, site and situation.

Summary

Here is a brief summary of the research process:
- The first step in the process is selection of the research topic.
- After an overview of previous research, the researchers identify the gaps in knowledge and define their own research focus.
- The specific topic area and the appropriate approach are selected.
- Following ethical guidelines, the researcher writes a research proposal and seeks access to gatekeepers and participants.
- It is essential that research in the healthcare arena is vetted by the relevant ethics committee.
- The researcher must obtain consent from participants, if possible, in writing.
- The study must be of importance for the people or setting under investigation.

References

Aveyard, H. (2019) *Doing a Literature Review in Health and Social Care: A Practical Guide*, 4th edn, Open University Press, McGraw Hill, London.

Bold, C. (2012) *Using Narrative in Research*, Sage, London.

Clancy, M.L. (2013) A guidebook and a research model: a review of doing excellent small-scale research. *The Qualitative Report*, **18** (15), 1–7.

Creswell, J.W. and Creswell, J.D. (2018) *Research Design: Qualitative and Quantitative and Mixed Methods Approaches*, 5th edn, Sage, Los Angeles, CA.

Glaser, B.G. (with the assistance of Judith Holton) (2004) Remodeling grounded theory. *Forum Qualitative Sozialforschung (Forum: Qualitative Social Research)*, **5** (2) (Article 4).

Hansen, E.C. (2020) *Successful Qualitative Health Research: A Practical Introduction*, Routledge, Abingdon, Oxon

Hart, C. (2018) *Doing a Literature Review: Releasing the Social Science Research Imagination*, 2nd edn, Sage, London.

Haverkamp, B.E. and Young, R.A. (2007) Paradigms, purpose and the role of the literature: formulating a rationale for qualitative investigations. *The Counseling Psychologist*, **35** (2), 265–294.

Holliday, A. (2016) *Doing and Writing Qualitative Research*, 3rd edn, Sage, London.

Holloway, I. and Brown, L. (2012) *Essentials of a Qualitative Doctorate*, Left Coast Press, Walnut Creek Chapters 2–5.

Jacobs, R.L. (2013) Developing a dissertation problem: a guide for doctoral students in human resources development and adult education. *New Horizons in Adult Education and Human Resources Development*, **25** (3), 103–117.

Kaba, E., Stavropoulou, A., Kelesi, M. *et al.* (2021) Ten key steps to writing a protocol for a qualitative study: a guide for nurses and health professionals. *Global Journal of Health Sciences*, **13** (6), 58.

Layder, D. (2013) *A Review of Doing Excellent Small-Scale Research*, Sage, Thousand Oaks, CA.

Locke, L., Spirduso, W.W. and Silverman, S.J. (2014) *Proposals that Work: A Guide for Planning Dissertations and Grant Proposals*, 6th edn, Sage, Thousand Oaks, CA.

Mantzoukas, S. (2008) Facilitating research students formulating qualitative research questions. *Nurse Education Today*, **28** (3), 371–377.

Metcalfe, M. (2003) Author(ity): the literature review as expert witnesses. *Forum Qualitative Sozialforschung (Forum: Qualitative Social Research)*, **4** (1). doi:10.17169/fqs-4.1.761.

Morse, J.M. (2003) A review committee's guide for evaluating qualitative proposals. *Qualitative Health Research*, **13** (6), 833–851.

Punch, K.F. (2016) *Developing Effective Research Proposals*, 3rd edn, Sage, London.

Wood, J. (2013) Qualitative strategies for health law evaluation, in *Public Health Law Research: Theory and Method* (eds. A.C. Wagenaar and S. Burris), John Wiley & Sons, Inc., San Francisco, CA.

Further Reading

Marshall, K., Rossman, G. and Blanco, L. (2021) *Designing Qualitative Research*, 7th edn, Sage, Thousand Oaks, CA.

Schneider, Z. and Fuller, J. (2018) *Writing Research Proposals in the Health Sciences: A Step-by-Step Approach*. Sage, London.

Shaw, R.L., Booth, A., Sutton, A.J. *et al.* (2004) Finding qualitative research: an evaluation of search strategies. *BMC Medical Research Methodology*, **4** (5).

Willig, C. (2022) *Introducing Qualitative Research in Psychology*, 4th edn, McGraw-Hill, London, selected chapters.

Chapter 4

Ethical Issues

This chapter will present issues of ethics in qualitative research as well as problems and dilemmas which the researcher might encounter. All forms of inquiry include these issues, be they quantitative or qualitative research, and they are of particular importance in health research.

Health researchers apply the principles that protect participants in the research from harm or risk and follow professional rules laid down in codes of conduct and research guidelines. Guidance for ethical conduct of research also include safeguarding participants and additionally thinking about the impacts and context of the research for the researcher, particularly concerning the range of places and space that the research data collection may be undertaken but also vulnerabilities that arise as a result of engaging in sensitive and emotionally demanding human topics. The issue of protecting participants and researchers alongside acting ethically for every stage of the research process is an important aspect of the quality of research, especially in health research. For the purposes of this chapter, we begin with a UK policy focus but much of the chapter content is transferable to other countries. A range of policy frameworks guide research internationally but all are underpinned by a foundational ethical framework for research.

KEY POINT

Doing no harm is one of the most important principles of health research.

In the United Kingdom, since January 2015, NHS Research Governance has been the responsibility of the Health Research Authority (HRA) that has articulated four research governance frameworks for England, Scotland, Wales and Northern Ireland. Standards for ethical research are comparable between UK nations (despite the fact that health/social care provision is devolved) and HRA also deals with research governance for most social care research.

Qualitative Research in Nursing and Healthcare, Fifth Edition.
Immy Holloway and Kathleen Galvin.
© 2024 John Wiley & Sons Ltd. Published 2024 by John Wiley & Sons Ltd.

The ethical framework guiding UK health and social care research has been in longstanding development with the Health Research Authority recently launching a new UK Policy Framework for Health and Social Care Research which is available online.

The UK Policy Framework for Health and Social Care Research (2020) (see https://www.hra.nhs.uk/planning-and-improving-research/policies-standards-legislation/uk-policy-framework-health-social-care-research/) uses 12 principles to underpin all health and social care research and outlines responsibilities for individuals, teams, organisations, employers and funders. Specific guidance for interventional research in Health and Social Care is also provided. The framework applies to health and social care research that is within the responsibility of the HRA and includes:

– … Research concerned with protection and promotion of public health;
– Research undertaken in or by (including health or social care research funded by any of the UK Health Departments) a UK health Department, its non-Departmental public bodies or the NHS (References to the NHS include Health and Social Care (HSC) in Northern Ireland) and social care providers (Reference to NHS and social care providers include contractors providing services under contract with care providers or commissioners (including services purchased by service users from their own resources or their 'personal budget'), e.g. general practitioners (GPs), privately run treatment centres, care homes, magnetic resonance imaging (MRI) services); and
– clinical and non-clinical research, research undertaken by NHS or social care staff using the resources of health and social care providers and any research undertaken within the health and social care systems (including research involving prison health services) that might have an impact on the quality of those services (2020, section 3.2).

The framework followed a scoping exercise and public consultation to provide a deeper understanding of the varied systems in place for research governance for social research also and included policy leads, research governance leads, ethics leads and other stakeholders. As research governance is a dynamic field it is advisable to check resources online at the time of planning research (see Research Ethics Service – Health Research Authority, hra.nhs.uk) The standards for all those involved in the conduct of research is not restricted to one professional group, and current policy framework in the UK builds on the historical *Research Governance Framework for Health and Community Care* of the Department of Health (2006) which although long standing, remains pertinent and can be organised into the following useful domains:

• *Ethics:* the dignity, right, safety and well-being of participants
• *Science:* the quality and appropriateness of research
• *Information:* the requirements for free access to research information
• *Health, Safety and Employment:* taking account of the safety of participants and of researchers and other staff

- *Finance and Intellectual Property:* financial probity and compliance with the law for research activity
- *Quality Research Culture:* application of principles and standards in an open and visible form, and promotion of expert management and leadership (Department of Health, 2006).

In addition, the fields of sociology and psychology also have developed their own disciplinary focused ethics guidelines, as have most universities, funding bodies, such as research councils (see for example, UKRI, 2021) and professional bodies. The British Psychological Society has recently provided ethical guidance for internet-based research (Ethics Guidelines for Internet-mediated Research. pdf, bps.org.uk). Most health professions bodies also regularly update their own ethical guidelines which reflect the same core principles and which are evolved as the research ethics field develops.

The foundational ethical framework for research

Many of the principles for doing ethical research are the same for all types of research. Historically, attempts at establishing international rules for ethical research stem from the time after the Second World War, as a result of the criminal trials in Germany. The Nuremberg Code contained guidelines for consent or discontinuation of studies and advised on the balance between risks and benefits.

Most of these rules were, however, concerned with experimental research. The World Medical Association's Declaration of Helsinki (2013, WMA) lists the basic principles for all medical research (the first version appeared in 1964 and has been amended several times). In 2014, the WMA produced a celebratory publication to mark the 50th anniversary of the adoption of the Declaration of Helsinki. '*The World Medical Association Declaration of Helsinki: 1964-2014 50 Years of Evolution of Medical Research Ethics*' and in 2016, the Declaration of Taipei on Ethical Considerations regarding Health Databases and Biobanks has complemented the Declaration of Helsinki. Although the terminology concerns medical research and human 'subjects' (*sic* – see Chapter 8), the declaration contains guidance for all research investigators and research participants. The latest revision (2016) strengthens the aspects of informed consent and new developments in the research field such as biobanks.

Ethics in research has its basis in certain philosophical assumptions (which cannot be discussed here). The term originates in the Greek word 'ethos' which, according to Aristotle, means 'character' and refers to the credibility of a speaker or writer. It is a branch of philosophy concerning value – and there are two approaches in ethics: the *normative* approach (what we should do) and the *descriptive* approach (what we actually do).

Ethics for health professionals/researchers is concerned with guiding professionals to protect and safeguard the interest of clients (for instance, see NMC Policy for Safeguarding and Protecting People (updated 2020)). The researcher needs to draw on ethical principles and rules and balance these in the research process. Key ethicists in this field are Beauchamp and Childress in their foundational work *Principles of Biomedical Ethics,* with a new edition in 2019. They view ethics as a generic concept for both understanding and examining moral life. Although the seminal book considers bio-medical ethics in particular, it is useful for all health professionals. The authors emphasise a framework of moral norms that encompass principles, rules, rights, virtues and moral ideals and outline four basic principles as pivotal to this framework. Although this 'principlism' has found critics – in particular social scientists – it emphasises some essential human rights important for all health and social care researchers:

1 The principle of *respect for autonomy* (respecting the decision-making capacities of autonomous persons)
2 The principle of *nonmaleficence* (avoiding the causation of harm)
3 The principle of *beneficence* (providing benefits and balancing benefits against risks and costs)
4 The principle of *justice* (distributing benefits, risks and costs fairly)

Respect for autonomy (from the Greek *autos*, self; *nomos*, law) means that the participants in the research must be allowed to make a free, independent and informed choice without coercion. The counterpart in law of this principle is the right of self-determination, and it underpins the notion of informed consent and refusal. The concept of respect for autonomy includes advice to the researcher to consider the social nature of individuals, the impact of their choices and actions on others and the emotions involved in the process of research (Butler, 2003).

A prime motive for healthcare research is to benefit individual patients and service users, care professionals and the public. The Department of Health (2006: 15) foundational statements make clear that the primary consideration in any research study is to protect the dignity, rights, safety and well-being of participants. As informed consent is at the centre of all research, studies must have appropriate arrangements for obtaining informed consent (see later in this chapter).

The principles of *beneficence* and *nonmaleficence* (do good, do no harm) demand that benefits outweigh the risks for the individual and the wider society. The principles set up by the World Medical Association (WMA) add that risks must be carefully assessed and weighed against benefits not only for the population as a whole but also for the individual; these risks should be kept to a minimum.

The principle of *justice* implies that the research strategies and procedures are fair and just. In a multicultural society, this includes proper representation in research samples (Department of Health, 2006) and respect for diversity (age, gender, disability and sexual orientation). In their ethical framework, Beauchamp and Childress (2019) also discuss ethical rules, and there is a loose distinction between rules and principles in the operation of these rules. They argue that rules are more specific, giving more precise guides to action. These are related to research as set out below:

- Veracity (truth-telling)
- Privacy
- Confidentiality
- Fidelity

Veracity in healthcare involves an accurate flow of information that is comprehensive and takes account of the participant's understanding. These features are important for gaining informed consent for participation in research. The rule of 'truth-telling' links to the principle of respect for autonomy. Dishonesty would not respect the autonomy of the individual and impede the decision-making process. Similarly, considerations of veracity are necessary in terms of disclosure and nondisclosure of information. An individual cannot make a fully informed decision about participation in research if some information is withheld. Giving full initial information, however, can be problematic with respect to the flexibility of qualitative research methods as shown later.

Privacy is also part of the principle of respect for autonomy. Researchers must respect privacy of the research participants which is closely linked to confidentiality. The Declaration of Helsinki (WMA, 2013: 3) states that 'every precaution must be taken to protect the privacy of research subjects (*sic*) and the confidentiality of their personal information and to minimize the impact of the study on their physical, mental and social integrity'.

Confidentiality in healthcare generally is recognised as underpinning the patient–practitioner–researcher relationship. Without such confidentiality there would be no basis for trust in these encounters. Information can only be given to a third party with the consent of the research participant. All those involved in research need be aware of their ethical and legal duties and ensure that systems are in place to protect confidentiality (Department of Health, 2006).

Finally, the ethical rule of *fidelity* concerns notions of faithfulness or loyalty. Beauchamp and Childress (2019) argue that traditionally professional loyalty concerns giving priority to the participant's interests but third-party interests such as institutional interests and the changing health professions also need consideration, and conflict might occur between these differing priorities. Beauchamp and Childress specifically examine aspects of conflicts of fidelity and stress that fidelity conflicts can occur in both therapeutic and non-therapeutic research. The Declaration of Helsinki (WMA, 2013: 3) states that research participants must be informed of any institutional affiliations or potential conflicts of interest of the researcher. All of the guidance from NHS Health Research Authority (HRA), professional bodies and academic disciplines share the principle *that it is the researcher's duty* to protect the dignity, rights, safety and well-being of participants.

All health and social care researchers have to justify the research not only to research ethics committees (RECs) but also to participants, superiors and gatekeepers. They must recognise the right of participants to decline participation in the project or to withdraw from it if they wish. In Britain, the NHS Health Research Authority (HRA) under whose aegis RECs operate, helps to safeguard patient rights. It also guides and advises research applicants, be they students or other researchers. Its purpose and functions can be found on the web and include all application forms and guidance notes. The Integrated Research Application System (IRAS) under the aegis of the HRA is an online system for preparing regulatory and governance applications for health and social care research in the United Kingdom. It includes detailed guidance for research applications.

The United States has the National Institute of Health (NIH) which has an ethics manual and provides training.

Hammersley and Traianou, as far back as 2012, maintained that there has been a major increase in the attention given to ethical issues in research, which they ascribed to the rise of new technologies and data protection issues in the United Kingdom and other countries and this field has since been rapidly developing.

Ethics in qualitative research

Many aspects of the sections below would apply to all types of research, but for practical reasons they are integrated with issues particularly concerning qualitative research.

Introduction

Van den Hoonaard (2008) indicates that ethical guidelines for bio-medical research have – problematically in his opinion – shaped the ethical guidelines for social research, an area which encompasses qualitative health research. He suggests that the traditional medical view of the human 'subject' is inadequate in social research when compared to the holistic understanding of the World Health Organization (WHO). For qualitative researchers a holistic view of 'participant' as an active and interactive human being is of major importance, and researchers need to be aware of the social and cultural context. While this is the case for social and medical research, these issues must be considered at depth, especially in qualitative research, as it is context bound and usually interactive (see also Van den Hoonard, 2002, 2008; Van den Hoonard and Hamilton, 2016). The following section is a discussion of research with patients which includes the particular concerns of qualitative researchers. Several useful texts are concerned with the specific pursuit of qualitative ethical research, such as Hammersley and Traianou (2012); Miller *et al.* (2012), Van den Hoonard and Van den Hoonard (2016) and Tolich and Iphofen (2019).

Ethics in research with patients

Patients are in a particularly endangered position for two main reasons: the perceived imbalance of power in their relationship with health professionals and the special vulnerability of being ill. Participants are in a situation in which they have limited power, and they may feel a lack of control. They are not always aware of their rights to decline participation in the research, particularly if it lasts over a long period of time, and when unexpected issues arise. The researcher must understand the feeling of obligation that participants might have. Often, they can feel powerless to deny the researchers access to their world. This may be because the person who has asked them to take part, or the service/institution that this person is perceived to represent, has provided (or will provide) a service to the patient. Or they may feel they are being rude if they decline, the patient may feel an obligation to help other patients; they may feel their care may in some way be compromised by declining to take part. While official documents focus on the rights of patients, research in healthcare often deals with people who have little real power in their situation. The power balance is perhaps more equal in the patients or service users own home than in the healthcare or residential care home setting.

Timing is an important issue in qualitative research (Cowles, 1988; Magnusson and Marecek, 2015). This refers to timing of invitation to participate, the timing of the consent process, length of time given to make a decision, formal recruitment to the study, the timing and frequency of data collection. Poor timing can inhibit participants, especially when they have recently been through a personal challenge or experienced a traumatic episode. They might feel threatened at this particular time and too emotionally involved to make rational decisions about taking part or continuing the research. This can lead to the problems involved in interviewing patients. All of these issues are also transferable to social care contexts.

Interviews and observations

Interviews, in particular, may deeply affect participants who do not just reveal their experiences and deep thoughts to the researcher but also might become aware of hidden feelings for the first time. Interviews might provoke distressing memories and strong emotions and the researcher should be prepared to allow the participant to work through these. It can be harmful to participants to begin to talk about an emotive issue, but to lack the skills to follow through on properly addressing the issue in a supportive way in the interview for example. Concurrently, the researcher also needs to reflect and remain aware of their own role and limits in the context of the issues that may be or are surfaced. Specialist training in preparation for data collection alongside bespoke supervision specifically to support and debrief the researcher may be necessary in some circumstances. Interviewers often find conversations potentially distressing and stressful, and they too might need peer support or even counselling; for example, a health researcher (mental health nurse) explored the perspectives of people whose relatives had committed suicide. In addition, it is important to 'be in touch' with the skills one is using, researchers with specific expertise in for example, counselling and psychotherapy, and mental health nursing, need to be reflective and aware of their boundaries in their research interactions with patients, and be clear with themselves and with participants about whether (and how much) they will draw on their other professional skills in research interactions. Apart from the major ethical dilemmas and problems involved in the research which have to be resolved, the researcher can also become distressed and has to think through the impacts of the interviews and their own role in the research and put in place strategies to manage distress for both participants and themselves. Additionally, research participants may view researchers as experts, and expect that if they mentioned, for example, a symptom for which they had not yet sought advice and access to services, then the researcher would have confirmed to them if they needed to do so. Another example concerns the ethical problem of people agreeing to participate in research in order to access counselling and help, particularly because such help is unavailable to them. Therefore, the qualitative researcher has to constantly reflect on their role and skills, and in the course of data collection inform participants what their specific role in the research is, and is not. One strategy that forms good practice is to always sign-post participants to their general practitioner, to other services or back to regular healthcare provider as a matter of course as part of the research process, in case of participant distress, or in case of health concerns. It is important to think about these kinds of impact and how they will be managed before the data collection commences.

Towards the end of the research project, another problem may arise: the continuous, intimate nature of the interviewer–participant relationship generates trust and sometimes friendship; therefore, it is difficult for both researcher and participants to extricate from it. A sensitive researcher does not leave the patient anxious or worried. The 'debriefing' of participants and the provision of emotional support, if needed, is important. If health researchers find strong distress in patients, there is need for debriefing and a mechanism for following up the participants and this may include support for safeguarding.

Example 4.1 Managing Distress

A nurse might wish to interview patients who suffer from severe chronic back pain about their experiences, emotional well-being, feelings and treatment. The research will probably help other people in the future because new knowledge and insights about the depth and details of what it is like to live with chronic back pain might be gained. Patients, however, might feel upset to find the professional probing into their everyday life, emotions and thoughts when they are already anxious about their future, and all they want is an end to their pain. The interview may also surface past negative experiences and perhaps, for example, feelings of not being taken seriously in the past. The researcher will not only consider how to mitigate distress in participants but also debrief them with a view to helping them with emotional impacts of the interview. Strategies to support participants to obtain the help they need from the most appropriate health professional are needed and it is recommended to plan these in advance, and to be able to offer other support at the end of the interview.

In extreme circumstances, participants may become disturbed, or where there are mental health considerations referral to a professional counsellor or high-level emotional support skills might be needed beyond the research interview. However, in all studies, researchers should reflect on the impacts and plan what they will do in data collection circumstances and provide a guide for safeguarding participants for their own study. This is often explicitly required by bodies providing ethical approval. In addition, when undertaking qualitative research, participants may share information that indicates a risk or a safeguarding issue that requires action from a professional perspective, thereby breaking confidentiality, and these complexities and possibilities require reflections and planning in advance.

It has been a longstanding consideration (Mander, 1988) that patients are particularly vulnerable because they are 'a captive population'. Patients are obviously more vulnerable when they are very young or very old or considered frail. Interviews must take into account the difficulty they might have in sustaining long in-depth interviews; the researcher might consider several short interviews instead. Children, people with learning difficulties and those who have a mental or terminal illness need particular protection. For children and some people with learning difficulties, researchers are obliged not only to gain permission from the participants but also from parents or legal guardians as ethical issues are particularly complex in this case. Even experienced health professionals should undertake research with these groups only after careful consideration of all the complexities and also balance this with including groups with particular needs and vulnerabilities so that they are not inadvertently excluded from research altogether. Striving for inclusivity in research is also an important consideration (Specific guidance exists for research with those who cannot give consent for themselves), and innovative processes to facilitate inclusion have been developed, see for example Hall *et al.* (2019) and Usher and Arthur (2002), including using digital methods (Braun *et al.*, 2017).

There are particular issues to be considered when carrying out research with frail older people or people who may have cognitive difficulties or speech impediments as much qualitative research now focuses on these groups. It is difficult for some, though by no means impossible for members of these groups to give fully informed consent, but they might be constrained from doing so by ill health, chronic disease or fatigue. Even factors such as size of writing in the information sheet or consent form or the clarity of the researcher's voice are important, as is the potential participant's ability to understand the information and to concentrate on it. Good practice examples can guide consent processes successfully even when there are challenges (Cowdell, 2013).

Very similar issues are taken into account in research with children. Researchers also need special consideration for marginalised groups as there is often a tension between using people as sources of data and respecting the rights of individuals to be heard. Researchers must give reasons for focusing on or excluding minority or marginalised groups.

Ethical questions arise in *observation*, too. Covert observation brings with it complex problems and its ethical aspects are controversial in healthcare. Researchers in the field of healthcare most often disclose their presence as observers and are required to reveal the purpose of the observation. This may generate the observer effect – the change that observers may bring about in the setting through their presence. However, Patton (2014) suggests that the effect can be overestimated, as participants are immersed in the setting and get used to their presence. In any case, clients and colleagues generally trust the health professional to behave ethically. The ethical dilemmas in undertaking research in a health setting need careful consideration, reflection, justification and planning.

Permission for observation must always be obtained. Rogers (2008) gives the example of midwifery research where a researcher might wish to observe the empathising skills of midwives during the labour process. This means that clients and others in the setting have to be asked for permission and not only midwives.

Informed consent and voluntary participation

Informed, voluntary consent means that research participants are fully informed about the research and give their voluntary agreement to take part in it. There should be neither implicit or explicit pressure from researchers nor any inducement. The Royal College of Nursing (RCN, 2005) gives guidance about informed consent in health and social care research and states: 'Informed consent is an ongoing agreement by a person to receive treatment, undergo procedures or participate in research, after risks, benefits and alternatives have been adequately explained to them' (RCN, 2005: 3). When working with children, researchers can consider 'Gillick Competence'; in the United Kingdom, children aged 16 and older are normally considered capable of consenting to research participation (as well as healthcare). In the United Kingdom, for younger children parent/guardian consent may be required, but not always. For example, subject to appropriate research governance and ethical approval, if undertaking research with sexual health clinic users, the research team may be permitted to gather data from under 16s without parental consent, on the basis that requiring consent from their parents would disclose their service use to their parents and that Gillick competence would already have been assessed routinely by the service.

KEY POINT

Informed consent and voluntary participation are at the heart of all health research.

The nature of qualitative research is its flexibility, the use of unexpected ideas arising during data collection (emergent designs with open ended approaches) and the exploratory prompts that are used during interviews. Qualitative research focuses on the meanings and interpretation of the participants. The developing concepts are grounded in the data rather than in a previously established framework; hence, qualitative researchers have inherent problems with informed consent. When the research begins, they have no specific objectives for pre-defined findings and research outcomes, though they have a general aim, focus and detailed purpose. Shaw (2008) discusses this problem: the participants cannot always have full and detailed information about the project as the ideas of the researcher might change during its process. This is a dilemma of which participants must be informed. Researchers must often make difficult decisions after balancing advantages and disadvantages of giving full information from the beginning of the research. The initial lack of complete information is only justifiable because it produces data without harming the participants. By the end of the research, participants need full disclosure of details, so they can make an informed decision on the use of their data; consent given before the interview cannot be taken for granted and must be confirmed throughout without putting pressure on the participants.

Consent in qualitative research is an ongoing process. Whilst consent may be implied in one phase of the research, it cannot be assumed at another stage when the researcher's ideas change on the basis of the information provided, or indeed, when participants change their minds. Thus, consent is not a once and forever agreement by participants but requires ongoing consent. For a discussion of the complexity of these staged issues in relation to negotiating the journey of a qualitative research study, see Redwood and Todres (2006).

The process of informed consent is located within the principle of respect for autonomy. This principle demands that participation is voluntary and that participants are aware not only of the potential benefits of the research for the population but also of the personal and individual risks they take. First-time researchers, in particular, should take care that there is no major risk involved, though all research involves some risks. Participants then must be informed throughout about the voluntary nature of participation in research and about the possibility of withdrawing at any stage. This should be shown in the written consent form required in most health research. Van den Hoonaard and Hamilton (2016) (also see Van den Hoonaard, 2002), however, think that written consent is inappropriate in qualitative research, and Green and Thorogood (2018) even believe that the research relationship might be damaged through this. They argue that, although individuals are usually willing to participate, they often reconsider when asked to sign forms. However, in all health and social care research to ask for consent forms; otherwise, they would not generally gain permission from ethics committees, however ethical their behaviour is. Ethics committees generally request a consent form (see later in this chapter). There are of course, exceptions to this. When people are illiterate, researchers cannot give out written consent forms. They might record the verbal consent of the participants as an audio recording. In circumstances of remote data collection, written consent might be substituted by video recorded consent. There is an ethical issue with switching on the recording button before obtaining consent to audio/video record. Therefore, the researcher may document consent (researcher signs the form) and then sends a copy of the consent form to participants. Requiring ink signatures to be returned by post risks losing potential participants due to delays, and a video recording of consent may be easier for participants. Therefore, it is valuable to reflect on the research administrative demands on potential participants and ways that this can be made easier for participants while still complying with good ethical practice and the requirements for formal ethical approval from external bodies.

It is useful to anticipate potential problems in the course of the research and consider their solutions. The researcher must be aware that the research might threaten participants, superiors or institutions, even if it is intended to have a positive effect. Sim (1991) identifies a major very longstanding dilemma of researchers: they experience conflict between the recognition of the rights of human beings and the wish to advance professional knowledge. E-mail and Internet inquiry also pose particular problems as it is difficult to ascertain that the consent is truly given by the participants (see important reflections from Kralik *et al.* (2005)). Special measures need to be taken to safeguard people when the Internet is used for research (see Further Reading section).

Anonymity and confidentiality

Qualitative healthcare research might be seen as more emotionally intrusive than quantitative research; however, all research is intrusive and therefore, the researcher needs sensitivity and communication skills. Usually in research, anonymity is guaranteed, and a promise is given that identities will not be revealed. Qualitative researchers work with small samples and use thick description (see Glossary); it is not always easy to protect identities and the challenges of anonymity require reflection (Saunders *et al.*, 2015). Even a detailed job description or an unusual occupational title of a participant may destroy anonymity.

Researchers sometimes change minor details about the participants so that they cannot be identified. For instance, researchers may change the age of all participants by 2 or 3 years when age is not an important factor in the research (Archbold, 1986). This of course must be reported in the research account without giving exact particulars. Only the researcher should be able to match the real names and identities with the recordings, report or description; participants are given numbers or pseudonyms. Recordings, notes and transcriptions – important tools for the qualitative researcher – must be kept secure and confidentiality agreements made with external transcribing services. The research team might be familiar with names in the transcripts to help manage data but personal details and personal information and contact details, and signed consent forms must not be located near the recordings beyond the research team. If other people, superiors, supervisors or typists have access to personal information – however limited this might be – the reason for their access to this information must have a rationale and permission sought. If in doubt, when planning the research and management of data, researchers can consult the data protection officer for their organisation. In general names should not be disclosed, even names can be sensitive information in particular circumstances, participants' identities must be disguised and they should always be asked for permission. It is also worth noting that, although undertakings of confidentiality are given, participants need to know that others might have access to the recordings for peer or supervisor reviews. Additionally, special consideration of these issues in dyadic research is needed. For example, where a patient and family carer might be interviewed separately, and the researcher has responsibility of protecting the confidentiality of both (from each other), including in research interactions, and in research dissemination.

The researcher's dilemma is to decide what information can be made public; if there is doubt or ambiguity, the decision depends upon the participant's wishes – and of course, ethical guidelines.

Patton (2014) suggests that recordings should be erased a year after the research has been finished, but many ethics committees demand that recordings are destroyed as soon as anonymised transcripts are available and checked. How long transcripts are kept is determined by local policies and archiving requirements of funding bodies and universities. This can be as long as 10 years. When engaged in remote data collection, with online interviewing, the researcher needs to consider whether they really need to video-record the interview, or whether an audio-recording would suffice. Visual data such as films, photos or video recordings are treated in the same way as other data. Covert image taking is not only unethical, it is also illegal (see Further Reading section).

Confidentiality is a separate issue from anonymity but also important. In research where words and ideas from participants are used, full confidentiality cannot be promised, especially as qualitative research contains quotes from the interview data. In these studies, confidentiality means researchers keep confidential that which the participant does not wish to disclose to others. Patients, in particular, sometimes disclose intimate details of their lives which the researcher cannot divulge, although the information could be useful for the research. Hammersley and Traianou (2012) discuss the issue of privacy in particular as qualitative research often involves inner feelings and thoughts of participants. (They also discuss the issue of confidentiality in their Chapter 5.)

The following are some examples of ethical issues in research with patients.

Example 4.2 Non-Disclosure of Identity

Here are some examples of ethical issues in research with patients.

1 Ruth, a physiotherapist and Ph.D. candidate, wanted to show her supervisor some of her interview transcripts and the way she had analysed the interview data. The supervisor asked if she could also listen to her recordings to hear the voice and intonation of the participants' narratives. The researcher sought permission from the people involved and ensured them of the discretion of the supervisor and the non-disclosure of their identities.

2 Sunil, a nurse, wanted to have his interview transcripts typed by a typist as he believed that instead of typing these himself, he could use his time better by listening to the recordings several times to really immerse himself in the data. He realised that he had to gain the typist's written confirmation not to divulge the data or any details gleaned from transcribing the interviews. Also, to let participants know of how data would be handled and by whom with reference to formal data protection frameworks.

3 When Parveen, a medical registrar, completed their data analysis, they decided to use 'peer reviews' of research informed colleagues to see whether they arrived at similar results of the analysis. They had taken this into account when writing the consent sheet by asking patients' permission to show the data to two or three of their colleagues without identifying the participants.

The participant information sheet

The information for research participants needs to be clear, unambiguous and written in lay language. The researcher must confirm that the participation is voluntary. (Details for these can be obtained from the Health Research Authority and RECs. Some of the elements in the information below are specific for qualitative research.)

The information sheet consists of a *short* summary:
- The title of the research
- Invitation to take part
- The purpose of the study
- Detail about the research
- Why the participant has been asked to take part (how the participant was chosen, how many others in the research)
- Voluntary participation (voluntary, right to withdraw at any time, no effect on standard of care)
- What happens if the participant takes part (how long is the research and the involvement of the participant, how often attendance is needed and how long, what will happen to the data, security and confidentiality of tape-recorded material)
- What will happen if the researcher has concerns about the participants' well-being based on information that emerges, and in what circumstances others or support services will be contacted

- What are the disadvantages, benefits or risks
- What happens after the study (what happens to data such as recordings or fieldnotes)
- Issues of confidentiality, anonymity (permission for use of quotes without identifying participant and who has access to the data)
- Any involvement of others in the study (in qualitative research: the involvement of supervisors, peers for peer review, typists of interview scripts)
- What happens to the results (will participants want to know about these dissemination, publication)
- Who is funding and reviewing the study (self, funding body, university, etc.)
- Who is leading or supervising the research with full contact details

In the interest of clarity, the information sheet should be understandable by lay persons and not too long.

The researcher also presents a consent form for signature when giving out the information sheet. This form is not the same for all participants but depends on the individual (adult, child, colleague, etc.) and the type of research. An example taking account of qualitative research is given below. (Information Sheets and Consent Forms of the HRA specify more details for research in general.)

Example of Consent Form

Title of Research

Name and status of researcher (student, nurse, doctor and professional researcher)
Institutional affiliation
Contact address with telephone number.
Date

Permission for Research

I have read and understood the information sheet, I have had the opportunity to ask
   questions about the research and have received satisfactory answers.
I know that the participation is voluntary and that I can withdraw at any time without
   giving a reason (and, for patients: without my care being affected).
I agree to take part in the interview (focus group, observation, etc.) and give my permission
   for recording this.
I give my permission for the use of quotes, without my name being disclosed.
I give consent for anonymised data to be used in other future research (Open access data
   archive)
I understand that the data might be looked at by the researchers' supervisors or peers for
   reviewing without my identity being revealed.
I agree to take part in the research.
Name of participant
Name of researcher
Institution logos

Information sheets for children, young people and guardians are of course developed with attention to the needs of these groups.

Researching one's peers

When carrying out research with one's peers, different problems arise. Although Platt (1981) suggests that in interview situations participants are often in a position of inequality, this is not necessarily so for colleagues, unless the researcher is in a position of authority as manager or senior colleague. When researchers interview and observe their peers, a more reciprocal relationship exists which makes it easier for participants to become equal partners in the research enterprise – the aim of most qualitative research relationships. Work colleagues and peers of the researcher can, however, become vulnerable. The relationship of trust that they have may be broken through unintended disclosures or subtle pressure 'for the sake of colleagueship'. Wiles *et al.* (2006: 294) put forward the idea that peers already know some of the 'tricks of the trade' when they take part in the research while patient participants do not have this knowledge or information. The peers' awareness of these issues might endanger honest disclosure. There may be common preconceptions which the researchers share with their peers; moreover, 'researching one's peers' may mean that researchers impose a framework which is based on their *assumption* of shared perceptions, and this does not allow participants to develop their own ideas. Coghlan and Brannick (2005) advice researchers not to become rigid in their views but be open to 'disconfirming' and challenging evidence.

The research relationship

Influence in research means a process of changing something whilst studying it. Researchers influence the research and its findings. Qualitative researchers acknowledge their subjectivity and make this explicit in their report. Thus, nurses and other health researchers must account for the influences of their own perspectives in the process and outcome of the research. They need to scrutinise their own actions throughout the research process and this includes the interpersonal and interactional aspects of the research (Guillemin and Gillam, 2004). This also suggests a quick response to 'ethical moments' which means managing critical issues when they arise.

The dual role

Health professionals have dual roles and responsibilities, that of professional and researcher, and they may experience problems of identity. On the one hand, they are committed to the research as they wish to advance health knowledge for the good of their clients and recognise that research is needed for the advancement of knowledge. On the other hand, as professionals they are dedicated to the care and welfare of clients. Nurses in particular who care so intimately for patients, and also other health professionals, cannot close their eyes to distress and pain because their professional training guides them towards caring and being advocates for their clients. If participants are threatened by the research or feel that they are, then the professional has to give up the researcher role.

In their professional role, health researchers recognise the person as patient or client while in their researcher role they see the person as informant, as participant in the research. The different elements of the researcher identity – researcher/professional – cannot always be reconciled. West and Butler (2003) state that role conflict or confusion might prevent the researcher from performing either role well. Clients, too, do not always understand this duality and dichotomy in the health worker's role. They expect care and help from the person whom they perceive as a career and who professes to be a researcher. Clients might recognise that professional intervention by the researcher is not always possible. Nevertheless, health professionals cannot completely detach themselves from their participants, particularly in the close relationship of the qualitative research process. They respond to distress and need, especially in emergency situations, or call on colleagues who perform appropriate roles in the setting. RECs will usually require a strategy for providing ongoing support, for example, carrying the names and addresses of self-help groups.

A research study requires both the closeness of an empathic stance and distancing. These traits at first appear contradictory. On the one hand, researchers are asked to be non-judgemental and must be aware of personal values that could influence the research. On the other hand, professionals often have empathy and feeling for their clients. The researcher, however, cannot allow preconceived attitudes or over-involvement to influence the data. This might be problematic because of the close relationship between researcher and participant.

Researchers must be able to put themselves into the participant's place; this helps to establish the rapport that is important in this type of approach but might also generate intense emotions in both. Qualitative research into sensitive topics generates these problems to a greater extent than any other type of inquiry. The qualitative interview can in some cases resemble a counselling session in that the researcher is a non-judgemental listener. However, researchers who are also health professionals need to be careful to distinguish between research and therapeutic roles and to reflect upon this as the research proceeds. In some very sensitive cases, it is advisable to put in place a particular kind of research supervision to confidentially reflect and discuss tensions, conflicts and success as the data collection unfolds.

Research in the researcher's workplace

Writers on ethics always include a caution on carrying out research in one's own setting because it can be complex and difficult. As early as 1986, Archbold suggested that health professionals do not do research with people directly in their care, particularly because of the power relationship between the researcher and the researched. Nevertheless, many health researchers are interested in their own setting in particular and wish to understand the issues and solve the problems specific to their workplace. Qualitative researchers will experience some of the same dilemmas to those who carry out other types of inquiry, although some of the problems differ. Butler (2003) discusses some of these issues, such as recruitment, role conflict and issues of confidentiality.

The main problems are linked to the following:

Access and recruitment

The intimate nature of the relationship between participants and researcher

The dual role of the researcher

Gatekeepers and ethics committees sometimes deny access if they can foresee problems. Even if gatekeepers understand the research and are sympathetic towards it, dilemmas remain, as many are in a position of authority or care directly for the patient. Butler (2003) warned of the danger of implicit or subtle coercion and pressure; even if participants are assured that their participation is voluntary, they might feel obliged to take part because they know the researcher as a professional on whom they are dependent to an extent. They might give different answers to a professional whom they know well, to avoid endangering their future care and relationship than to a researcher who is a stranger to them. The participants often disclose more about their lives than is necessary for the research. Not only might this special knowledge and information influence the researcher but it also adds to the danger of inadvertent disclosure in the research account. Researchers need special awareness and reflexivity always being conscious of and examining their own actions.

The role of research ethics committees

We have acknowledged the existence of RECs in the health service earlier in this chapter. Health Services and universities usually have their own ethics committees to scrutinise students' research to safeguard the participants, the researchers and the institution. (Different countries have different names for their ethics committees; for instance, in the United States there are institutional research ethics review boards (IRBs) – independent ethics committees ethics review boards.)

Guillemin and Gillam (2004) differentiate between 'procedural ethics' and 'ethics in practice'. Procedural ethics is linked to the process of gaining permission from ethics committees and review boards for the research. Ethics in practice is related to the considerations which arise in the process of carrying out the research such as day-to-day dilemmas that occur (see above). In this section we shall consider procedural ethics.

Procedural ethics includes completion of ethics forms which are requested by committees. Researchers try to convince these committees that they are competent and trustworthy from the very beginning of the research when submitting the proposal. This means using language which is clear to readers (the committee includes lay members). Ethics Committees, which in the past were not always well informed about qualitative research, are now usually knowledgeable about this type of inquiry.

West and Butler (2003) describe the review process of one such ethics research committee, and while this is over 18 years old, provides relevant useful process guidance for qualitative researchers. It focuses on general ethical issues and those specific to qualitative research just as relevant today, such as its emotional impact – on both researcher and participant – and the demands the researcher might make. The conflict or tension between the roles of researcher and health professionals should also be considered. More recently, Stevenson *et al.* (2015) discuss challenges and critique of current health care approach to ethics and make an interesting case for an iterative approach which is useful contextual reading.

Ethics committees are also concerned with the safety of the researcher and participants. Many of these committees see interviews in people's homes as potentially problematic for the researcher and only permit them if particular safeguards are in place (such as contact through mobile phones, information about timing of interviews and return to base, address left with colleague or supervisor). Indeed, committees advise researchers not to travel to dangerous locations and to undertake work in public places of safety.

An awareness of the emotional response helps researchers to deal with distress, stress or grief of the participants and indeed their own. Most ethics committees look for strategies that can potentially help in the management of surfacing emotional issues. Not all researchers are aware of the inconvenience or burden they place on participants, especially on those who may be vulnerable. Qualitative interviews in particular can be very demanding in time and concentration and emotionally. Ethics committees will mainly focus on the ethical elements of the research, but there are expectations for every application to be accompanied by a peer review (and the latter looks at the research in terms of 'good' science, that is, that the research design and procedures are appropriate and its aim worthwhile and credible). Indeed, the *Research Governance Framework for Health and Community Care* (Department of Health, 2006) demonstrates a historical and longstanding demand for quality standards in research; a poorly designed research project could be considered unethical.

Ells (2011) claims that the main challenge is the quality of the research design, which contains an effective and ethical research plan and can justify each step of the research. This is especially so when the ethics committee guidelines are geared towards quantitative research. For example, interview questions in grounded theory studies evolve but cannot be specified at the very beginning of the research because of the strategy of theoretical sampling. We suggest to our own students that they write the types of questions which might be asked and make explicit that these questions are potentially changeable. (Ells speaks of the 'dynamic' aspect of qualitative research.)

KEY POINT

It is a requirement to follow the formal rules of ethics and RECs; however, it is equally important to act ethically throughout the research.

Reviewing the research project

Walker *et al.* (2005) suggest some useful key ethical questions on which ethics committees will focus. Researchers themselves might reflect on these not only to get through the ethics committee review process but also to improve their own chances of acting within an ethical framework. Not all these questions have unambiguous answers but researchers reflect on them and are prepared to justify their actions. The following ethics checklists are underpinned by Walker *et al.* (2005: 93–95).

Key ethical questions: audiotaped interviews

Informed Consent and the Principle of Respect for Autonomy
1 Is the recruitment strategy appropriate and acceptable?
2 Is the participant information sheet (PIS) presented in a user-friendly way that reflects the person-centred nature of the interview process?
3 Does the PIS include information about the following?
  • The approximate length of the interview.
  • Where and when the interview is arranged and how contact is to be made?
  • What is expected of the participant?
  • The possibility of eliciting distressing thoughts or memories and the availability of safeguards and follow-up supports in the event of this.
  • Full details about confidentiality and possible limits to confidentiality.
4 Does the application make it clear that consent is ongoing and will be reconfirmed at each stage of the research process?

- Does the application include consent to use personal information once it has been collected/analysed? Are data protection issues dealt with (a data protection officer's advice is helpful to ensure compliance with **General Data Protection Regulation** (EU) 2016/679 (GDPR) requirements?
- Where focus groups are used, what action will be taken if one participant withdraws his or her consent following data collection (i.e. will all the data be discarded)?

Right to Privacy/Confidentiality

1 Does the research location allow for privacy?
2 Does the applicant have appropriate strategies for dealing with the following potential problems or issues?
   - Legitimate complaints made during confidential disclosures.
   - Concerns about the health, safety and/or well-being of the patient, based on confidential disclosures.
   - Concerns about the safety or well-being of others, based on confidential disclosures.
   - The protection of anonymity during writing-up/publication.
3 Where the GP or other health professional is to be informed at any stage, will participants be asked for their consent?

Nonmaleficence/Beneficence

1 Is there any possibility that the interview might prompt distressing thoughts or memories?
   - If so, is this recognised and adequately addressed?
2 Do the interviews involve sensitive topics or potentially psychologically vulnerable groups?
   - If so, do the CVs of the research team indicate that the researcher is suitably qualified and adequately prepared to deal with the possible consequences?
   - Is the researcher adequately supported to deal with this?
3 How does the researcher intend to deal with participants' distress?
   - During interview
   - Following interview
   - For example, is there provision for professional support and/or follow-up services (including voluntary organisations), as appropriate?
4 Where a maximum time limit is imposed on the interview, has the researcher allowed sufficient time to deal with all possible eventualities, such as distress and questions, and achieve closure?

Fairness/Justice

1 Does the information provided indicate that the power relationship between researcher and participant is suitably balanced to favour the needs of the participant?
2 Where applicable, is the involvement of the researcher as research tool adequately justified in terms of the potential for bias?

3 Is the exclusion of those from minority groups justified?

4 Is the sample adequately justified in terms of diversity according to such criteria as age, gender, disability and sexual orientation?

Safety of the Researcher

1 Are provisions in place to protect the safety of the researcher, particularly when interviewing in the home?

2 In the case of a sensitive topic, is support available to protect the emotional well-being of the researcher?

Safety of the Participant

1 Are provisions in place to ensure safety and safeguarding of the participant?

2 Is there a safeguarding plan in place for the research study approved by ethics committee?

Data Protection

1 Are adequate steps identified to preserve confidentiality during transcribing and data storage?

- Will transcribing be undertaken by someone outside the research team?
- Does the storage of recordings/transcripts conform to local R&D policies and, where necessary, education institution requirements?
- Are open access requirements considered for data archives or open access data management?
- Has advice of local data protection officer been sought?
- Is there a data management plan and is it approved at institution level?
- Has consideration been given to General Data Protection Regulation (EU) (GDPR) (2016/679) requirements?

Key Ethical Questions: Observation Studies Informed Consent

1 How will informed consent be obtained from all participants, particularly when observation is undertaken in a public setting?

- Will information be provided individually or by public notice?
- Is there a copy of the PIS and/or public information sheet, and is this suitable?
- Is written or verbal consent obtained from each participant, or is consent presumed in the absence of dissent (this is very rare) with a clear rationale for this?
- How will the researcher support those who fail to give, or subsequently withdraw, their consent?
- How will the researcher deal with or discard the data for those who subsequently withdraw consent?
- What special measures will be taken to gain consent from vulnerable groups and those with communication difficulties?

2 How will informed consent be obtained from consenting participants in closed (institutional) settings?

- Will consent be ongoing?

- Will participants have an opportunity to withdraw their consent to the use of the data after they have been collected?
- What undertakings of confidentiality are given and are these realistic?

3 Are there any plans to use video extracts for demonstration or teaching purposes? (These data can afford a powerful educational tool.)

- If so, is this made explicit in the information sheet?

Rights to Confidentiality

1 What steps will be taken to preserve the confidentiality of the observation data, particularly *in vivo* data?

2 Does the applicant have an explicit strategy for dealing with observations that might require breach of confidentiality, such as malpractice, criminal behaviour, or concerns about the health, safety or well-being of participants?

Nonmaleficence

1 Is there the potential to cause distress, embarrassment or other form of harm to an individual or organisation and how do the researchers intend to deal with this?

2 Are the research team members suitably qualified to undertake this type of work?

3 What mechanisms are there to deal with any observed malpractice or professional misconduct?

Fairness/Justice

1 Is there any danger that participants might be under coercive influences to participate or maybe unaware that they are participating?

2 Is the study setting appropriate for the research question or aim?

3 Is consideration given to inclusivity?

Safety of the Researcher

1 Are provisions in place to protect the safety of the researcher if making observations in potentially insecure environments?

Data Protection

1 What measures are in place to store the data?

2 Does the storage of data conform to local R&D policies and, where necessary, education institution requirements?

3 Has consideration been given to implications of open access data?

Although consideration of these questions helps researchers to decide on the ethical content of their research, the answer does not automatically guarantee ethical behaviour throughout.

It can be seen that health researchers who attempt qualitative projects in clinical or social settings have to construct a complex ethical framework for the research which is all the more important when dealing with patients and clients who have a range of needs. In all research situations the needs of the participants take precedence over those of the researcher and inclusivity has to be balanced with the focus of the research question.

Summary

- Researchers adhere to the principles and rules of the ethical framework.
- The 'dignity, rights, safety and well-being' of participants are paramount.
- Participation in research is voluntary.
- The researcher respects the rights to anonymity, confidentiality and privacy.
- In qualitative research the process of consent is ongoing.
- Vulnerable individuals and groups such as children, frail older or disabled individuals require particular ethical and legal considerations.
- The researcher should seek permission from the appropriate ethics committees.
- Ethical issues concerning sharing of data, open access data and publication considerations and location of findings beyond life of the study require consideration
- Formal application through Research Governance systems with approval and local formal agreement processes is usually a requirement
- Data protection is essential following legal requirements and frameworks. We always advise researchers consult the Data Protection Officer for the organisation that the research will take place within and the organisation where the researcher is based. The ownership, storage and management of data is complex and needs expert guidance.

References

Archbold, P. (1986) Ethical issues in qualitative research, in *From Practice to Grounded Theory* (eds. W.C. Chenitz and J.M. Swanson), Addison-Wesley, Menlo Park, pp. 155–163.

Beauchamp, T.L. and Childress, J. (2019) *Principles of Biomedical Ethics*, 7th edn, Oxford University Press, New York, NY.

Braun, V., Clarke, V. and Gray, D. (2017) *Collecting Qualitative Data*. A Practical Guide to Textual, *Media and Virtual Techniques*, Cambridge University Press.

Butler, J. (2003) Research in the place where you work. *Bulletin of Medical Ethics*, **185**, 21–22.

Coghlan, D. and Brannick, T. (2005) *Doing Action Research in Your Own Organization*, Sage, London.

Cowdell, F. (2013) *That's How We Do It … We Treat Them All the Same*. Cambridge Scholars Publishing.

Cowles, K.V. (1988) Issues in qualitative research on sensitive topics. *Western Journal of Nursing Research*, **10** (2), 163–179.

Department of Health (2006) *Research Governance Framework for Health and Social Care*, 2nd edn, Department of Health, London. (This is often updated. Available at http://www.hra.nhs.uk/resources/research-legislation-and-governance/research-governance-frameworks/).

Ells, C. (2011) Communicating qualitative research study designs to research ethics review boards. *The Qualitative Report*, **16** (3), 881–891.

General Data Protection Regulation (EU) (GDPR) (2016/679) Regulation (EU) 2016/679 of the European Parliament and of the Council of 27 April 2016 on the protection of natural persons with regard to the processing of personal data and on the free movement of such data (United Kingdom General Data Protection Regulation) (Text with EEA relevance). legislation.gov.uk.

Green, J. and Thorogood, N. (2018) *Qualitative Methods for Health Research*, 4th edn, Sage, London.

Guillemin, M. and Gillam, L. (2004) Ethics, reflexivity and 'ethically important moments' in research. *Qualitative Inquiry*, **10** (2), 261–280.

Hall, A., Brown Wilson, C., Stanmore, E. and Todd, C. (2019) Moving beyond 'safety' versus 'autonomy': a qualitative exploration of the ethics of using monitoring technologies in long-term dementia care. *BMC Geriatrics*, **19** (1), 145. doi: 10.1186/s12877-019-1155-6.

Hammersley, M. and Traianou, A. (2012) *Ethics in Qualitative Research: Controversies and Contexts*, Sage, London.

Kralik, D., Warren, J., Koch, T. and Pignone, G. (2005) The ethics of research using electronic mail discussion groups. *Journal of Advanced Nursing*, **52** (5), 537–545.

Magnusson, E. and Marecek, J. (2015) *Doing Interview Based Qualitative Research*. A Learners' Guide, Cambridge University Press.

Mander, R. (1988) Encouraging students to be research minded. *Nurse Education Today*, **8**, 30–35.

Miller, C.E., Birch, M., Mauthner, M. and Jessop, J. (eds.) (2012) *Ethics in Qualitative Research*, 2nd edn, SAGE Publications Ltd., London.

Patton, M.Q. (2014) *Qualitative Evaluation and Research Methods*, 4th edn, Sage, London.

Platt, J. (1981) On interviewing one's peers. *British Journal of Sociology*, **32** (1), 75–91.

RCN (Royal College of Nursing) (2005) *RCN Guidelines for Nurses*, revised edn, RCN, London.

Redwood, S. and Todres, L. (2006) Exploring the ethical imagination: conversation as practice versus committee as gatekeeper. *Forum Qualitative Social Research*, **7** (2). Available at http://www.qualitative-research.net/index.php/fqs/article/viewArticle/129.

Rogers, K. (2008) Ethics and qualitative research: issues for midwifery researchers. *British Journal of Midwifery*, **16** (3), 179–282.

Saunders, B., Kitzinger, J. and Kitzinger, C. (2015) Anonymising interview data: challenges and compromise in practice. *Qualitative Research*, **15** (5), 616–632. doi: 10.1177/1468794114550439.

Shaw, I. (2008) Ethics and the practice of qualitative research. *Qualitative Social Work*, **7** (4), 400–414.

Sim, J. (1991) Nursing research: is there an obligation on subjects to participate? *Journal of Advanced Nursing*, **16** (11), 1284–1289.

Stevenson, F.A., Gibson, W., Pelletier, C. *et al.* (2015) Reconsidering 'ethics' and 'quality' in healthcare research: the case for an iterative ethical paradigm. *BMC Med Ethics*, **16**, 21. doi:10.1186/s12910-015-0004-1.

Tolich, M. and Iphofen, R. (2019). Ethics of qualitative research, in *SAGE Research Methods Foundations* (eds. P. Atkinson, S. Delamont, A. Cernat *et al.*). doi:10.4135/9781526421036745030 9.

UKRI (2021) Ethics review application forms and protocols, *Ethics Reviews*, UKRI.

Usher, K.J. and Arthur, D. (2002). Process consent: a model for enhancing informed consent in mental health nursing. *Journal of Advanced Nursing*, **27**, 692–697.

Van den Hoonaard, W.C. (2002) Introduction: ethical norming and qualitative research, in *Walking the Tightrope: Ethics for Qualitative Researchers*, University of Toronto Press, Toronto, pp. 1–16.

Van den Hoonaard, W.C. (2008) Re-imagining the "subject:" conceptual and ethical considerations on the participant in qualitative research. *Ciência Saúde Coletiva*, **13** (2), 371–379. Available at http://www.scielosp.org/scielo.php?script=sci_arttext&pid=S1413-81232008000200012&lng=en&nrm=iso.

Van den Hoonaard, W.C. and Hamilton, A. (eds.) (2016) *The Ethics Rupture: Exploring Alternatives to Formal Research-Ethics Review*, Oxford University Press, New York.

Van den Hoonard, W.C. and Van den Hoonard, D.K. (2016) *Essentials of Thinking Ethically in Qualitative Research*, Routledge, Abingdon.

Walker, J., Holloway, I. and Wheeler, S. (2005) Guidelines for ethical review of qualitative research. *Research Ethics Review*, **1** (3), 90–96.

West, E. and Butler, J. (2003) An applied and qualitative LREC reflects on its practice. *Bulletin of Medical Ethics*, **185**, 13–20.

Wiles, R., Charles, V., Crow, G. and Heath, S. (2006) Researching researchers: lessons for research ethics. *Qualitative Research*, **6** (3), 288–299.

WMA (World Medical Association Declaration of Helsinki) (2013) *Ethical Principles for Medical Research Involving Human Subjects*, WMA, The World Medical Association, Seoul.

Further Reading

Alderson, P. and Morrow, V. (2011) *Ethics of Research with Children and Young People*, 2nd edn, Sage, London.

Jelstrup Balkin, E., Geil Kollerup, M., Gåre Kymre, I. *et al.* (2023) Ethics and the impossibility of the consent form: ethnography in a Danish nursing home. *Journal of Aging Studies*, **64**. doi:10.1016/j.jaging.2023.101110.

Li, J. (2008) Ethical challenges in participant observation: a reflection on ethnographic field-work. *The Qualitative Report*, **13** (1), 100–115. Available at http://www.nova.edu/ssss/QR/QR13-1/li.pdf.

McCarron, M.C.E. (2013) Negotiating responsibility for navigating ethical issues in qualitative research: a review of Miller, Birch, Mauthner and Jessop's (2012) *Ethics in Qualitative Research*, 2nd edn. The Qualitative Report 18 (Review 29), 1–4. Available at http://www.nova.edu/ssss/QR/QR18/mccarron29.pdf.

Prior, L. (2008) Qualitative research design and ethical governance: some problems of fit. *Northern Ireland Forum for Ethics and Healthcare*, **4**, 53–64.

Wiles, R., Prosser, J., Agnoli, A. *et al.* (2008) Visual ethics: ethical issues in visual research. ESRC National Centre for Research Methods Review Paper, Southampton ESRC National Centre for Research Ethics.

World Medical Association (2016) Declaration of Taipei on ethical considerations regarding Health Databases and Biobanks, 53rd WMA General Assembly, Washington, DC.

Hall, V., Conboy-Hill, S. and Taylor, D. (2011) Using virtual reality to provide health care information to people with intellectual disabilities: acceptability, usability, and potential utility. *Journal of Medical Internet Research*, **13** (4), e91. doi:10.2196/jmir.1917.

Harris, R. and Dyson, E. (2001) Recruitment of frail older people to research: lessons learnt through experience. *Journal of Advanced Nursing*, **36** (5), 643–651.

NMC (Nursing and Midwifery Council) (2015) *The Code: Standards of Standards, Performance and Ethics for Nurses and Midwives* (Revised Code), NMC, London.

Chapter 5
Supervision of Qualitative Research

The supervisor is an important support, critic and mentor during the research process. Supervisors oversee the dissertation or thesis and give advice on the research topic, methodology and other research issues as well as guiding and supporting students through the process and the regulations of the university.

Although supervision may differ according to circumstances – the type of research, the topic as well as the level of study and experience of students – the principles remain similar for different students and types of research; the experience and expertise of the supervisors and their relationships with students will affect the success of the project. Delamont *et al.* (2004) stress the importance of the relationship between supervisor and researcher in the process; it can become close over the time of study but should stay within professional boundaries. After the research is fully completed, researchers, particularly when they are mature professionals, sometimes become friends with their supervisors, and this is appropriate as long as the research– or tutor–student relationship has finished.

Supervisors have some responsibility for the quality and completion of the research project for ensuring that students define and achieve their aims, and an obligation to the student to support and advise as well as constructively criticise when necessary. On completion, it is important only to submit the work when the supervisors have given their approval for this. Although this is not mandatory in all institutions, it is advisable, because an experienced supervisor will be able to judge whether the study has been satisfactorily completed and will stand a chance to be seen as successful by the examiners.

Students, however, have and take responsibility for their research. While examining externally, the authors found that occasionally when students were questioned about an issue, they defended themselves by referring to the supervisor (I did this because my supervisor said ...), but this is never a good idea, as students have to demonstrate that they can think for themselves and see the reasons for their arguments rather than following the supervisors' advice slavishly.

Sometimes students can choose their own supervisors from a given list of potential tutors after deciding on the research topic, but usually supervisors are allocated according to expertise in method and topic. There should be a match

Qualitative Research in Nursing and Healthcare, Fifth Edition.
Immy Holloway and Kathleen Galvin.
© 2024 John Wiley & Sons Ltd. Published 2024 by John Wiley & Sons Ltd.

between student and supervisors, and they need to feel comfortable with the topic and the relationship. Support and willingness to advise are useful criteria. Postgraduate students in particular will become experts in their own research and their knowledge will, towards the end of their research, sometimes super-sede the expertise of the supervisors, but undergraduates too will be able to speak authoritatively about the topic of their projects if they take time and effort to analyse the data carefully and link the relevant and appropriate literature to the findings.

The style of supervision will depend on student, supervisor and the research process. Some students, for example, like having a highly structured timetable and want to be strictly guided or organised by their supervisors, others are self-directed and see supervisors as an informal sounding board. The style of supervision has to be negotiated during the stages of the research. The stage and level of the research will make a difference – both for undergraduates and postgraduates. The stage determines the amount of guidance and structure necessary; usually students need more guidance at the beginning and towards the end of the process. Also, undergraduates and novice researchers obviously need more guidance, while experienced researchers or doctoral students might need less, as one of the goals of the work is to develop independence in thinking and managing the day-to-day process of the research. It is not advisable to start the data collection too early and before the supervisors have discussed it.

KEY POINT

It is important for researchers to be familiar with the institution's rules and regulations.

The responsibilities of supervisor and student

Supervisors and students have a common aim: to achieve a study of high stand-ard that will be completed on time. Both student and supervisor(s) should be committed to the contract of respectively carrying out and supporting the research. The supervisor generally guides and advises rather than directs, except in circumstances where the student acts contrary to ethical or research guide-lines. Doctorates in health many of which have clinical relevance, are more specific in a variety of areas, a topic that Jackson *et al.* (2021) explored in their research.

Supervisor and student will have to negotiate the relationship from the beginning of the study. The frequency of contact depends on the student's needs and the stage in the research process. This can be discussed at the beginning of the research and revised at intervals. As suggested before, generally the student needs most help and support at the start and then again at the stage of writing up. Nevertheless, it is necessary for students to be in touch regularly rather than erratically. Some people need to see the supervisor often; others enjoy working on their own, although they too need feedback and constructive criticism. There should be a systematic and structured programme of work that forms the basis for the student–supervisor work relationship, but the instigation for this programme should come from students themselves unless it is their very first piece of research.

The responsibility for contacting supervisors, rests largely with students; indeed, Cryer (2006) suggests that legally the responsibility to inform the supervisor of problems and getting in touch with them is likely to be the student's. Telephone and e-mail contact can be useful, especially when a student experiences an academic or a personal problem that affects the smooth process of the research.

Students should inform supervisors about problems that have occurred, preferably in advance of a meeting. This means that both student and supervisor are prepared for the meeting, saving precious time. Many students and supervisors keep written notes on the supervision meetings; this is useful as a basis for further appointments and makes meetings more systematic and methodical. The supervisor generally advises the student to come with questions and problems. Most supervisors become involved and interested in the students' research topics; students have the right to expect this interest.

Often students are so enthusiastic about the research that they start data collection and analysis before becoming acquainted with the research methods. We have, on occasion, had students who immediately started collecting data, even before they had chosen an approach to their inquiry; this is not good practice and must be avoided. It can lead to inadequate interviewing and observation, because methodological and ethical considerations have been neglected, and this threatens any coherence between the research question, approach, methodology and methods. Students must make sure that they are fully aware of the strategies, techniques and problems of their chosen research method, sometimes needing a break so they can reflect on methods and topic.

Students, in particular, do not always want to start writing after the start of the data collection; they believe that much of the research is 'in their head'. In our experience this is a fallacy, and it is useful to start writing early. We see no reason why an initial literature review and methodology should not be written up before entering the field to collect data, and consider this best practice. In the methodology section, the examples for the specific study can be added later. The supervisor will often ask for reflections or chapters on background, literature review and methodology, depending on the type of research. This ensures that students both understand the process and produce ideas that generate fresh motivation and interest, even though sections of the writing might have to be changed at a later stage. This way, students immerse themselves in the methodology; some of the problems and pitfalls of the research become obvious and can be resolved at an early stage.

How then does the qualitative research supervision process differ from that in other studies? One of the common issues that arise is linked to data collection and analysis: In much qualitative research, data collection and analysis are managed in parallel, or interact, which both students and supervisors need to take into account. For instance, there are particular distinctions between the schools of qualitative enquiry regarding the data collection and analysis process and these must be made explicit and understood; one way to fully grasp these complexities is talking at length with your supervisor about them. From an ethical perspective, permission is not given once and for all, and therefore a staged perspective may be needed since any ethical issues are ongoing throughout the research journey. Again, such complexity benefits from ongoing discussion with the supervisor throughout the process. Regarding the time element, although all research is time-consuming, the participants need to be even more aware of the 'labour-intensive nature' of their studies, which need careful time management (Madill *et al.*, 2005). Like all research, qualitative research requires careful planning and each stage of the research needs to be thought through in advance. In particular, the analysis stage is likely to be intense and also much slower than one may anticipate, postgraduate students should plan accordingly.

The supervisors might be experts in the field of research but not in the very specific area, because the study explores 'uncharted waters'; the exact focus might not be determined at the very beginning of the research. Although the initial literature review is not as extensive as that for quantitative studies, participants (researchers and supervisors alike) have to know that the researcher conducts a dialogue with the literature in relation to the findings, and this takes more time towards the end the study (see relevant chapters). Overall, to rush qualitative research is to risk superficiality, and this is to be avoided; a core hallmark of good quality qualitative research is that it uncovers depth and reveals new insights. This requires time, immersion and reflective dialogue.

Writing and relationships

Students often find the writing up at the end an insurmountable task. The advice to start writing early will reduce this problem. The introduction, research strategies and writing up of ethical issues might give direction to later chapters, and can be written quite early. If written work is sent to supervisors before a meeting, they are then able to give feedback and encouragement more easily. Students can expect that their supervisors have read the written work when they come for their prearranged supervision sessions, and that it will be criticised constructively. Sometimes supervisors e-mail their comments to students before the meeting. Phillips and Pugh (2015) see the script as a basis for discussion. It is inadvisable to leave writing to the last stage of the research for two reasons: interesting and stimulating ideas will be forgotten and students might run out of time and hence panic. Seeing a chunk of the report in writing will motivate the student to proceed. All through the process, researchers make fieldnotes and memos as often as possible. The usefulness of carrying a small writing pad (as well as a field diary) to jot down ideas that arise cannot be underestimated.

Supervisors are not always gentle and diplomatic in their criticism; some students are hurt by this. The advice is best taken without seeing it as a personal attack but as an academic argument. In any case, the relationship between supervisor and student develops over time as they learn about each other's weaknesses, strengths and idiosyncrasies, and both sides negotiate the process. The best supervisors are able to provide a supportive environment for students, draw out their ideas and are flexible and approachable (Phillips and Pugh, 2015), but direct and explicit in their critique of the research. Even if students lack this type of supervisor, they can still learn. As in everyday life, sometimes it is necessary for students to work with individuals to whom they cannot relate on a personal level. This does not mean that the professional relationship needs to be problematic. Students do have some responsibility to try adapting to a style of tutoring with which they might not be familiar, just as supervisors need to do their best even for students with whom they have no particular friendly relationship.

Supervisors cannot always help their students because they do not have unlimited knowledge about all the facets of the research, especially as it develops over time. Researchers often find other experts who can advise them, and on whose knowledge, they can draw without offending the supervisor; experts in the field of healthcare might be very useful. Supervisors often know their own limitations and help students find other experts or advisors. It is useful and appropriate, however, that students inform their supervisors when they seek advice from persons outside the supervisory relationship. Students build up relationships with their supervisors on a one-to-one basis. Janssen *et al.* (2020) found in their research, that expectation of fulfilment of basic needs 'contribute to student satisfaction and success'. These are among others, the need for autonomy, competence and relatedness (p. 10).

KEY POINT

Eventually the student becomes an independent researcher and expert in the field of study.

Practical aspects of supervision

There are some other practical points that must be remembered. Students should make an appointment before coming to see their supervisors, if this is at all possible. Of course, open access to supervision is sometimes necessary and always valuable, but supervisors are busy with many other commitments, and an appointment system helps to save time for all parties. Students (and supervisors) should be available and punctual for a pre-arranged meeting, but if appointments have to be cancelled, the cancellation should be made as early as possible. If no other time for necessary supervision can be found, an occasional telephone session might do in an emergency. The main stress should be on regular and quality time of contact. One of our highly motivated students worked independently for some time before contacting the supervisors. By that time, he had lost his direction and had used valuable time recovering older ground in order to go back to find it again.

To keep in contact, e-mail addresses and telephone numbers need to be exchanged. Sometimes supervisors are reluctant about revealing their home number, and the student should only use this in an emergency – and this is the same for the home telephone number of the student. University e-mails, however, can be very useful for academic exchanges between student and supervisor. The supervisor's role is to act as a critical friend, and as the relationship is long term, it is helpful to discuss with each other roles and expectations within the supervisory relationship at the beginning of the process.

KEY POINT

Regular contact between student and supervisor is essential.

The following is a summary of the roles and tasks of supervisors and students (adapted from Holloway and Walker (2000)).

The Responsibilities of Supervisors
- They support and advise students.
- They help to ensure that students adhere to ethical principles.
- They give feedback such as constructive criticism and motivating praise.
- They produce progress reports (if required).
- They introduce students to other experts or advisers (if needed).
- They make students aware of problems relating to progress and quality of the project.
- They encourage students throughout the research process.

The Responsibilities of the Students

* They negotiate the process and style of supervision with the supervisor.
* They regularly submit written work to the supervisor (as negotiated), generally well before supervisory meetings.
* They give progress reports if required.
* They negotiate major changes and modifications in the research with the supervisor.
* They inform the supervisor of any problems which might interfere with the research project.
* They observe ethical principles (which include not plagiarising the work of others).

In addition to the above, postgraduates attend agreed research sessions or training programmes.

Single or joint supervision

Students have either one, two or indeed several supervisors for their research studies. One supervisor could be an expert in research method, the other(s) might have specialist knowledge in the field of study. Supervisors generally differ in their skills and knowledge but complement each other. Too many supervisors could be problematic for the student.

There are a number of arguments for joint supervision. For the student, continuity is ensured when one supervisor is absent or ill. The student's experience can be enhanced by the support of several supervisors. For the supervisors there is support from colleagues who can discuss the appropriateness of advice about which they are uncertain. New supervisors gain from the guidance of experienced colleagues.

Taught master's degrees in the health professions have proliferated and tend to recruit large numbers of students. Most part-time students work in the clinical setting and wish to carry out research in this environment in order to examine a problem or a major issue relevant to their work. Therefore, the supervisors' experience and knowledge in the clinical setting can be useful but not especially necessary for methodologists.

Single supervision avoids the danger of the conflicting guidance from different people, however most universities see dual supervision in MPhil and PhD studies as important, although undergraduates and MSc/MA students often have a single supervisor.

When examining an educational problem, a student needs at least one supervisor with expertise in the educational field. Undergraduates, as novices to the research process and relatively inexperienced in the clinical setting, need guidance to the principles of research while the topic is of lesser importance, although it should reflect the student's interest and advance knowledge in a more limited subject area.

In PhD and MPhil research, students often have a supervisory team to assist continuity in supervision when one supervisor is absent for any reason. To avoid conflicting advice to students, it is, of course, important that joint supervisors have a common ideology about supervision, a similar view about the particular method and topic, and that they stay in contact with each other. Students must be aware of the pitfalls and problems in supervision, because ultimately the responsibility is theirs.

Students often propose ambitious projects in which they intend to use both qualitative and quantitative methods. For short student projects that take less than a year, mixed-methods study might be too time-consuming and the student is often advised to carry out single-method studies.

Supervisors have the task of asking questions about the particular circumstances, settings and people the students want to take into account when investigating the topic. Often, they are able to advise students on relevant and useful method texts. Although students cannot be forced to listen to their supervisors, they will usually find it profitable to do so.

Trust and honesty are very important in establishing a supervisory relationship as supervisor and student are working collaboratively and in partnership (Rugg and Petre, 2020). In this process, truth-telling is essential. There is an obvious duty for both to recognise the need to share all aspects of the study phases, be it positive or negative.

Supervisors are usually able to help because they have inside knowledge of the research and/or are experts in the chosen method. In general, supervisors have lengthy experience of a variety of student projects. This knowledge helps students to trust the advice given and be guided appropriately. Students have responsibility to the discipline and their profession to report the findings as truthfully and accurately as possible.

Many universities have introduced team supervision for continuity and practical reasons. More than two supervisors are necessary for students who are carrying out interdisciplinary studies or want very specific advice (Guerin and Green, 2013).

KEY POINT

Students themselves have the ultimate responsibility for their work.

Problems with supervision

Students might have problems with their supervisors. Some are due to their own actions or inactions; others are the responsibility of the supervisor or the interaction between student and supervisor. Occasionally, there may be a personality clash. The problems are more easily resolved at the beginning of the study, and it is important not to leave them for too long. Fortunately, there is rarely a major problem between researcher and supervisor. If it does occur, researchers, and particularly novices to research, can obtain advice from other members of the department or seek help from a senior staff member (such as the departmental research director, the departmental research degrees committee for research students or the course tutor in the case of undergraduates) who will advise on an appropriate course of action. In most cases, negotiation with the supervisor(s) is not only possible but also desirable, and it resolves small problems. However, Bock *et al.* (2013) suggest that, if there are concerns, they should first be discussed between the supervisor(s) and the student; if they go to senior people, it may create difficulties, conflicts and disruptions.

Academic problems

The following problems may arise from time to time:
1 The supervisor is inaccessible or lacks time to see the student.
2 The supervisor gives too little guidance or is uncritical.
3 The supervisor is too directive or authoritarian (although in programmatic research there may be a protocol that the researcher is required to follow).
4 The student cannot keep to the agreed timetable.
5 The supervisor leaves the university or is allocated a different role.
6 Some mature students in the health field have much prior knowledge and expertise in their field, and sometimes supervisors do not realise this.

   Students' most common complaints concern inaccessibility of supervisors. Supervisors are busy people who do not always consider the student and supervision as their priority. Students can avoid this problem by making an appointment well before the supervisory session or by deciding on a future date at each meeting. It is important to inform the supervisor of cancellations. Students might supply supervisors with their home and (for part-time students) work telephone numbers so that the latter can cancel well before the meeting if they cannot attend.

   When novice researchers have little guidance, feedback or criticism, they feel uninformed and unsure about their progress or the standard of their work. They should not be afraid to ask for help. Most supervisors are willing to assist students in any way they can and have their interests at heart. It's their task!

   Students sometimes complain about too much guidance and over-direction. They may feel that the supervisor never allows them to make their own decisions and guides the work in a direction they do not wish to go. If the researcher is a novice, it is generally advisable to listen to the advice of the supervisor, particularly in the early stages. At a later stage, supervisors are generally open to academic argument and do not object to changes in direction as long as the student can justify these.

A problem sometimes occurs in joint supervision when supervisors have conflicting ideologies and different ideas about the research. Sometimes this is the outcome of misinterpretation. The situation can usually be negotiated. However, academic conflict can also be productive as it might stimulate discussion. It is important for both researcher and supervisors to keep notes on meetings. It is also advisable for all parties to get together to discuss the research, but of course, this is not always possible.

One of the main problems is the timetable that has been negotiated with the supervisor and that the institution demands. Many students neglect this issue until it becomes urgent. It is most important to look at the date for completion at the very beginning and plan the research carefully so that the timetable can be kept. This means that students and supervisors have to be realistic (Delamont *et al.*, 2004). Qualitative research is particularly demanding during the analysis and writing stages, and takes more time than the student might have originally envisaged. Also, during this stage, students have to gain access to the literature connected with their themes or categories, and the articles often take much time to arrive at the library.

Occasionally, supervisors change their roles or move on during the student's time at the university. They might be promoted and have little time for the student. They may have a sabbatical or a serious illness. In this case, joint supervision is valuable, and the department can add another supervisor if necessary. Also, telephone and e-mail tutorials Skype and zoom tutorials are often possible, and we have used these successfully. Face-to-face contact is, of course, desirable.

Final notes

Throughout the study, the student must keep in mind some major points linked to supervision.

1 *Consulting the Supervisors:* Some students write many chapters of their study in well-motivated but misplaced haste before consulting their supervisors, which means that occasionally they take an inappropriate path for the study.

2 *Consulting the Regulations:* Each university, college or grant-giving body has its own regulations. Many students only consult these at the very end when most of the work has been completed. It is important to have an occasional read of the regulations from the very beginning of the study, so that they will be remembered throughout.

3 *Consulting the Latest Literature Relevant to the Study:* The student must be up-to-date with the latest research and important discussion on the research topic and also about the methodology.

Summary

The supervision process can be summarised as follows:
- Student and supervisor(s) have responsibility for, and collaborate on, the research project, but the main responsibility for the research lies with the student.
- Supervisors are chosen because of their knowledge in the area of topic and methodology.
- Negotiation between students and supervisors takes place early in the research when the ground rules are established.
- It is essential that close and regular contact is maintained between the student and the supervisor(s), and that they share ideas throughout the research.

References

Bock, E.M., Kwonowe, O. and Chikte, U.M.E. (2013) Research supervision needs and experiences of Master's students in nursing. Article from a Master's Dissertation. Stellenbosch, SA. Available at http://scholar.sun.ac.za.

Cryer, P. (2006) *The Research Student's Guide to Success*, 3rd edn, Open University Press, Maidenhead.

Delamont, S., Atkinson, P. and Parry, O. (2004) *Supervising the Doctorate: A Guide to Success*, 2nd edn, Open University Press, Maidenhead.

Guerin, C. and Green, I. (2013) They're the bosses: feedback in team supervision. *Journal of Further and Higher Education*, **39** (3), 320–335.

Holloway, I. and Walker, J. (2000) *Getting a PhD in Health and Social Care*, Blackwell Science, Oxford. (Now old with the rules of its time, some of which are now obsolete; however, general points still apply.)

Jackson, D., Power, T. and Usher K. (2021) Learning to be a doctoral supervisor: experiences and views of higher degree research students. *Journal of Clinical Nursing*, 2021, 1–10. doi:10.1111/jocn.15651.

Janssen, S., van Vuuren, M. and de Jong, M.D.T. (2020) Sensemaking in supervisor-student relationships. *Studies in Higher Education*. Available at https://srhe.tandfonline.com/loi/cshe20.

Madill, A., Gough, B., Lawton, R. and Stratton, P. (2005) How should we supervise qualitative projects. *The Psychologist*, **18** (10), 616–618.

Phillips, E.M. and Pugh, D.S. (2015) *How to Get a PhD*, 5th edn, Open University Press, Maidenhead.

Rugg, G. and Petre, M. (2020) *The Unwritten Rules of PhD Research*, 3rd edn. Open University Press, London and New York.

Further Reading

Holloway, I. and Brown, L. (2012) *Essentials of a Qualitative Doctorate*, Left Coast Press, Walnut Creek, CA.

Jackson, D., Power, T. and Usher, K. (2021) Understanding doctoral supervision in nursing: 'it's a complex fusion of skills', *Nurse Education Today*, doi:10.1016/j.nedt.2021.104810.

Lee, A. (2012) *Successful Research Supervision*, Routledge, Abingdon.

Oliver, P. (2014) *Writing Your Thesis*, 3rd edn, Sage, London.

Yona, L. (2020) *Masters and PhD Students Handbook*, AuthorHouse, Bloomington, IN

Part Two

Data Collection and Sampling

Chapter 6

Interviewing

Interviews as sources of data

In qualitative health research, interviews are the most common form of data collection, though many experts advise on combining them with observation. Novice researchers often rely on interviews as the main form of data collection because they want to gain the inside view of a phenomenon or problem by asking people about it and also because they find observation difficult. Nevertheless, most experienced researchers agree that a combination of both is the better way of doing research though the choice also depends on the purpose of the research, its specific aims and research design.

It is understandable why health professionals wish to interview clients and colleagues. In their professional lives, too, they have conversations with patients in order to obtain information. They counsel their clients and already possess many interviewing skills. Professional assessment, for instance, relies on skilful questions and includes interviewing to elicit information from patients or clients. Interviewing is, however, a complex process and not as simple as it seems.

Beatrice and Sidney Webb who undertook social research around the turn of the last century used the term 'conversation with a purpose' when discussing interviews, but the research interview has only some of the characteristics of a conversation. Research interviews differ from ordinary conversations because the rules of the interview process are more clearly defined.

The one-to-one interview consisting of questions and answers is the most common form of research interview. Other types include focus group and narrative interviews (discussed more fully in other chapters).

Interview studies have contributed to the understanding of participants and of the wider culture. In health research, interviewing provides the basis for exploring both colleagues' perspectives and clients' interpretations. It is necessary, however, to warn researchers of 'anecdotalism' when they accept 'atrocity stories' from participants and do not always explore cases which contradict these (Silverman, 2020). If researchers apply high standards and rigour to the research, and search for contrary occurrences in the analysis of the interview data, their studies will represent – at least to some extent – the reality of most of the

Qualitative Research in Nursing and Healthcare, Fifth Edition.
Immy Holloway and Kathleen Galvin.
© 2024 John Wiley & Sons Ltd. Published 2024 by John Wiley & Sons Ltd.

participants' perceptions and a description of the phenomenon under study. There are a number of ways for the researcher to interview participants, in person with one participant or a group of people, by telephone, email or through Skype, Zoom, Microsoft Teams, etc., especially in times when a personal interview is not possible.

The interview process

Unlike everyday conversations, research interviews are set up by the interviewer to elicit information from participants. The purpose of the interview is the discovery of informants' feelings, perceptions and thoughts. Marshall and Rossman (2015) state that interviews focus on the past, present and, in particular, the essential experiences of participants. The interview can be formal or informal; often informal conversations or chats with participants generate important ideas for the project. Depending on the response of participants, researchers formulate questions as the interview proceeds rather than asking pre-planned questions. This gives participants some measure of control over the agenda. It also means that each interview differs from the next in sequence and wording, although distinct patterns common to all interviews in a specific study often emerge in the analysis. Indeed, for many research approaches, it is necessary that researchers discover these patterns when analysing data.

One interview, however, does not always suffice. In qualitative inquiry it is possible to re-examine the issues in the light of emerging ideas and interview for a second or third time. Seidman (2019) sees three interviews as the optimum number, but these require much planning in the short time span available to undergraduates for their project, so this is only possible for postgraduates. Many novice researchers use one-off interviews although postgraduates and other more experienced researchers sometimes carry out more than one with each participant.

Pilot studies are not always used in qualitative inquiry as the research is developmental, but novice researchers could try interviews with their friends and acquaintances to get used to this type of data collection. We found that we lacked confidence when we started, and a practice run proved very useful. In our experience, students become more confident as interviews proceed.

Most qualitative research starts with relatively unstructured interviews in which researchers give minimal guidance to the participants. The outcome of initial interviews guides later stages of interviewing. As interviews proceed, they become more focused on the particular issues important to the participants and which emerge throughout the data collection. Most qualitative studies not only explore commonalities and uncover patterns but also describe the unique experiences of individuals, particularly in one-to-one interviews.

One-to-one interviews are the most common form of data collection, although researchers also use group interviews (see Chapter 8).

Preparing for the interview

Interviews need careful preparation, unless they are informal or on-the-spot conversations. We have adapted the valuable list by McNamara (2005) who advises researchers to do the following:

1 Elect a setting where you would not be disturbed.
2 Tell the participants about the aim of the interview.
3 Describe its framework.
4 Tell participants how long (approx.) it might last.
5 Provide your contact address or phone number.
6 Offer opportunities for participants to ask questions.
7 Take notes or record the interview.

Types of interview

Researchers have to decide on the structure in the interview. There is a range of interview types on a continuum, from the unstructured to the structured (not used in qualitative research). Qualitative researchers generally employ the unstructured, open-ended or semi-structured interview. In these interviews there are no, or few, predetermined factual questions except at the very beginning where researchers need to find out factual matters such as for instance, occupation, the length of the condition, and for professionals, length of service or any relevant facts. These also help to put the participant at ease. This tends to be followed by one or two broad-ranging opening questions and a series of prompts. Roulston (2010) calls the qualitative interview 'the reflective interview'.

The unstructured, non-standardised interview

Unstructured interviews start with a general question in the broad area of study. Even unstructured interviews are usually accompanied by an *aide mémoire*, an agenda or a list of topics that might be covered.

Example 6.1 Unstructured Interview Aide Mémoire

Starter questions: How did you first find out about your condition?
Can you tell me more about this?
Aide mémoire (**or aide memoir**)
Feelings and thoughts
Interaction with health professionals
Coping with symptoms
Feelings about treatment
Social support from family and friends
Practical help
(These are merely examples and the researcher follows up on the words of the participants.)

This type of unstructured interviewing allows flexibility and makes it possible for researchers to follow the interests and thoughts of the informants rather than their own assumptions. Interviewers freely ask questions from informants in any order or sequence depending on the responses to earlier questions. Warm-up and simple questions are generally asked first; however, if the interviewer leaves the essential questions till the end of the interview, the participant may be tired and reluctant to discuss deeper issues.

Researchers also have their own agenda. To achieve the research aim, they keep in mind the particular issues which they wish to explore. However, direction and control of the interview by the researcher is minimal. Generally, the outcomes of these interviews differ for each informant, though usually certain patterns can be discerned. Informants are free to answer at length, and great depth and detail can be obtained. The unstructured interview generates the richest data, but it also has the highest 'dross rate' (the amount of material of no particular use for the researcher's study), particularly when the interviewer is inexperienced. Charmaz (2014) calls this type of interview 'the intensive interview'. (For advice on interviewing, see p. 55.)

The semi-structured interview

Semi-structured or focused interviews are often used in qualitative research. The questions are contained in an interview guide (not interview schedule as in quantitative research) with a focus on the issues or topic areas to be covered and the lines of inquiry to be followed. The sequencing of questions is not the same for every participant as it depends on the process of the interview and the responses of each individual. The interview guide, however, ensures that the researcher collects similar types of data from all informants. In this way, the interviewer can save time, but more importantly a well-planned interview, where the researcher has reflected on the research question, helps to reach meaning as led by the participant (Kvale, 2007). Researchers can develop questions and decide for themselves what issues to pursue, but give primacy to the participant in the conversation.

Example 6.2 Interview Guide for Semi-Structured Interview

Tell me how you found out about your condition.
What did you think at that stage?
Can you describe what it was like?
What did the health professionals do?
What about your treatment?
What did you think at that stage?
How did your family and friends react?
How did you cope with your work?
Tell me more about that.
Can you describe some examples of that?
(Obviously, these are only example questions. There needs to be a follow-up of the answers.)

The interview guide can be quite long and detailed although it need not – should not – be followed strictly so that the participant has control and prioritises what they want to discuss. It focuses on particular aspects of the subject area to be examined, but it can be revised after several interviews because of the ideas that arise. Although interviewers aim to gain the informants' perspectives, the former need to keep some control of the interview so that the purpose of the study can be achieved and the research topic explored. Ultimately, the researchers themselves must decide what interview techniques or types might be best for them and the interview participants. Our students and other researchers preferred good questions of medium length combined with the use of prompts and reported better results.

The structured or standardised interview for demographic data

Qualitative researchers in general *do not use* standardised interviews as they are contradictory to the aims of qualitative research. In these, the interview schedule contains a number of pre-planned questions. Each informant in a research study is asked the same questions in the same order. This type of interview resembles a written survey questionnaire. Standardised interviews save time and limit the interviewer effect. The analysis of the data seems easier as answers can be found quickly. Generally, knowledge of statistics is important and useful for the analysis of this type of interview. However, this type of pre-planned interview directs the informants' responses and is therefore inappropriate in qualitative approaches. Structured interviews may contain open questions, but even then, they cannot be called qualitative.

Qualitative researchers use structured questions only to elicit socio-demographic data, that is, about age, duration of condition, duration of experience, type of occupation, qualifications and so on. Sometimes research or ethics committees ask for a predetermined interview schedule so that they can find out the exact path of the research. For the purpose of gaining permission, a semi-structured interview guide is occasionally advisable for health researchers.

Types of questions in qualitative interviews

When asking questions, interviewers use a variety of techniques. Patton (2015) states that there are specific strategic themes for qualitative research and lists particular types of questions, for example *experience, feeling* and *knowledge* questions. The sequencing of the questions is also important.

Spradley (1979) distinguishes between grand-tour and mini-tour questions. Grand-tour questions are not specific but broad, for instance: Tell me about a typical day in your clinic (on your ward, in your profession, etc.). Tell me about your condition (to a patient). Mini-tour questions are more specific, for instance: What did you do when you were questioned about your decisions (to a health professional)? What were your feelings when you first came to the clinic (to a patient)?

Example 6.3 Experience Questions, Feeling Questions, Knowledge Questions and Follow-up Questions

Experience questions
Tell me about your experience of caring for terminally ill patients.
Tell me about your experience of working with sick children.

Feeling questions
How did you feel when your first patient died?
How did you feel when you were first diagnosed?

Knowledge questions
What did you do to cope with this?
What treatment did you receive?
What services are available for this type of patient?

Follow-up questions
You told me about the time when you went to hospital, can you tell me more about that, please?
     You used the term 'I was thrown into the deep end' when you started working in your profession, what did you mean by that?
     (All questions can be followed up to explore the participants' thoughts more fully.)

KEY POINT

The skilled interviewer is non-judgemental, flexible and listens rather than talks in the interview.

Charmaz (2014) advises interviewers to consider the differences between open-ended questions, which allow flexibility for participant and researcher, and others that might just be answered by 'yes' or 'no'. She demonstrates the need for the researcher to ask explorative questions.

Practical considerations

In qualitative studies, questions are as non-directive as possible but still guide towards the topics of interest to the researcher. Researchers should phrase questions clearly and aim at the various participants' levels of understanding. Ambiguous questions lead to ambiguous answers. Double questions are best avoided; for instance, it would be inappropriate to ask: How do you feel about this condition, and what did you think about your treatment?

The researcher must be aware of practical difficulties in the data collection phase, particularly when interviewing in hospital. The routine of the hospital is disrupted by the presence of the health researcher whose activities might be viewed with suspicion by colleagues. A quiet place for interviews cannot always be found, and therefore the privacy of patients may be threatened. The ward might be full of noise and activity, and the researcher does not always find a convenient slot for interviewing without being interrupted by nursing activity, consultant round, cleaners, meals and so on. In the community, interviews are often interrupted by children or spouses and by the visits of friends or relatives. Mainly however, the interviewer listens carefully and attentively without prejudice.

Probing, prompting and summarising

During the interviews, researchers can use prompts or ask for examples and descriptions. These also help to reduce anxiety for researcher and research informant. The purpose of probes is a search for elaboration, meaning or reasons. Seidman (2019) suggests the term 'explore' and dislikes the word 'probe' as it sounds like an interrogation, and is the name for a surgical instrument used in medical or dental investigations and stresses the interviewer's position of power.

Exploratory questions might be, for instance: What was that experience like for you? How did you feel about that? Can you tell me more about that? Can you describe an example of when that happened? That's interesting, why did you do that? Questions can follow up on certain points that participants make or words they use. The researcher could also summarise the last statements of the participant and encourage more talk through this technique. For a discussion of the issues of achieving both breadth and depth in interviews, see Todres and Galvin (2005).

Example 6.4 Interviews and Telephone Interviews

Nguyen *et al.* (2020) conducted research in Germany on 18 men who lived with breast cancer, a rare occurrence in this gender. They investigated these participants' experiences over time face-to-face or by semi-structured telephone interviews which lasted between 18 and 85 minutes. They found among other results that men need male-specific information, support and care.

Participants often become fluent talkers when asked to tell a story, reconstructing their experiences, for instance a day, an incident or the experience of an illness. Unfortunately, the data from interviews are sometimes more fluent or extensive when the participants are articulate, and occasionally researchers may choose those who have language and interaction skills. This may create bias in the interviews, however, and choosing only articulate participants is therefore not a good strategy.

The social and language skills of the researcher often make a difference to the outcome of the interview. Non-verbal prompts are also useful. The stance of the researcher, eye contact or leaning forward encourages reflection. In fact, listening skills, which some nurses, midwives and allied health professionals already possess from the counselling of patients, will elicit further ideas. Patients often give monosyllabic answers until they have become used to the interviewer, because they are reluctant to uncover their feelings or fear that judgements might be made about them. When participants do not understand the interview question, the researcher can rephrase them in the language they understand. Researchers find that articulate people are easier to interview, but the research would be skewed if they only talk to these people; others too have a need to be heard. The interview planning should include reflection on these issues and include strategies to help people describe and share their views and experiences.

The social context of the interview

Interviews must be seen in the social context in which they occur; this affects the relationship between researcher and research as well as the data generated by it (Manderson *et al.*, 2006). The setting is of particular importance; if interviews take place in the home of the participants, they are more relaxed, the researcher might gain richer data and the participant is in some position of control. On the other hand, this setting can be a difficult choice for the researcher as there might be many distractions such as children or spouses who interrupt the proceedings. Sometimes a neutral place such as a corner in a café or park or an academic environment can be appropriate.

The researcher has to reflect on time and location and the persons involved in the interaction. Experience, background and characteristics of the researcher, as well as the participants' group membership such as age, gender, class or ethnic group might also influence the interaction. Manderson *et al.* (2006) suggest that changes in any of these factors might generate different interview data as the social dynamics of the interview vary; indeed, Roulston *et al.* (2003: 654) stress 'the socially constructed nature of interview talk'. When sensitive topics are discussed, researchers have to use their own judgement whether their gender or ethnic membership might interfere with the research relationship. In some situations, it is more sensitive and even useful when researcher and participant are of similar background. This is by no means always so. One of our students, a very young woman, interviewed older people about their lives. This study elicited more data than would be usual. The participants provided very rich data and deep thoughts – perhaps because they did not feel threatened.

When patients are interviewed, they might ask the researcher about advice on their condition or treatment. It is best to separate the researcher and professional roles, although this cannot always be done. It is best to point out a professional source of information or put the participants in touch with an expert who can answer their questions. In the case of very vulnerable people and sensitive topics, the researcher might seek advisors or experts before the research starts and ask for permission to contact them if necessary. If an emergency occurs during the interview, the researcher has to adopt the best way to assist the patient. It is important to consider the setting of the interviews carefully so that both the participant and the researcher are safe during the interview process.

Unexpected outcomes: qualitative interviewing and therapy

Certain commonalities exist between qualitative and therapeutic interviews. However, researchers and therapists have different aims; the researcher's aim is to gain knowledge while the therapist's aim is to assist in the healing process. Several studies have shown, however, that qualitative interviews might be beneficial for the participants, especially after they have gone through a traumatic experience. Brinkmann and Kvale (2015) argue that among other elements of interviews, interaction with others and remembering the past might be therapeutic. The researcher, however, should not lose sight of the original purpose of the interview.

Length and timing of interviews

The length of time for an interview depends on the participants, the topic of the interview and the methodological approach. Of course, the researcher must suggest an approximate amount of time – perhaps an hour and a half – so that participants can plan their day, but many are willing or wish to go beyond this, some as much as 3 or 4 hours. Others, particularly elderly people or physically weak informants may need to break off after a short while, say 20 minutes. Children cannot concentrate for long periods of time and special considerations are needed when research involves children. Health researchers have to use their own judgement, follow the wishes of the participant and take the length of time required for the topic. One of our colleagues suggests that 3 hours should be the absolute maximum because concentration fails even experienced researchers or willing participants.

Phenomenological interviews focus on one phenomenon or a limited number of very specific phenomena by using 'experience near' questions. Because of the reflective character of the interviews, the participants may become tired as they recount their experiences and importantly describe and illustrate with examples; hence the researcher may not be able to continue the interview for long. Also, as the questions concentrate on the specific phenomenon, extraneous matters are not always significant for the study, in contrast to ethnographic research for instance.

Stating an approximate time length for the interview can ensure that the interview can be closed comfortably, coming to a natural ending point for the researcher who is pressed for time, although it is advisable to leave plenty of time for interviewing, at least 90 minutes. For hard-pressed professionals, this type of data collection is very time-consuming, however useful and therapeutic it may be for the participant. It is also trying and can be stressful for participants who willingly give their time. As stated before, researchers can, of course, re-interview one or more times, and often this is recommended for methodological reasons or for practical reasons.

KEY POINT

Interviewers should take account of the age and vulnerability of the participants.

Recording interview data

A number of techniques and practical points must be considered so that the data are recorded and stored appropriately.

Interview data are recorded in three ways:
1 Digital recording of the interview
2 Note taking during the interview
3 Note taking after the interview

Digital recording

Before analysing the data, researchers must preserve the participants' words as accurately as possible. The best form of recording interview data is by using a digital recorder or tape recorder. Recordings contain the exact words of the interview, inclusive of questions. When recording, researchers do not forget important answers and words, can have eye contact and pay attention to what participants say.

Researchers must ask for permission before recording. Some participants do not wish to be recorded, and researchers have to respect this and either take notes or remember the gist of the interview and record it in writing in their fieldnotes shortly after the interview. Occasionally, participants change their minds about recording, and their wishes should be paramount. The principle of respect for autonomy includes choice and free decision and must be considered first in terms of consent. This allows for the participants' right to refuse participation in research. This right can be exercised at any stage of the research process. Video recording is more problematic, and many participants may refuse to be recorded on film; this is their right. Some large-scale research programmes depend on video recording, but again, the recording depends on the participants.

Initially the participants may be hesitant, but they will get used to the digital recorder; a small unobtrusive recorder is easier to forget than a large one, but a larger recorder can be placed further away so it is not necessarily always visible or disturbing. In addition, special microphones can be placed around the room if necessary and where resources allow. By asking factual questions first, researcher allows the participants to relax and help make them feel more secure. Some interviewees have soft and quiet voices, particularly if they feel vulnerable. Interviewers therefore place the recorder near enough, but not so prominently that it intimidates the hesitant person. Lapel microphones allow a better quality of sound, and there are specially designed microphones available that can rest on a table which are useful for focus groups. A room away from noise and disturbances enhances not only the quality of the recording but also the interview itself; participants feel free to talk without interruption.

We have experienced some problems with recorders. They sometimes run low on battery power or can break down, and it is advisable to try them out at the beginning of the interview and after it has been recorded. Researchers should remember to pack some extra batteries. A range of good digital recording devices are now available, although expensive, but they can download audio files directly onto a computer. Check out how you will listen to the recording for transcribing before you invest in equipment. Generally, it is much better to use recorders with conference facility, although we know that students often find them too expensive and have no access to them. The university often can supply digital recorders to staff and students for the duration of the data collection.

The recording is dated and labelled. Only pseudonyms should appear on the digital file or its transcription, and participants' names must be stored in a different place from the recordings. The transcription of data will be discussed in Chapter 17.

There was a charity organisation formerly called DIPEx – Data Base of Individual Patient Experience – which is now called 'health talk online'. (The website is http://www.healthtalk.org/peoples-experiences.)

This is an internet-based multimedia resource, which records and disseminates research into the health experiences of people. The qualitative interviews on the website were undertaken by the Health Experiences Research Group of the Department of Primary Care Health Services at the University of Oxford.

From this developed an umbrella organisation, DIPEx International, which is an affiliation of all the countries carrying out this type of research.

Note taking

Note taking is important but might disturb the participant during the interview. It is also difficult to listen attentively if taking notes. Contextual notes can be made before the interview; others immediately afterwards when events and thoughts are still clearly in the mind of the researcher. Note taking is further discussed in Chapter 17.

The interviewer–participant relationship

The relationship between researcher and participant is based on mutual respect and a position of equality as human beings. The fallacy exists, however, that the interviewer and the person interviewed work together in a relationship of complete equality. Health researchers, by virtue of their professional expertise and skill in interviewing, are in a position of some power, however much they attempt to achieve a relationship of equality with the participant. Researchers can empower patients and colleagues by listening to their perspective and giving voice to their concerns. In our experience, often participants report that they have not had an opportunity to fully reflect on their experience or their health condition until the qualitative interview. The interviewer also respects the way in which participants develop and phrase their answers (Marshall and Rossman, 2015); they are, after all, not passive respondents but active participants in an important social encounter. Trust is built up through involvement, attentiveness and interest in the perspectives of the patient. It must also be remembered, however, that the interviewer is not a blank screen (*tabula rasa*) but also an active participant in the interview and thus takes part in co-constructing meaning.

Often, though not always the conversational participants have similar, though not the same, understandings of it and base interview questions and answers on shared meanings, but different ideas of both also must be taken into account. Interviews can be enjoyable for the participants: Lofland *et al.* (2004) suggest that there is often a *quid pro quo* in research. The researcher gains knowledge from informants who, in turn, find listeners for their feelings and reflections, and many indeed state that this is the first time for a disclosure of these thoughts.

Peer interviews

Many health professionals have an interest in the views and ideas of their colleagues. There are advantages and disadvantages in interviewing one's peers. Shared language and norms can be advantageous or problematic. A researcher who is involved in the culture of the participants more easily understands cultural concepts. Although there is less room for misinterpretation, misunderstandings can arise from the assumptions of common values and beliefs.

Researchers do not always question ideas that are uncovered or constructs that arise from interviews with colleagues, or they make unwarranted assumptions. This can be overcome by acting as 'cultural stranger', or 'naïve' interviewer, asking participants about their meaning and clarification of their ideas.

In many peer interviews, researcher and informant are in a position of equality (Platt, 1981), and the researcher is not distant or anonymous. The close relationship has the advantage that the participants will 'open up' and trust researchers, but there is the danger of over-involvement and identification with colleagues.

Coar and Sim (2006) reported on a study which included peer interviews and found that professionals often saw these as a test of their professional knowledge and felt vulnerable. The authors described the methodological issues involved in these peer interviews and showed that the interviews depended on the research relationship and the view of the professional identity of participants.

Students, however, sometimes interview friends and acquaintances for pragmatic and opportunistic reasons. Although this is useful to overcome the hurdles of getting to know informants and forming relationships, the selection from this group might create unease or embarrassment if the topic is a sensitive one. Participants and interviewers might hold assumptions about each other, which might prejudice the information. Great care needs be taken in the choice of participants, and there needs to be awareness of the implications of undertaking an inquiry in a context where one is an insider, colleague or friend.

Problematic issues and challenges in interviewing

Interviews are often seen as easy by novice researchers. Roulston *et al.* (2003) give four specific challenges: unexpected participant behaviour, consequences of the researcher's own actions and subjectivities, phrasing and negotiating questions and dealing with sensitive issues. We shall give examples here: The people in the research are sometimes less articulate than the researcher assumes; it may be hard to bring to words the depth of the experience; they may be in an environment not conducive to interviewing, or they might not be able to concentrate. The researchers might not have explained their behaviour, and the participant is confused or worried; they might be too controlling in the interview and take over the talk or speak far too much. Sometimes this is linked to enthusiasm and interest, but nevertheless, too much talk from the interviewer is not appropriate. The questions might not be focused on the core of the study, or not open-ended enough. New researchers, in particular, often do not know how to phrase questions to put the participants at ease. People feel awkward to discuss sensitive issues, and particular skills are needed; whilst the participants might be willing to answer a nurse, they might feel uncomfortable being interviewed by a student or a senior professional. On the other hand, one of the richest data sets were obtained by one of our third-year students, because the participants felt able to disclose details to somebody who did not judge them and had great ability to communicate empathy. Dealing with emotional situations is easier for some researchers, while it is more difficult for others, and this is also the case for participants.

Interviewing through electronic media

E-mail and other online research as well as telephone interviews have become more popular in all research in recent years. Computer-mediated research entails the direct use of computers in research. So far, not many health research studies exist which have used this form of inquiry but they are increasing, and telephone interviews are quite popular. Occasionally, some of these interviews are used to supplement face-to-face interviewing. Orgad (2005), for instance, carried out e-mail as well as face-to-face interviews with women who had breast cancer, and she also analysed websites about this topic.

Online research and e-mail interviews

The use of computers for research is increasing. It is important to know about the possibilities of qualitative interviewing online and through e-mail correspondence where the researcher and the participant do not meet each other face to face. As in conventional one-to-one or focus group interviews, researchers seek special interest groups or individuals with similar experiences or conditions, such as for instance a group of people in pain, supervisors of postgraduate students or patients with epilepsy and so on. Chat rooms and newsgroups can also be observed and their contents analysed. Denzin (1999), for instance, obtained access to a newsgroup of people recovering from alcoholism to examine the 'gendered narratives of self'.

There are two types of online one-to-one interviews: synchronous and asynchronous (Mann and Stewart, 2000). The synchronous interview takes place in real time and can be carried out with one participant or a group at the same time. This type of interview can proceed when researcher and participants read and write messages at the same time, using computers with software such as Internet Relay Chat (IRC). The researcher can ask questions and will receive an immediate response. The organisation of synchronous interviews is difficult because of differences in the time zones of various countries. It also limits the sample to those who own computers and use technology confidently and without fear.

Morton Robinson (2001) suggests chat rooms as a source of data as dialogues and multiple conversations can take place; this type of interactive discussion might be seen as a focus group interview; it is shared by a number of participants. As more than one conversation often proceeds at the same time, chat rooms can be confusing. Bulletin boards are also useful as messages and replies are posted there, and they stay in place for a time. Online discussion groups are also researched, but this needs permission from participants. There is the advantage, however, that patients can stay anonymous. Kaufman and Tzanetakis (2020) argue that research with the internet community is particularly useful, because researchers can adopt strategies and technologies that allow the participants not to be seen and have anonymity. This means the researcher is able to access vulnerable and hard to reach participants.

Ethically, access to chat rooms and bulletin boards is problematic unless the messages are completely public. It is more ethical in every case that the researcher uncovers his or her research identity to those who write the messages. The researcher also has to be careful about the trustworthiness of the data, as they are often provided anonymously.

Often virtual focus groups are purposively established by a researcher. Kralik *et al.* (2006) discuss the use of computer-mediated communication with groups of participants on e-mail, which was the result of research with people who had chronic illnesses. The advantage of these types of conversations is 'regular, reflective contact' over a period of time (p. 214). This and other types of e-mail conversation afford the participants anonymity if they want it, and this is particularly important in research with vulnerable people.

Asynchronous or non-real-time interviews are e-mail conversations. Data generation by e-mail correspondence entails asking a purposive sample of people with similar experiences to get in touch by e-mail and share these experiences with the researcher. These interviews enable correspondents to choose the best time for their writing. This technique is less intrusive than face-to-face interviews, but the researcher can still obtain the same rich data. Because correspondents never meet the researcher, they can be more open and honest about their condition or experiences. Status issues and hierarchical positions have less influence in this type of interview because the contact is not face to face. The procedure will only work fully, however, if the research is a process of ongoing dialogue over an extended period of time, sometimes as short as 3 months, sometimes as long as a year.

The advantage for the researcher is the instant availability of typed text that can be accessed at any time after the interview. Researchers can respond to questions or seek more answers when they find time and have considered the correspondents' narratives. Participants are able to enter the correspondence from an environment of their choice, often their homes. Bodily presence is not essential for a 'good' interview. Mann and Stewart (2000) showed that it can be useful for making emotions explicit in writing and being reflective. Researcher and participant are able to get to know each other quite well over a period of time. These types of interview save travel, time and money. The e-mail interviewer can also avoid lengthy transcriptions as the message can be printed out immediately. In a geographical sense, the e-mail interview can widen the access to participants.

Seymour (2001) lists several elements as important features of online research. She claims that 'the release of the interview from its imprisonment in time and space' makes it deeper, because the sites are open for longer periods of time and the response need not be immediate. Researchers can gain access to the participants in an ongoing process and clarify issues that are unclear, while participants too have the time to ask questions throughout the research process. The ongoing interaction, suggests Seymour, makes the position of the participants more egalitarian. There are also practical implications: The interviews need not be transcribed but are instantly available with little cost involved. Both researcher and participants have time to reflect on their answers. From a practical point of view, Internet research is cheaper and more convenient in some ways, as it does not necessitate travelling costs or room booking and has fewer time constraints as the research is ongoing and fits into the time frame of both researcher and participant. Also, there is a lack of assumptions that researchers have about the participants. As the latter are not visible and cannot be identified as members of particular groups with specific group membership, personality or outside appearance, they cannot be instantly labelled.

These interviews are not, of course, as spontaneous as face-to-face or even telephone interviews but they give the participants time to reflect on the questions. It must be remembered, however, that researchers who use this form of inquiry automatically exclude those who have no access to computers, although they might be important groups.

Another, now more common, type of interview takes place on 'Skype', 'Face time' or other conferencing facilities. It has some of the advantages of face-to-face interviews, and others are shared with e-mail interviewing. Some practical aspects, such as being disconnected or unclear in picture or sound, can become problematic however. Occasionally, and now more frequently, contacts for interviews are obtained via Facebook or by MSN Messenger.

Telephone interviews

Telephone interviews are another effective way of interviewing. The telephone interview is immediate, and researchers and participants are able to respond spontaneously to each other.

Telephone interviews are more convenient for health professionals and patients with little time for interviews but also save travel time for researchers who sometimes have to travel long distances and spend money on travel.

The advantages of telephone interviews are obvious. They include the immediacy of response, anonymity of participants and the effective use of time. Researchers need not travel to the participants' home or work location; they have access to a wider area and hard-to-reach populations (Mann and Stewart, 2000). The disadvantage is the lack of deeper interaction, as the interviewer does not get to know the participants and the social cues of facial expression or gestures are absent. A telephone discussion must be more structured, and this is in contrast to the tenets of qualitative research which is designed to elicit rich and deep data. It is, however, a useful way of obtaining data when other types of interview are not possible.

Ethical issues in interviewing

Ethical rules and principles that are considered in conventional forms of inquiry must also be considered in e-mail and other electronic research, for instance informed consent, confidentiality, the right not to be harmed or identified and the possibility of withdrawal at any time. Ethical issues are, however, particularly problematic in spite of the data protection law, as outsiders can gain access to the correspondence more easily than to tape-recorded interviews. It is therefore necessary that researchers inform the participants about the potential lack of security, and it is advisable to obtain written permission by post. Using e-mail, other online research and telephone interviewing means that the interviewer's words need to be more carefully considered and phrased, as they cannot be modified or accompanied by gestures and facial expressions like face-to-face conversations. Those obtaining access to a group site do not always ask for permission to 'listen in' or to use observations for research purposes, but we would suggest that health researchers inform the participants about the research and ask for this permission. In short, researchers must consider ethical issues most carefully and keep to ethical principles and procedures in all electronic media and forms of inquiry. (See also Chapter 4.)

Strengths and weaknesses of interviewing

There is an ever-increasing use of interviewing as data collection. Atkinson and Silverman (1997) spoke of 'the rhetoric of interviewing' two decades ago where the assumption exists that researchers gain full access to inner feelings and thoughts, uncovering the private self. These writers have questioned the overuse of the interview and claim that it is often seen naïvely or uncritically by researchers who take the words of the informants at face value and do not reflect or take an analytical stance; interviews do not have more privileged status than other forms of data. They should not be presented simply as 'experiences' but they have to be closely examined and analysed. Indeed, Silverman (2020) still argues, that these data depend on analysis. They often need to be complemented by other forms of research such as observations, as Hammersley and Atkinson (2019) also suggest. These writers criticise researchers' over-reliance on the use of interview data, indeed they believe that interviews are not necessarily the default method of collecting data (they elaborate this on p. 108).

There might also be inconsistency between words and actions – the old dilemma of 'what they say and what they do'. Therefore, researchers often need to observe situations and behaviour, so that they can collect data about social action and interaction. Observation not only is complementary to interviewing but is also a form of within-method triangulation.

Complex issues exist in interviewing. Researchers cannot know with certainty whether participants are telling the truth or if their memories are faulty. Generally, however, they 'tell the "truth"' as seen from their perspective even if their memories are selective. These are still useful data and context. The factual accuracy of the interview data is not as important as the motivations and thoughts of the participants (Holloway and Freshwater, 2007). Rarely the participant might tell lies but even these demonstrate their perspectives with roots in time and culture.

Researchers who interview will have to be aware of these issues to avoid the pitfalls in interviewing.

Advantages and limitations

One of the main features of qualitative interviewing is its flexibility. Researchers have the freedom to ask for more information, and participants are able to explore their own thoughts as well as exert more control over the interview as their ideas have priority. This also includes opportunities for participants to react spontaneously and honestly to questions or to articulate their ideas slowly and reflect on them. Researchers can follow up and clarify the meanings of words and phrases immediately, but they can also take time so that trust can develop.

On the other hand, the collection and especially the analysis of interview data is time-consuming and labour-intensive. Students who are very enthusiastic during the early data gathering process only realise when they are involved in transcribing and analysing how much time they need for the work.

KEY POINT

The in-depth analysis of interviews is of major importance.

The interviewer effect and reactivity

Participants sometimes react to the researcher and modify their answers to please or to appear in a positive light, consciously or unconsciously. For these reasons, a monitoring process is necessary so that researchers recognise the interviewer effect and minimise it (Hammersley and Atkinson, 2019). This means spending time with the participant so that trust can develop. The interviewers too react to the words they hear. Within the framework of the research, the researcher has different priorities from the participant. This has to be recognised so that both the insider's and the researcher's perspective can be made explicit in the research report. After all, health professionals are experts in care, informed about many health and illness issues and have their own perception of the phenomenon under study. Creswell and Poth (2018) suggest that the researcher stay as close as possible to the ideas of the participants but warn against the possibility of misinterpreting their words.

The interviewer effect is less noticeable in online interviews as interviewer and researcher do not see each other. Labelling or stereotyping is not likely, although it cannot be ruled out completely.

Summary

The in-depth interview is the most common form of data collection.
- Interviews can be face-to-face, online or by telephone.
- Through the interview, the researcher obtains the insider's view directly.
- The qualitative interview is guided, not directed.
- It is dependent on the participants whose ideas and thoughts are paramount.
- A detailed analysis is necessary.

References

Atkinson, P. and Silverman, D. (1997) Kundera's immortality: the interview society and the invention of the self. *Qualitative Inquiry*, **3** (3), 304–325.

Brinkmann, S. and Kvale, S. (2015) *Qualitative Interviews*, 3rd edn, Sage, Thousand Oaks, CA.

Charmaz, K. (2014) *Constructing Grounded Theory*, 2nd edn, Sage, London.

Coar, L. and Sim, J. (2006) Interviewing one's peers: methodological issues in a study of health professionals. *Scandinavian Journal of Primary Care*, **24** (4), 251–256.

Creswell, J.W. and Poth, C.N. (2018) *Qualitative Inquiry and Research Design: Choosing Among Five Traditions*, 4th edn, Sage, Thousand Oaks, CA.

Denzin, N.K. (1999) Cybertalk and the method of instances, in *Doing Internet Research* (ed. S. Jones), Sage, Thousand Oaks, CA.

Hammersley, M. and Atkinson, P.A. (2019) *Ethnography: Principles in Practice*, 4th edn, Routledge, Abingdon, Oxon.

Holloway, I. and Freshwater, D. (2007) *Narrative Research in Nursing*, Blackwell, Oxford.

Kaufman, M. and Tzanetakis, M. (2020) Doing Internet research with hard to reach communities: methodological reflections on gaining meaningful access. *Qualitative Research*, **20** (6), 927–944.

Kralik, D., Price, K., Warren, J. and Koch, T. (2006) Issues in data generation using email group conversations in nursing research. *Journal of Advanced Nursing*, **53** (2), 213–220.

Kvale, S. (2007) *Doing Interviews*, Sage, Los Angeles, CA.

Lofland, J., Snow, A., Anderson, L. *et al.* (2004) *Analysing Social Settings*, 4th revised edn, Wadsworth, Belmont, CA.

Manderson, L., Bennett, E. and Andajani-Sutjahjo, S. (2006) The social dynamics of the interview: age, class and gender. *Qualitative Health Research*, **16** (10), 1317–1334.

Mann, C. and Stewart, F. (2000) *Internet Communication and Qualitative Research: A Handbook for Researching Online*, Sage, London.

Marshall, C. and Rossman, G.R. (2015) *Designing Qualitative Research*, 6th edn, Sage, Thousand Oaks, CA.

McNamara, C. (2005) General guidelines for conducting research interviews. Adapted from the Field Guide for Consulting and Organizational Development. Available at http://managementhelp.org/businessresearch/interviews.htm#anchor1689211.

Morton Robinson, K. (2001) Unsolicited narratives from the Internet: a rich source of data. *Qualitative Health Research*, **11** (5), 706–714.

Nguyen, T.S., Bauer, M. Maas, N. and Kaduszkiewicz, H. (2020) Living with male breast cancer: a qualitative study of men's experiences and care needs. *Breast Care*, **15**, 6–12. doi:https://doi.org/10.1159/000501542.

Orgad, S. (2005) *Storytelling Online: Talking Breast Cancer on the Internet*, Peter Lang International Academic Publishers, New York, NY.

Patton, M. (2015) *Qualitative Evaluation and Research Methods*, 5th edn, Sage, Thousand Oaks, CA.

Platt, J. (1981) On interviewing one's peers. *British Journal of Sociology*, **32** (1), 75–91.

Roulston, K.J. (2010) *Reflective Interviewing: A Guide to Theory and Practice*, Sage, London.

Roulston, K.J., de Marrais, K. and Lewis, J.B. (2003) Learning to interview in the social sciences. *Qualitative Inquiry*, **9** (4), 643–668.

Seidman, I.E. (2019) *Interviewing as Qualitative Research*, 6th edn, Teachers College Press, New York, NY.

Seymour, W.S. (2001) In the flesh or online: exploring qualitative research methodologies. *Qualitative Research*, **1** (2), 146–148.

Silverman, D. (2020) *Interpreting Qualitative Data*, 6th edn, Sage, London.

Spradley, J.P. (1979) *The Ethnographic Interview*, Harcourt Brace Johanovich College Publishers, Fort Worth, TX.

Todres, L. and Galvin, K.T. (2005) Pursuing breadth and depth in qualitative research: illustrated by a study of the experience of intimate caring for a loved one with Alzheimer's disease. *International Journal of Qualitative Methods*, **4** (2), 20–31.

Further Reading

Fielding, N.G., Lee, R. and Blank, G. (2017) *The Sage Handbook for Online Research Methods*. Sage, London, Chapters 24 and 25 are of particular interest for this chapter.

King, N., Horrocks, C. and Brooks, J. (2019) *Interviews in Qualitative Research*, 2nd edn, Sage, London.

Chapter 7
Observation and Documents as Sources of Data

Participant observation

Observation provides a rich source of data. It is used in many research approaches but always forms part of ethnography as fieldwork. Through observation, researchers look at and try to understand the group or culture under study. It is not included formally in approaches based on narratives or textual analysis such as descriptive phenomenology, narrative research or conversation analysis. Although interviewing is a more popular strategy for those undertaking qualitative inquiry, many qualitative researchers believe that observation should complement interviews (Corbin and Strauss, 2015; Hammersley and Atkinson, 2019) or even precede them. It provides access not only to the social context of the inquiry but also to the ways in which people act and interact. In any case, for health professionals, it is important to observe patients, and this everyday practice in clinical settings might help them use participant observation in research. There are many opportunities to do so – perhaps on a ward, in a reception area, in the emergency department, a clinic or any other relevant location inside the hospital, the community, in the doctor's surgery or any other healthcare settings. (See also the critique of the 'interview society'.)

Savage (2000), a nurse researcher, sees parallels between observation and clinical practice two decades ago, and they are still valid:

1 *Reliance on Physical Involvement:* The researcher is present in the setting. This means that health professionals need to be familiar with the location and learn about the behaviour and activities of the participants.
2 *Claims to Experiential Knowledge:* Whether they act as researchers or as professionals in clinical practice, health professionals experience the situation in similar ways although they interpret the situation differently when carrying out research or when performing their professional activities.
3 *Sharing of Theoretical Assumptions:* Similar underlying theoretical assumptions are shared both in research and clinical practice.

Qualitative Research in Nursing and Healthcare, Fifth Edition.
Immy Holloway and Kathleen Galvin.
© 2024 John Wiley & Sons Ltd. Published 2024 by John Wiley & Sons Ltd.

4 *Reciprocity of Perspectives:* In both roles, health professionals attempt to empathise with patients and put themselves in their place. This is perhaps easier for the researcher than for the busy professional in clinical practice carrying out routine business. The relationship between observer and observed in a health setting is strong, and much meaning is shared.

When researchers decide to observe, they do not set up artificial situations but look at people in their natural settings. Qualitative researchers generally use the term 'participant observation', a phrase originally coined by Lindeman (1924) which he described as the exploration of a culture from the inside. Jorgensen (2020) suggests that participant observation provides access to the meaning and experience of the insider, though one might add that the observer who could be familiar with the setting might not necessarily be an outsider. The researchers will become an integral part of the setting they enter and, to some extent, a member of the group they observe.

There has been a debate about the nature of participant observation. Some see it as a research approach or methodology, others merely as a complementary procedure for collecting qualitative data and an additional data source. The discussion here centres on observation as a data collection strategy within particular approaches to qualitative research such as ethnography, grounded theory, action research and others. A major critique in qualitative research concerns the lack of observational strategies in many studies, particularly ethnography, and more generally: there is still not enough use of observation in qualitative health research.

The origins of participant observation

Participant observation has its origins in anthropology and sociology. Travellers in ancient times wrote down their observation of cultures they visited, often as participants in those cultures, making it probably the earliest of all forms of data collection. From the early days of fieldwork, anthropologists and sociologists became part of the culture they studied, and examined the actions and interactions of people in their social context, 'in the field'.

Immersion in culture and setting

Immersion in a setting can take a long time, often years of living in a culture. DeWalt and DeWalt (2011) stress that researchers need to be involved in the context for a prolonged period of time; they should learn the language used in the setting. For health professionals, this is an easy task as they are already familiar with language, routines and people in the setting, although they must be aware that these vary for context and situation. Extraordinary occurrences and critical events must also be observed as they are specific to the setting. DeWalt and DeWalt advise attention to detail which includes 'mapping the scene', observing patterns, arrangements and activities.

Participant observation sometimes proceeds over one or several years, although some observation does not take as long. Health professionals, of course, are already members of and familiar with the culture they examine. For these reasons, they may not need a long introduction to the setting; they might, however, miss significant events or in the locale because of familiarity. This also means that they should suspend prior assumptions, so as not to miss important aspects or misinterpret the situation. In smaller qualitative research studies, the observation is sometimes much shorter.

KEY POINT

To observe, researchers need to immerse themselves in the setting for a period of time.

Prolonged observation generates more in-depth knowledge of a group or subculture, and researchers can avoid disturbances and potential biases caused by an occasional visit from an unknown stranger. Observation is less disruptive and more unobtrusive than interviewing. However, participant observation does not just involve observing the situation, but also listening to the people in the setting.

The classic studies by Becker *et al.* (1961) and Atkinson (1995) demonstrate what immersion and prolonged engagement in healthcare settings mean.

Example 7.1 Immersion in the Setting

In the classic American study by Becker *et al.* (1961), the participants, medical students, were observed long term in their interaction with patients, colleagues and teachers, and the researchers then asked questions about what they saw and heard.

Focus and setting

The dimensions of social settings, according to Spradley (1980), focus on the features which catalogue some ideas about the foci of observation, although these depend on the particular research question.

Spradley (1980) classified the dimensions of social situations:

- Space: the location in which the research takes place.
- Actor: the participants in the setting.
- Activity: what is being done.
- Objects: the material objects in the setting.
- Act: single actions that persons in the setting carry out.
- Event: happenings and related activities.
- Time: sequencing and length.
- Goal: people's intentions.
- Feeling: what people feel and how they express their emotions.

(Adapted from Spradley (1980: 78 and 82)

Nurse researchers and other health professionals centre particularly on the interaction of patients and professionals as well as the actions and activities of both groups. Not only are there descriptions of physical actions and interactions but also of the dialogue that goes on in the setting. The dimensions of the situation and context need detailed description and, eventually, interpretation by the researcher which often can only be developed through asking people about their behaviours and about the meanings of objects, routines and events. Hammersley and Atkinson (2019) argue that interviewing is part of participant observation.

Examples 7.2 Observation Research

Thompson *et al.* (2020) published a study of observations – complemented by other methods – in a Canadian nursing home to examine intimate care. The 'complex process' explored found that quality care involved successful interaction at three major levels, the resident/care giver, the health care organization and health policy.

Danish nursing research was carried out by Sørensen *et al.* (2013) in three different sites with patients who had chronic obstructive pulmonary disease. This included participant observation during the treatment with non-invasive ventilation. To supplement observation of nurse–patient collaboration during treatment and care, Sørensen also interviewed patients and had informal conversations with nurses.

The above examples of observation studies are based on participant observation. A non-participant observation study reported by Dunford *et al.* (2013) examined parents' behaviour when dealing with their adolescent children who suffered from chronic pain. The observations described both non-verbal and verbal behaviours of parents in interaction with their children.

Any appropriate setting can become the focus of the study. Participant observation varies on a continuum from open to closed settings. Open settings are public and highly visible such as street scenes, corridors and reception areas. In closed settings, access is more difficult and has to be carefully negotiated;

personal offices or meetings in wards can be considered closed settings. It is useful to examine how people in the setting go about their routine and everyday business, how they act and interact with each other and how they relate to the space and the environment in which they are located. Rituals, routines and ways of communication can also be uncovered. Gobo and Molle (2017) discuss the questions of how to observe and what (whom) to observe. The first dilemma is one of familiarity and distance. Closeness to the setting can focus researchers and they know already some of the areas which they wish to observe. Distancing, however (being a naïve observer), will generate surprise and add a 'new lens' through which settings and people can be observed. The question of what to observe can be answered more easily: Marginal groups are appropriate for observation; for instance, those who are ill are isolated from ordinary social interaction, here researchers may find it easier to suspend their assumptions. Some researchers, for instance, might study the adaptation of immigrant nurses to a new culture; others observe novice learners on the hospital ward.

Researchers often observe critical incidents, dramatic events and examine language use, depending on location or topic, but they can also observe in detail exits and entrances of group members, body language, facial expressions and even choice of words and typical conversations (Abrams, 2000).

Observation provides a holistic perspective on the setting. Health researchers can observe as insider and ask questions, which an outside spectator could not do. If they become deeply engaged and stay for a considerable time, participants will become used to their presence, and the observer effect will be minimal. The problems and unexpressed needs of the participants also can be observed. Although participants describe their experiences in interviews and reflect on events and actions, researchers will not have to rely only on participants' memories; they will be able to distinguish between 'words and deeds', 'what we say and what we do', which are not always the same (see Deutscher, 1973). Also, observation, however useful and appropriate, is time-consuming; hence, it is not generally used in undergraduate research, while postgraduates and health professionals in the clinical arena have more scope to include observational periods of data collection.

Types of observation

Participant observers enter the setting without wishing to limit the observation to particular processes or people; consequently, they adopt an unstructured approach. Occasionally certain foci crystallise early in the study, but usually observation progresses from the unstructured to the more focused until eventually specific actions and events become the main interest of the researcher.

Gold (1958) identified four types of (overlapping) observer involvement in the field which most qualitative researchers still describe:

1 The complete participant
2 The participant as observer
3 The observer as participant
4 The complete observer

The complete participant

The complete participant is part of the setting, a member of a group within it and takes an insider role that often involves covert observation.

Example 7.3 Classic Research

Example of Classic Research with Complete Participant

Roth (1963), an American sociologist, was a patient in a tuberculosis hospital. While being part of the setting, he observed the interaction of patients with the health personnel, focusing on negotiation concerning time spent in and out of hospital. This is an early, classical observation study.

Pope and Allen (2020) argue that covert observation might be justified in research with participants to whom access is difficult, or when investigating sensitive topics. In spite of the value of some of these studies, complete participation generates a number of ethical problems. First of all, one would have to question seriously whether covert observation in care settings, without knowledge or permission of the people observed, is ethical. After all, this is not a public, open situation such as a street corner or rally, where individuals cannot be identified. In the public domain, observation is permissible and may produce valuable data. For health professionals who advocate caring and ethical behaviour, covert observation in closed settings would be inadvisable. We would not advocate this type of observation, and undergraduates or novice researchers should never attempt it (see also Chapter 4).

The participant as observer

Here, researchers have negotiated their way into the setting, and as participant observers they are part of the work group under study. This seems a good way of doing 'insider' research, as they are already involved in the work situation. They might want to examine aspects of their own practice area, team, hospital or ward, for instance. The first stage is to ask permission from the relevant gate-keepers and participants and explain the observer role to them. The advantage of this type of observation is the ease with which researcher–participant relationships can be forged or extended. Researchers can move around in the location as they wish, and thus observe in more detail and depth, for example, they may follow particular occupational groups or 'patient pathways'. For new researchers, observation is more difficult and demanding than interviewing, mainly because of the time needed for 'prolonged engagement', but also the many ethical issues involved require careful thought through strategies and planning for a range of possible events. For ethical reasons, the participant observer discloses their research role.

The observer as participant

An observer, who participates only by being in the location rather than working there, is only marginally involved in the situation. In this case, researchers might observe a particular unit but not directly work as part of the work force; for instance, they might observe a location where they have not been previously. They must, however, announce their interest and their public role and go through the process of gaining entry and asking permission from patients, gate-keepers and colleagues. The advantages of this type of observation are the pos-sibility of asking questions and being accepted as a colleague and researcher but not called upon as a member of the work force. On the other hand, observers are prevented from playing a 'real' role in the setting. Restraint from involvement is not easy, particularly in a busy situation where professionals must be protected from intrusion when working.

The complete observer

Complete observers do not take part in the setting and use a 'fly on the wall' approach. Being a complete observer when the observer is not a participant is only possible when the researchers have some distance from the setting and observe through a window, in a corner or through a two-way mirror where they are not noticed and have no impact on the situation or when they use static video cameras fixed on the ceiling. Researchers might also use films or videos from observations made by others and analyse them. This kind of obser-vation opens up the possibility of more covert research but also offers opportu-nity for the presence of 'a bystander'. Complete observation is often used in quantitative studies, because numerical scores related to time and events can be collected. However, there are increasing examples of qualitative research using technologies in a variety of settings, where recordings can then be analysed qualitatively.

There is no clear distinction, however, between these types of observation; they overlap, it is useful to think of a continuum of observer as participant and participant as observer when considering the observational stance for a study.

Specific ethical issues in observation

As usual permission from participants should be requested for observation in healthcare settings. Access and permission to observe is more difficult to achieve than in other forms of data collection. All within the setting are included for this permission and also those who have power to withhold and gain access, such as service managers. When researchers have achieved the initial contact, it is important to establish rapport with the group or cultural members. Researchers must make it quite clear that they are not 'spies' for organisations in any of these situations. People feel more vulnerable in observational or any research situations, and they worry about their identification, the longevity, ownership and sharing of observational records. Hence it is unusual – though not impossible – to record films in healthcare settings; however, we would not advise this for novice researchers. Often documentary programmes are made by television channels, and sometimes these are somewhat lax about ethical issues, though lately film makers have become more aware. There are sensitive and important issues and challenges in any observational strategies and particularly as health researchers have a great responsibility to vulnerable people in any setting.

Progression and process

In his classic text, Spradley (1980) claims that observers progress in three stages; they use *descriptive, focused* and finally *selective* observation. Descriptive observation proceeds on the basis of general questions that the observer has in mind. Everything that goes on in the setting provides data and is recorded, including colours, smells and appearances of people. Description involves all five senses. As time goes by, certain important areas or aspects of the setting become more obvious, and the researcher focuses on these because they contribute to the achievement of the research aim. Eventually, observation becomes highly selective, centring on very specific issues only. Researchers adopt the strategy of progressive focusing.

LeCompte *et al.* (1997) give guidelines for observation, which we will summarise here as they are still valid.

The 'who' questions

Who and how many people are present in the setting or take part in the activities? What are their characteristics and roles?

Health professionals observe the situation and specifically focus on the many role performances and interactions.

The 'what' questions

What is happening in the setting, what are the actions and rules of behaviour? What are the variations in the behaviour observed?

Health professionals focus on the activities and behaviour of those involved.

The 'where' questions

Where do interactions take place? Where are people located in the physical space?

For health professionals this means looking at the ward, the clinic, the GP's surgery or meeting. Even discussions at the bedside or handovers are of importance.

The 'when' questions

When do conversations and interactions take place? What is the timing of activities?

Events, discussions and interactions take place at different times. Health professionals must ask whether there is any significance in the timing of these.

The 'why' questions

Why do people in the setting act the way they do? Why are there variations in behaviour?

The 'why' questions are self-explanatory. Researchers examine the reasons for the activities, behaviour or critical incidents. This does, of course, often include interviewing participants.

Process

Mini-tour observation leads to detailed descriptions of smaller and more intimate units, while *grand-tour observations* are more appropriate for larger settings. After the initial stages, certain dimensions and features of observation become interesting to the researcher who then proceeds to observe these dimensions specifically. 'Progressive focusing', which was discussed earlier, is not a feature just of interviewing but also of observation.

The study becomes more focused as time progresses, because the observer notices important behaviours or interactions. Focused observations are the outcome of specific questions. From broader observations, researchers might proceed to observing a small unit. They could look for similarities and differences among groups and individuals. For this type of observation narrow focus and specificity are useful and necessary.

Marshall and Rossman (2015) argue that observation means systematic exploration of events and actions as well as noting the use and position of artefacts (objects) in the setting under study. Researchers observe social processes as they happen and develop. Participant observations can focus on events, processes and actions, but they cannot explore past events and thoughts of participants; this has to be done in interviews. Hammersley and Atkinson (2019) see interviewing as part of participant observation. The previously cited work by Becker *et al.* (1961) shows this clearly. Hammersley and Atkinson (2019), in fact, propose that one might see all social research as participant observation to the extent that the researcher actively participates in the situation.

Researchers may be reluctant to carry out formal participant observation because of time and access problems; for instance, it is easier to interview colleagues or clients than to observe them. Observation might change the situation, as people act differently in the presence of observers, although they often forget being observed in long-term research. The latter, however, takes more time than is available in student projects and therefore it is more often used by postgraduates and experienced researchers who have a longer time span for their research.

When observations are successful, they can uncover interesting patterns and developments, which have their basis in the real world of the participants' daily lives, and the task of exploration and discovery is, after all, the aim of qualitative research.

Researchers sometimes triangulate within method, for instance, they use qualitative analysis of observation *and* interviews *and/or* documents; triangulation enhances the trustworthiness and authenticity of the study (see Chapter 18). Most of the examples above are triangulated within method.

The data gained from observation and other data sources might be serendipitous and generate unexpected findings.

Problems in observation

Observation, through familiarity with the culture under study, generates much information about settings and situations. However, there are also some problems and disadvantages particularly for researchers who have time constraints; indeed, interviewing is particularly popular in health research because it is not quite as time-consuming.

It is difficult to record the data during observation as scribbled notes take time and might cause reactivity from the people who are being observed. We would advise careful consideration of digital-recording as participants might become embarrassed or worried, and many professionals and patients would not wish their actions to be on record, as discussed earlier. Often researchers have to base their recollections on memory rather than notes, and memories decrease over time. This means that notes which are not recorded on the location need to be written immediately after the observation. As other types of data collection, observation relies on the researcher as 'the tool' in the research whose assumptions can intrude. Indeed, the researcher leaves assumptions and expectations behind when entering the setting. Ethical issues are paramount – as in all health research. The researcher must fade into the setting, show sensitivity and not be too obvious so that there is little observer effect. The presence and intentions of the researcher need to be disclosed to all participants in healthcare settings unless they are in a public domain such as a corridor or reception area where they cannot be identified (and even that could present problems). McNaughton Nicholls *et al.* (2014: 245) suggest that observation 'sits a little messily on the continuum between generated and naturally occurring evidence'. This means there is a varied range of researcher immersion and participation. It might mean actively focusing on particular issues or indeed letting important issues emerge.

Technical procedures and practical hints

- A series of steps need to be taken, some of which are also described by Creswell and Poth (2018).

  1 The setting for the observation is selected and permission for access obtained from gatekeepers.

  2 The researcher obtains informed consent from participants.

  3 Exact location, details and the most useful time and length of observation will be chosen and other decisions made about fieldwork and note taking.

  4 Researchers decide on the roles which they will adopt, from outsider to insider.

  5 Physical settings, behaviours such as actions, interactions and reactions are observed and noted.

  6 The researchers also note down their own feelings and reactions of the research by being reflexive.

  7 The researcher disengages from the site and debriefs the participants while assuring anonymity.

Researchers might use cameras and digital equipment to catch movements and expressions of participants more accurately, although cameras could intimidate or disturb the participants and change their behaviour. If digital recording is used, it can be viewed over and over again so 'nothing is lost' (Abrams, 2000: 58). This also means, of course, that the tapes must be kept secure and confidential, and they cannot be shown to colleagues or friends (for student projects, only to supervisors with permission of the participants).

Taking fieldnotes is an important task. Observations in the form of field notes are translated into written records which researchers take while observing or immediately afterwards. These are detailed descriptions of the setting and the behaviour of participants. The researchers' own reflections on the situation and their feelings about it are also recorded in fieldnotes (see Chapter 10). Writing might be difficult at the time of observation, and participants might object. If not possible during observation, researchers need to write them soon afterwards. Mulhall (2003: 311) suggests that 'recording events as they happen' means that the memory of the researcher is fresh and details are not lost. In the first instance, of course, fieldnotes consist of jotting down quick notes which become expanded at a later stage.

Health researchers who are actively involved in patient care may not be able to observe as well as take notes at the same time. It is important to record impressions as soon as possible after the observation. Diagrams and charts also help in recording how people act and interact in the setting under observation.

Once researchers have collected the initial observational data, they start analysing them so that the collection and analysis of data interact and go in parallel. This way the observation can become progressively focused on emerging and interesting themes that are important to the research. Drawing maps of the location or indicating interaction through diagrams can be useful devices to help observation. (Some of the analysis of observation will be discussed in Chapter 16, but in general, it progresses in the same way as other types with the fieldnotes and memos as documents for analysis.) After creating ethnographic records, collecting interview answers, documents, images or other sources of data, Gobo and Molle suggest that the researcher goes through stages those of deconstruction, construction and confirmation which are similar to the coding steps in grounded theory. When deconstructing, researchers break down the events that occur; in constructing they link the concepts found and generate stories about the phenomenon which is being studied; and confirmation follows particular core concepts in the data collection and confirms their presence in the observation, reports them and connects them to the theoretical ideas. This phase is more abstract and of higher generality than earlier stages (see also Chapter 17).

Researchers sometimes choose not only one but several locations for observation. McNaughton Nicholls *et al.* (2014) state that procedures or services which take place over a number of sites are best observed in a range of locations. If the researcher wants to examine a specific setting, only one site might be necessary.

KEY POINT

Depending on the specificity or generality of the location researchers wish to observe, they choose either one, or a range of sites.

Documentary sources of data

Documents which are written texts and records are also useful sources of data. Prior (2018) asserts that it is important to examine how they are assembled and used. It is not enough to focus on their content. They can only be understood within their context, such as time and locality. Hammersley and Atkinson (2019) suggest multiple documents such as records, rules, personal or policy documents as well as many others; they add that they could be paper-based or electronic (p. 125). Documentary sources contain added knowledge about the group being studied, and discuss that which cannot be observed. Typically, they consist of autobiographies and biographies, official documents and reports, the latter ranging from informal documentary sources to formal and official reports such as newspapers or minutes of meetings. Timetables, case notes and reports can become the focus of nurses' investigation. The researcher treats them like transcriptions of interviews or detailed descriptions of observations; that is, they are coded and categorised. They may act as 'sensitising devices' and make researchers aware of important issues. Documents may be primary or secondary sources of data. Primary sources comprise documents which have been generated by researchers themselves about the participants' experiences. They could be interview transcripts or diaries, photographs and other data.

Examples 7.4 Documents as Data

Brassolotto *et al*. (2014) showed how the analysis of a variety of different documents could be usefully employed in a study which examined epistemological barriers to dealing with the social determinants of public health professionals in Canada. Complementing the 18 interviews with professionals from public health units, the researchers analysed the units' websites, research reports, education materials, information sheets and other important documents to find key concepts and themes.

Dalglish *et al*. (2020) analyse documents in health policy. They discuss two case studies, one from Pakistan which explores the discussion of health issues in that country, and one from Niger which is an analysis of health policy on a national level.

Dalglish *et al*. also describe the way the documentary analysis might be developed. They describe their READ model: Extract data, analyse data, distil the findings and showed this in detail in their article.

Secondary sources are documents which have been produced by other researchers; these documents might be published articles or other people's studies. They are not often used in qualitative research, but when they are, they can save time and money.

Many of these texts exist before researchers start their work, others are initiated and organised by the researchers themselves, meaning that that there are pre-existing documents or researcher-generated sources. Historical documents, archives and products of the media exist independent of researchers while personal diaries might be written through their intervention or instigation.

Scott (1990) differentiates between types of document by referring to them as *closed, restricted, open-archival* and *open-published*. Access to closed documents is limited to a few people, namely their authors and those who commissioned them. As far as restricted documents are concerned, researchers can only gain access with the permission of insiders under particular conditions.

Private documents might include patient complaints, their GP's or hospital notes. Diaries and data belonging to specific people are 'closed' documents. Historical documents are archival, and these as well as published guidelines, policy papers or newspapers belong to the open-archival and open-published category.

Permission for access is asked from the living authors of diaries and keepers of other confidential documents. Open-archival documents are available to any person, subject to administrative conditions and opening hours of libraries. Published documents, of course, can be accessed by anybody at any time. There is no reactivity or observer effect in examining documentary data, although researchers, of course, come to the reading with their own assumptions. They are useful and rich sources of information for researchers.

Qualitative researchers most often seek access to diaries – which are people's own accounts of their lives – and letters, but also to historical documents or the products of the media. Some researchers encourage participants to keep a diary for analysis. Jones (2000) lists two different forms of diary: *solicited* and *unsolicited*. The former are accounts of conditions or treatments kept by patients at the behest of researchers. Unsolicited diaries are the personal and informal records patients keep about their stay in hospital, about their condition, illness or care. A researcher cannot easily access these documents.

Example 7.5 Diary Research

Three researchers published a study which used diary research in the North East of England during the COVID pandemic (Scott *et al.*, 2021). They wished to explore the young participants' experiences of this pandemic on health through diaries followed by interviews. Three major themes were found which illuminated the effects on these young people's mental health.

A different way of diary research was carried out in a study by French researchers who asked health workers (doctors, nurses and nursing assistants) in an intensive care unit to keep diaries about and for their patients. In conjunction with interviews, Perier *et al.* (2013) sampled these diaries to gain new insights into the perceptions of both health workers and patients to enhance the understanding of care.

Through documents, researchers in the health professions acquire a perspective on history which gives them insiders' views on past lives and attitudes; they can analyse contemporary documents – such as articles and comments in the press – and become aware of the significant features of issues or the dramatisation of particular events. Last, and most importantly, health professionals can trace the perspectives of diary or autobiography writers by collecting, reading and analysing these personal documents. Through this, researchers can gain knowledge of the experiences of others in a particular context and at a particular time.

Researchers must be concerned about four major criteria that determine the quality of the documents: *authenticity, credibility, representativeness* and *meaning* (Scott, 1990). To demonstrate authenticity for historical documents, questions about their history as well as their writers' intentions and biases must be asked. Credibility involves some of these questions too. Accuracy might be affected by the writer's proximity in time and place to the events described and also the conditions under which the information was acquired at the time. Representativeness of documents is difficult to prove because researchers often have no information of the numbers or variety of documents about a particular event.

Scott (1990) claims that the most significant aim of the document collection and analysis is their meaning and interpretation. It is far easier to analyse a personal document written in the recent past where the researcher is familiar with language and context than to assess the representativeness or authenticity of a historical document whose context can only be assumed. Therefore, the researcher can only try to interpret the meaning of the text in context, study the situation and conditions in which it is written and try to establish the writer's intentions.

As in other types of data, the meaning is tentative and provisional only and may change when new data present a challenge and demand reappraisal. Hammersley and Atkinson (2019) warn that documents may generate biases as they are often written by and for elites, or people in power. That in itself, however, might be useful because not many sources exist that give the ideas of these informants.

KEY POINT

Both content and context are important when analysing documentary data.

Images as sources of data

Images are increasingly becoming part of qualitative inquiry. Audiences sit in front of television or cinema screens or in the theatre; films and photos are taken by social researchers. Those individuals who work with visual data do not form a coherent group; however, because of the rise of social and other media, this type of research is becoming more and more important.

Loizos (2000) declares that images are important records of social reality. Visual information generates primary data or can be used to supplement other data collection methods, although care must be taken in its use. Videos in particular, can enhance and expand the data derived from initial observation (the ethical issues inherent in filming are problematic, however). Still photographs are not as useful – they freeze the situation in time and do not demonstrate its processual character.

Loizos gives some practical advice in his chapter on images, such as videos, photos or films. He also points to some essential reading for the use of images. He suggests, for instance, that researchers

1 Log recordings, files, photos and other images immediately with written details of locations, people and dates.
2 Get permission from informants to reproduce their images.
3 Make sure to get good quality sound.

4 Do not forget that the technology is just a means to an end.

5 Only use recordings and other images when they really enhance the research as they may be expensive and disturb the participants in the situation. (See Chapter 15 on performative social science.)

The advantages of documentary data are obvious. Green and Thorogood (2018) maintain that they are efficient, as many are easily available from official sources such as libraries or government agencies. It is also easier to use textual and visual analysis on these data, and they consume less time.

Summary

- Observation, documents and visual data are common sources of data and complement interviews.
- Observation, in particular participant observation is part of many qualitative approaches; it can stand on its own or used in conjunction with other methods.
- There are different types of observation and a multitude of documents that can be used.
- Researchers need to record their observations and use 'thick description' for writing up.
- Participant observation can pose specific ethical problems for the researcher.

References

Abrams, W.L. (2000) *The Observational Handbook: Understanding How Consumers Live with Your Product*, NTC Business Books, Chicago, IL.

Atkinson, P.A. (1995) *Medical Talk and Medical Work*, Sage, London.

Becker, H.S., Geer, B., Hughes, E. and Strauss, A.L. (1961) *Boys in White*, University of Chicago Press, New Brunswick, NJ.

Brassolotto, J., Raphael, D. and Baldeo, N. (2014) Epistemological barriers to addressing the social determinants of health among public health professionals in Ontario, Canada: a qualitative inquiry. *Critical Public Health*, **24** (3), 321–336.

Corbin, J. and Strauss, A. (2015) *Basics of Qualitative Research: Techniques and Procedures for Developing Grounded Theory*, 4th edn, Sage, Thousand Oaks, CA.

Creswell, J.W. and Poth, C.N. (2018) *Qualitative Inquiry and Research Design: Choosing Among Five Approaches*, 4th edn, Sage, Thousand Oaks, CA.

Dalglish, S.L., Kahid, S. and McMahon, S.A. (2020) Document analysis in health policy research: the READ approach. *Health Policy and Planning*, **35**, 1421–1431.

Deutscher, I. (1973) *What We Way/What We Do: Sentiment and Acts*, Scott, Foresman, Glenview, IL.

DeWalt, K.M. and DeWalt, B.R. (2011) *Participant Observation: A Guide for Fieldworkers*, 2nd edn, Altamira Press, Walnut Creek, CA.

Dunford, E., Thompson, M. and Gauntlett-Gilbert, J. (2013) Parental behaviour in paediatric chronic pain: a qualitative observational study. *Clinical Child Psychology and Psychiatry*, **19** (4), 561–575.

Gobo, G. and Molle A. (2017) *Doing Ethnography*, 2nd edn, Sage, London.

Gold, R. (1958) Roles in sociological field observation. *Social Forces*, **36** (3), 217–223.

Green, J. and Thorogood, N. (2018) *Qualitative Methods for Health Research*, 4th edn, Sage, London.

Hammersley, M. and Atkinson, P. (2019) *Ethnography: Principles in Practice*, 4th edn, Routledge, Abingdon, Oxon.

Jones, R.K. (2000) The unsolicited diary as a qualitative research tool for advanced capacity in the field of health and illness. *Qualitative Health Research*, **10** (4), 555–567.

Jorgensen, D.L. (2020) *Principles, Approaches and Issues in Participant Observation*, Routledge, Abingdon, Oxon.

LeCompte, M.D., Preissle, J. and Tesch, R. (1997) *Ethnography and Qualitative Design in Educational Research*, 2nd edn, Academic Press, Chicago, IL.

Lindeman, E.C. (1924) *Social Discovery: An Introduction to the Study of Functional Groups*, Republic Publishing, New York, NY.

Loizos, P. (2000) Video, film and photographs as research documents, in *Qualitative Researching with Text, Image and Sound* (eds. M. Bauer and G. Gaskell), Sage, London, pp. 93–107.

Marshall, C. and Rossman, G.R. (2015) *Designing Qualitative Research*, 5th edn, Sage, Thousand Oaks, CA.

McNaughton Nicholls, C., Mills, L. and Kotecha, M. (2014) Observation, in *Qualitative Research Practice* (eds. J. Ritchie, J. Lewis, C. McNaughton Nicholls, and R. Ormston), 2nd edn, Sage, London.

Mulhall, A. (2003) In the field: notes on observation in qualitative research. *Journal of Advanced Nursing*, **41** (3), 306–313.

Perier, A., Revah-Levy, A., Bruel, C. *et al.* (2013) Phenomenologic analysis of healthcare worker perceptions of intensive care unit diaries. *Critical Care*, **17**, R13.

Pope, C. and Allen, D. (2020) Observational methods, in *Qualitative Research in Health Care* (eds. C. Pope and N. Mays), Blackwell, Oxford.

Prior, L. (2018) Using documents in social research, in *Qualitative Research* (ed. D. Silverman), Sage, London.

Roth, J.A. (1963) *Timetables*, Bobbs Merril, Indianapolis, IN.

Savage, J. (2000) Participant observation: standing in the shoes of others. *Qualitative Health Research*, **10** (3), 324–339.

Scott, J. (1990) *A Matter of Record: Documentary Sources in Social Research*, Polity Press, Cambridge.

Scott, S., McGowan, V.J. and Visram S. (2021) I'm gonna tell you how Mrs Rona has affected me. Young people's experiences of the Covid 19 pandemic in the North East of England. *International Journal of Environmental Studies and Public Health*, **8** (7), 3837.

Sørensen, D., Fredriksen, K., Groefte, T. and Lomborg, K. (2013) Nurse–patient collaboration: a grounded theory study of patients with chronic obstructive pulmonary disease on non-invasive ventilation. *International Journal of Nursing Studies*, **50** (1), 26–33.

Spradley, J.P. (1980) *Participant Observation*, Harcourt Brace Johanovich, Fort Worth, TX.

Thompson, G.N., McClement S.E., Peters, S. *et al.* (2020) More than just a task: intimate care delivery in the nursing home. *International Journal of Qualitative Studies on Health and Well-being*, **16** (1), 1943123. doi:10.1080/17482631.2021.1943123.

Further Reading

Gorsky, M. and Mold, A. (2020) Documentary analysis, in *Qualitative Research in Health Care* (eds. C. Pope and N. Mays), 4th edn, Wiley Blackwell, Oxford.

Gum, L.F., Sweet, L., Greenhill, J. and Prideaux, D. (2020) Exploring interprofessional education and collaborative practice in Australian rural health services. *Journal of Interprofessional Care*, **34** (2), 173–183.

Wood, L.M., Sebar, B. and Vecchio, N. (2020) Application of rigour and credibility in qualitative document analysis: lessons learnt from a case study. *The Qualitative Report*, **25** (2), 456–470. Available at https://nsuworks.nova.edu/tqr/vol25/iss2/1.

Chapter 8

Focus Group Research (FGR)

The nature and features of focus group research

Focus group research (FGR) is a form of qualitative inquiry where small groups of people, who have common experiences and who are asked to participate in a discussion by a researcher/facilitator (sometimes assisted by a moderator) for the purpose of exploring ideas, thoughts and perceptions about a specific topic or certain issues linked to an area of interest. (The terms researcher, facilitator or moderator are sometimes used interchangeably although sometimes two or three of these are present in focus groups.)

Most methodologists broadly agree about the features of FGR. Morgan (2019: 5) expresses it as 'a research method that collects qualitative data through group discussion'. He stresses that the dynamics of group interaction is important in this type of inquiry. Krueger and Casey (2015: 6) see the features of a focus group as '(1) A small group of people who (2) possess certain characteristics, (3) provide qualitative data, (4) in a focused discussion and (5) to help understand the topic of interest'.

Focus groups can be employed if the research question demands that participants should be exposed to a range of viewpoints so that they can express their own view about a topic, or when a group of people with similar experience helps an individual to talk about the topic in a shared context rather than in one-to-one interviews. Undertaking FGR is not easy, because complex data are generated through this method, and they are difficult to transcribe and analyse.

In the past, researchers have employed focus group techniques in the area of marketing and business research, but in the last decades they have become increasingly popular in social science or the health and caring professions. The ideas generated are normally analysed by qualitative analysis methods. FGR can stand alone, or it can be an adjunct to one to one interviews and observation, or as a complement before and after quantitative research.

Qualitative Research in Nursing and Healthcare, Fifth Edition.
Immy Holloway and Kathleen Galvin.
© 2024 John Wiley & Sons Ltd. Published 2024 by John Wiley & Sons Ltd.

Example 8.1 Stand-Alone FGR

Aquino *et al.* (2018) conducted FGR about women's perspectives on maternity care and collaboration of health professionals in two children's centres in London, UK. The 12 women involved in 3 focus groups had given birth 8 months prior to the study. One of the important findings of the research was that collaborative care from midwives and health visitors was not routinely provided but valued by the participants when it occurred.

FGR as part of a larger study

Rachel Arnold (Arnold *et al.*, 2015) conducted ethnographic research in a Kabul hospital. This involved individual interviews, observation and focus group discussions. The focus groups took place with women in the community. One of these was carried out with women of an extended family, the other took place in a poor area of the town within a pre-existing self-help group.

The type and purpose of focus groups and the number of groups are determined by the research question. Researchers might use pre-existing groups whose members have the same experience – for instance a carer group of people with similar conditions or a support group – or they can establish their own group for which members are purposefully selected to achieve the functions of the particular type of research.

The use of focus groups is centred on the specific benefits of collecting data in a group context and how the principles of the qualitative approach are made explicit and are coherent with the research question and such benefits. Focus group discussions differ from one-to-one interviews. In some texts they are called focus group interviews but more recently the term focus group discussion is used (Finch *et al.*, 2014) which is more appropriate, as this type of research resembles conversations and discussions though it is guided by researchers/facilitators. (The term researcher or facilitator will be used interchangeably in this chapter, though several of these, also called moderators might be present during the discussions.)

KEY POINT

Focus groups in research are groups of people with common interests and experiences brought together and guided by a researcher and/or facilitator.to discuss a specific topic.

While one-to-one interviews are based on the personal experiences of individuals, focus group discussions are generated through interaction between participants, and this interaction is of major importance. However, Morgan (2010) warns that interaction, although important, is not data in itself. He advocates an agenda for enhancing the understanding of the part that interaction plays: First, he suggests that researchers examine how different ways of carrying out focus group discussions affect group dynamics; second, he recommends introducing a reflexive element to assess the value that different approaches bring to the analysis of interaction; third, he wants researchers to consider when and how reporting of interaction is important (p. 721).

Group discussions require more organization and larger rooms; they also need some geographical closeness (unless they take place on the internet – see later in this chapter).

The origin and purpose of focus groups

The first text on focus groups was written by Merton and Kendall (1946), as a result of these writers working with groups during and shortly after the Second World War. In 1956 they expanded their knowledge into a book (Merton *et al.*, 1956). Business and market researchers had used this type of in-depth group discussion since the 1920s. It became especially popular in market research in order to gather information about customers' thoughts and feelings about a product, though initially this type of research was not rooted in the qualitative tradition.

Today FGR is used by a wide variety of researchers in the area of communications, policy, marketing and advertising, as well as in social research and health research. Focus groups in the social sciences and health professions have become ever more fashionable since the growth of qualitative research methods in the 1980s. This approach does not rely merely on the ideas of the researcher and a single participant; instead, the members of the group generate new questions and answers through verbal interaction. According to Tausch and Menold (2016) the interaction encourages 'synergy and spontaneity'. Researchers are able to discover the insights, needs and multiple perspectives of their clients, the perceptions and attitudes of their colleagues, and they can also examine the thought processes and organisational rationale of decision makers. The cultural values and beliefs of people can also be explored this way.

Focus group research in healthcare

Focus groups produce thoughts and opinions about a topic relevant to health care, treatment evaluation and illness experiences. Many examples are reported in nursing and social science journals.

FGR in health is characterised by interaction between the participants from which researchers discover how people think and feel about particular issues.

It is not the intention to examine a wide variety of issues in one study; these groups are set up to explore a specific issue rather than general topics which are more often investigated in marketing or political focus groups.

Focus group members respond to each other. The discussion might be started with eliciting knowledge about a specific condition, the use of a new treatment, method of intervention or by facilitating the group members to be at ease, can evolve to a discussion of reactions to and perspectives on the topic at hand. Different reactions stimulate debate about the topic, because group members respond to each other, as well as to the questions of the researcher. Discussions in groups might help not only in the development of ideas about problems and questions which researchers have not thought about before but also by finding answers to some of these questions and solutions to problems.

In the health research field, focus groups are used for the following:
Exploring patients' experiences of their condition, treatment and interaction with health professionals.
Evaluating programmes, interventions and treatment.
Gaining understanding of health professionals' roles and identities.
Examining the perception and efficacy of professional education.
Obtaining perspectives on public health issues.

These are just some of the functions of FGR. The ultimate goal for the researcher is to understand the context of the participants, and not to make decisions about a specific issue, intervention or problem without attention to this context. Future actions and policy may be based on the findings of the focus group discussions. Focus group discussions differ from individual interviews in that they depend on the stimulus that participants gain from each other, and that they discuss both unique and shared perceptions and experiences.

Sample size and composition

As in any qualitative research, the sample is linked closely to the research topic. The people who take part in a focus group usually have similar roles or experiences. They may be colleagues who share the same speciality, use the same technical equipment or nursing procedures, or people who live in the same community, use the same service or patients who suffer from the same condition.

The purpose of the focus group generally determines its composition and size. A small group might be better for controversial or complex topics (Morgan, 2019), while larger groups tend to have lower levels of involvement with less highly intense topic areas. We have also found that in smaller groups individuals can be facilitated to express more opinions and heard more clearly, although groups with larger numbers of participants might generate more ideas.

Morgan also suggests well-defined criteria for the selection of participants. These might include demographic factors, gender, ethnic group membership and specific experiences or conditions. Participants in focus groups will have had common experiences, share the same condition or receive the same services. To give examples: if health professionals wish to explore the ideas of a group of people about diabetes or asthma, they obviously involve individuals with this condition in the focus groups. A midwife can obtain the views and thoughts of pregnant women or new mothers by small focus groups about a topic which involves pregnancy or motherhood. A physiotherapist might wish to evaluate a particular technique of improving chronic back pain by setting up of small focus groups to uncover their ideas. A nurse working in a public health context wishes to understand the barriers to healthy eating and sets up focus group discussions with people who use a particular community centre. Participants who are asked to take part, generally share common interests, work in similar settings, live in similar conditions or perform similar tasks. If a nurse researcher seeks the thoughts of colleagues from a psychiatric setting about the service to support people with anorexia nervosa, for example, then the sample has to be composed of nurses with experience of caring for people who have this condition. Students in the field of healthcare can be asked about perspectives on their professional education. Health promotion, too, is commonly a topic for FGR.

The choice of the members of focus groups depends on a condition or experiences that potential participants have in common. Although group members share these, it does not mean that they all have the same views, or that they come from the same background or organisation. It might be useful to recruit members from naturally occurring groups such as antenatal classes, patient support groups or carers' groups. While they have similar experiences, they are nevertheless heterogeneous in other ways, and so could illuminate the topic from many sides.

The number of focus groups depends on the needs of the researcher and the demands of the topic area. For one research project, the usual number is about 3 or 4, but the actual number depends on the complexity of the research topic and the range of people the researcher is aiming to reach to seek their perspective. If the sample of participants is heterogeneous, more groups are needed.

Research with large focus groups and many participants is more difficult. Group sessions can last from 1 to 3 hours. We must stress, however, that 3-hour discussions with patients would be far too long and demanding. In market research, participants are paid for their time and effort but this is not always the case in healthcare research, particularly in PhD and masters projects where there is no financial resource to support participant payment. Although there can be concerns that payment may implicitly coerce informants, it has become recommended practice to pay patients and the public for their valuable time, particularly in larger focus group studies funded by research councils, the health service or charities.

Example 8.2 Stand-Alone FGR

In a study with a fairly small number of participants, Usher-Smith *et al.* (2017) carried out FGR with health professionals (24 participants, including GPs and members of primary care teams) to explore their perspectives on service provision and funding, specifically concerning patients with cancer and their life styles.

A larger study in by Barnett *et al.* (2017) explored the perceptions of individuals, within the National Bowel Cancer screening programme, whose bowel cancer screening showed a negative result. The participants were recruited through seven GP practices, two in Scotland and five in England. The researchers were particularly interested in a wide range of perspectives; hence they chose 60 participants from inner and outer cities and from affluent as well as deprived areas. The group discussions were conducted in the GP practice, and the participants received a high street voucher as a small thank you.

In FGR, each group might contain between 4 and 12 people, but 6 is probably the optimum number as it is large enough to provide a variety of perspectives and small enough not to become disorderly or fragmented. Indeed, one of our colleagues found that in her experience, even a group of six was too large and that the optimum number of members in the group was three, but the number could of course vary depending on the topic or the background of group members. Greenbaum (1998), a market researcher, however, claims that group dynamics work better if the group is not too small. The groups by Schipper *et al.* (2014), for instance, included 12 participants. However, the larger the group, the more difficult the group facilitation and transcription of the discussion. When several people start talking together, and the group is lively and noisy, it can be difficult to distinguish voices, and therefore difficult to analyse consistent or contentious perspectives.

Much new information is gained in initial groups as the researcher can follow up the ideas obtained in subsequent discussions. As in other qualitative research, important themes emerge often at an early stage, although some serendipitous results might be found in a later phase.

There may well be a difference between groups who come together for market research purposes and those who gather for health research. The former will feel much less vulnerable, because the area of discussion is rarely threatening or sensitive. The nature of the topic area too is of importance: focus groups in which sensitive topics are discussed are more difficult to facilitate. A clear rationale for the purpose of focus groups is needed if the topic is sensitive or even potentially 'taboo'.

Members of the group, although sharing common experiences, do not have to know each other. In a group of immediate colleagues or friends, private thoughts or ideas might not be revealed, although the opposite could also be true. One individual, or an 'in group' can potentially dominate others, the past history and dynamic of the group may inhibit or lead individuals in a particular direction. In healthcare research, familiarity between participants, or participants and researchers could be useful, because the 'warm-up' time – the time where participants get to know each other to facilitate interaction – is shorter, and the researcher can focus on the discussion topic earlier in the process. Stewart and Shamdasani (2014), for instance, believe that compatibility among group members is more productive than conflict or polarization; this too depends on the topic; sometimes conflict can generate new and different ideas, although it has to be managed by an experienced group facilitator.

Gender and age of the group members affect the quality and level of interaction and through this the data. For instance, evidence shows greater diversity of ideas in single sex groups than in those of mixed gender according to Stewart and Shamdasani. Mixed gender groups tend to be more conforming because of the social interaction between males and females; both groups sometimes tend to 'perform' for each other. That said, it all depends on the topic and the benefits of single gender or mixed gender groups.

KEY POINT

Focus groups differ in number, size and length but their nature depends on topic, gender and age of the participants.

Conducting focus group discussions

FGR must be planned carefully. The participants are contacted well in advance of the discussion, usually in writing, and reminded a few days before they start. As in other types of inquiry, ethical and access issues are considered. The environment for a focus group is important as the room must be big enough to be comfortable for participants and the digital recorder and microphone(s) placed in an advantageous location, where they can all be heard and recorded. For focus group work, it is essential to have a top-quality recorder. Merton and King (1990) suggest a spatial arrangement of a circle or semi-circle, which seems the most successful seating arrangement.

The group discussions should have a clearly identified agenda otherwise they deteriorate into vague and chaotic discussions (Stewart and Shamdasani, 2014). Time management is one of the tasks of the facilitator as researchers and participants do not have unlimited time. Focus groups are more productive if the time for interchange is not too short. Usually focus group discussions last around 1½ to 2 hours but this might depend on age, vulnerability or power of concentration of participants.

From the beginning the researcher establishes ground rules, so that all group members know how to proceed. Researchers plan the initial questions and prompts. When the discussion starts, they put the group at ease and introduces the topic to be debated. Strategies such as showing a film or telling a story related to the topic sometimes stimulate interaction. Photographs or vignettes might act as stimuli; Barbour (2018: 86) even suggests such stimulus material as tabloid newspapers or sections of soap operas.

Researchers often adopt the strategy of asking stimulus questions and generally proceed from the more general to the specific, just as in one-to-one qualitative interviews. Involving all the participants, rather than letting a few individuals dominate the situation demands diplomacy and would be easier with a smaller group. Extreme views in a group of people are balanced out by the reactions of the majority when debating questions. As suggested before, focus groups can be combined with individual interviews, observation or other methods of data collection, but this is not essential. We recommend two people to facilitate focus groups, one acting as observer and facilitator who helps the lead researcher to manage the group, so as to ensure everyone has a say and in keeping the discussion to time.

In focus groups, as in all other research, ethical issues must be considered. Confidentiality, in particular, could be problematic in group settings as members of the group might discuss the findings in other settings and situations. They should be reminded to keep the discussions confidential. Anonymity cannot be guaranteed, as members of the group might be able to identify other participants even when researchers only use first names. Participants may make remarks that are hurtful to others, or show prejudice, and the researcher has to plan for this eventuality and find ways to deal with this.

Finch *et al.* (2014: 218) suggest five stages for focus groups researchers: that they set the scene and establish ground rules, introduce the participants, choose a neutral opening topic, discuss the area they wish to research, and end with debriefing the participants.

The involvement and tasks of the researcher/facilitator/moderator

Researchers must be able to stimulate discussion and have insight and interest in the ideas of the informants, but they also need to step back and open the forum to the participants. The leadership role of the moderators demands abilities above that of the one-to-one interviewer. First of all, they decide on the type of participant, the number of groups and the number of people in each group (Barbour, 2018). They must have the social and refereeing skills to guide the members towards effective interaction and sometimes be able to exert control over informants and topic without directing the debate or coercing the participants. If the group feels at ease with the facilitator, the interaction will be open and productive and the participants comfortable about disclosing their perceptions and feelings.

The researcher needs to let the participants talk to examine their real feelings, and much of the discussion evolves from the dynamics of group interaction. This means that the conversation does not always follow a clear structure (Morgan, 2019). The group needs guidance as this non-directive approach has particular importance in exploratory research where perceptions are examined. High involvement of the researcher leads more quickly to the core of the topic, but special facilitation skills are needed if the focus groups are going to be successful. Researchers should not express their own biases or assumptions in the focus groups. A special relationship with a specific individual, an affirmative nod at something of which the facilitator approves, or a lack of encouragement for unexpected or unwelcome answers may bias the discussion too. Again, group behaviour is an important factor.

Focus group discussions uncover both agreement and differences between participants, and these ideas need be elicited by the researcher. Often points of agreement are discussed; although conflicts of opinion can produce valuable data, the facilitator must defuse personal hostility between members, which demands good facilitating skills. Polarisation of views may generate a difficult group climate. Gestures and facial expressions have to be controlled to show members of the group that the researcher is non-judgemental and values the views of all participants. Streubert Speziale and Rinaldi Carpenter (2011) argue that a good facilitator can help the group to avoid 'group think' and offence to some participants.

Research with online or virtual focus groups

Although FGR usually takes place with face to face contact, in recent years, it has often been conducted online: discussions take place online to debate an area of interest for research purposes. To conduct these, of course, participants need be computer-literate which automatically excludes some sections of the population. The research can occur through text by emails, on Facebook, instant messaging, chatrooms or sometimes, though rarely, even Skype.

The groups might take place at the same time, which means they are synchronous, or they could be asynchronous and occur at different times.

Example 8.3 Synchronous Focus Groups

Wirtz *et al.* (2019) conducted a feasibility study for synchronous online group discussions about HIV concerning adult transgender women in the United States. Forty-one transgender women in seven synchronous focus groups, from six cities in the United States were involved. Each group contained between 5 and 10 participants, and the discussions lasted around 60–90 minutes. A facilitator and a notetaker were present for these discussions. This study is important as it showed the feasibility of synchronous focus group discussions and its technical challenges as well as advantages and problems of this type of research.

Asynchronous focus groups

Asynchronous focus group discussions and their feasibility were explored by Boateng and Nelson (2016) also in the United States. They set up this type of inquiry with adolescents post heart transplants and their parents.

It showed that asynchronous online FGR was feasible, cost effective and could be conducted with diverse populations.

The advantage of online focus groups allows researchers to gain access to hard-to-reach or vulnerable individuals, and that the group members can stay anonymous if they so wish. Hard-to-reach participants are those who live far apart from each other or the researcher, sometimes even in different countries. Sensitive topics too can be explored, because participants are able to discuss issues that they would not disclose face-to-face with others.

The disadvantage is that the researcher does not usually see the faces of the participants, and this means that they cannot attempt to interpret their gestures and facial expressions. Online focus groups often take place in pre-existing groups who share a common interest and experience which they discuss often, and researchers attempt to gain access to these existing groups on the net, although they might also ask for people on Facebook or Twitter. Examples might be pre-existing group of people who have had a stroke or participants who suffered some form of cancer as well as support or carers' groups.

Recording, analysing and reporting focus group data

The principles of group qualitative data analysis are similar to those of other non-structured or semi-structured interviews. Most often the discussions are recorded, and initially the researchers listen carefully several times to each tape before making transcripts. Although this method has been used in market research, it is difficult to identify individuals' voices on a tape. The problem of identification might be overcome with video recording, but Sim (1998) suggests that this might inhibit participants, particularly when they discuss a sensitive issue.

All recorded files, fieldnotes and memos are dated and labelled and transcribed. The transcription should include laughter, notes about pauses and emphasis, and the researcher makes fieldnotes on anything unusual, interesting or contradictory and writes memos about theoretical ideas while listening, transcribing and reading. It is important to be clear about who says what, because this can identify those individuals who try to dominate the discussion. The researchers could note this while listening to the tape. At the listening stage, major themes and patterns can already be found. It is important, however, that researchers focus on the context of group interaction not just on the comments of particular individuals but on all of them (Asbury, 1995). This interaction might stimulate thought in the participants but it could also intimidate some or encourage others.

The analyst codes paragraphs and sentences by extracting the essence of ideas within them and using labels which are placed into the margin of the transcript. Through a reduction of these codes into larger categories, themes and ideas will be found. The analyst repeats the process with each focus group discussion and compares the transcripts. The major themes arising from each discussion group are then connected with each other; themes in one discussion will overlap with those of other focus groups. Once these themes have been formulated, the patterns described and their meaning interpreted, the litera-ture connected with these ideas is discussed. The appropriate literature becomes confirmation or challenge to the researcher's findings as in other qualitative research.

As in other types of qualitative research, the frequency of themes that are found is not as important as their significance; some obviously have priority over others for the specific study. The method of analysis in focus groups is similar to those of other approaches; in fact, focus groups can be analysed by thematic analysis (see Chapter 17) or another form of qualitative analysis. If the study is phenomenological, the group discussion and subsequent analysis will follow the principles of phenomenological interviewing and analysis, seeking transferable meaning with rich description. In grounded theory, theoretical sampling needs to be used (see respective chapters). FGs are not 'traditionally congruent with phenomenological study (Jones, 2015: 566) indeed they were seen as incompat-ible with it (Bradbury-Jones et al., 2009). Lately focus groups discussions have been undertaken within a phenomenological approach, for instance, a large study with general practitioners in an area of Denmark, used FGR (Hvidt et al., 2017). This type of FGR may be a useful way to help people describe complex everyday experiences, or to gain access to complex universal human feelings. The analyses follow the principles of the specific approach.

To write up the study, the researchers develop a storyline, that is, they must produce an account that is readable and clear. The main concerns of the partici-pants have to emerge from the report as the most important parts of the story. The findings from the focus group discussions in health research are often used as a basis for action.

KEY POINT

The analysis of focus group discussions is similar to that of other qualitative inquiry, though the interaction of participants must be taken into account.

Advantages and problems of focus groups

In general, the advantages and limitations in this approach are those of all qualitative interviews, but there are a number of strengths and weaknesses specific to focus groups (Stewart and Shamdasani, 2014). The main strength is the production of data through social interaction. The dynamic interaction stimulates the thoughts of participants and reminds them of their own feelings about the research topic. Informants build on the answers of others in the group. Second, on responding to each other's comments, informants might generate new and spontaneous ideas, which researchers had not thought of before or during the discussion. Through interaction participants remember forgotten feelings and thoughts. Third, all the participants, including the researcher/ facilitator, have the opportunity to ask questions, and these will produce more ideas than individual interviews. Kitzinger (2005) suggests that group interaction gives courage to the informants to mention even sensitive topics. The discussion might empower participants, because as group members they often feel more able to express their views.

The researcher has the opportunity for prompts and questions for clarification just like the other members of the group. These probes will produce more ideas than individual interviews, and the answers show the participants' feelings about a topic and the priorities in the situation under discussion. The researcher can clarify conflicts between participants and ask about the reasons for these differing views. Focus groups produce more data in the same space of time; this could make them cheaper and quicker than individual interviews. Some people dislike opening up their inner thoughts in public and may be reluctant to answer some questions – one of the reasons for careful selection of participants. Though the presence of others might inhibit disclosure, which is a disadvantage in these settings, it can also allow individuals to be quiet and obviate the need to respond if they do not wish to disclose something.

There are also some disadvantages. The researcher generally has more difficulty managing the debate and less control over the process than in one-to-one interviews. As group members interact throughout the discussion, one or two individuals may dominate the discussion and influence the outcome or perhaps even introduce bias, as the other members may be merely compliant. The group effect may, as Carey and Smith (1994) warn, lead to conformity or to convergent answers. They use the term 'censoring', by which they mean the critical stance of group members towards each other. The participants affect each other, while in individual interviews the 'real' feelings of the individual informant may be more readily revealed. A person who is unable to verbalise feelings and thoughts will not make a good informant in focus groups. Indeed, Merton and King (1990) stress the importance of educational homogeneity of the group. If group members have similar educational backgrounds, the chance for contribution from all members is greater. The status of a few well-educated individuals would inhibit the rest of the members in the group and might even silence them, and therefore similarity of social background is useful. If the group members might know each other before the meeting, it is important to take this into account. Sampling procedures which determine the composition of the group, are of paramount importance.

KEY POINT

FGR might not be appropriate for certain groups of people, for instance for those who are frail, very young or those who need privacy, but online group members are often able to keep their anonymity if they live in different locations.

The group climate can inhibit or fail to stimulate an individual or it can, of course, be stimulating and lively and generate more data. Where a researcher feels certain that confrontation and conflict is likely to occur between potential group members, she or he has to be sensitive to group feelings and reconcile their ideas. Conflict can be destructive but can also generate rich data. In any conflict situation, ethical issues must be carefully considered. Sim (1998) identifies some problems with focus groups.

1 It cannot be assumed that there is conformity and consensus between the individual members of the group, although it may seem so.
2 Although some inferences may be drawn about the absence or presence of certain perspectives or feelings, the strength of the individual's emotions cannot be measured or assumed.
3 Focus group findings based on empirical data cannot be generalised, though theoretical generalisation is feasible as in other qualitative research.

In research with nurses and other health professionals, it is always difficult to establish focus groups because of the differences in time when they can be available or in the lack of a suitable location which has to be large enough to accommodate more than just two people. This is easier in the community than in hospitals.

Transcription can be much more difficult than in one-to-one interviews because peoples' voices vary, and the distance they sit from the microphone influences the clarity of individuals' contributions. As there are certain dangers of group effect and group member control, it is useful to analyse the discussions both at group level and at the level of the individual participants. The researcher must remember that the data must be seen within the context of the group setting (Carey and Smith, 1994). Fieldnotes should be made immediately after the session.

Critical comments on focus group research in healthcare

Although FGR in healthcare is a useful form of inquiry because ideas from a number of people can be gained at the same time, it might be more superficial than one-to-one interviews. Also, if people are vulnerable, they might not like to disclose personal information in a group. This type of research is not always appropriate.

There is other criticism about the use of focus groups in healthcare research. We would suggest that sometimes these types of discussion are used because researchers feel this is an easy and popular way of gaining access to a larger sample, and funding agencies seem to welcome the convenience of focus groups. The complexities of setting up and facilitating focus groups are often forgotten. In a search through the Cumulative Index of Nursing and Allied Health Literature (CINAHL), Webb and Kevern (2001) found rather unsophisticated and uncritical uses of FGR in the years 1990–1999. Although this type of research has much improved, it can still be problematic. Few articles from the past contained empirical research, and furthermore, some of the discussions were superficial and non-analytical. The writers suggest that researchers discuss the theoretical and methodological assumptions in their work and become more rigorous in their use of methodology. Since the late 1990s, Webb and Kevern's claim that the input from other disciplines, the social sciences in particular, would enhance and develop knowledge has been built upon. There is now a vast array of FGR in many varied fields of health and allied social science research with developments in procedures, analysis and theoretical perspectives with several focus group methods texts, guides and handbooks available.

Summary

- A focus group consists of a number of people with common experiences or areas of interest which is guided by a researcher/facilitator in a discussion for research purposes.
- Several focus groups with a number of individuals are involved in each study.
- Whilst the discussions are carefully planned, the researcher must at the same time be flexible and non-judgemental.
- The dynamics of the group situation is intended to stimulate ideas and elicit feelings about the focus of the study.
- It is important that an open climate exists so that group members feel comfortable about sharing their thoughts and feelings.
- The data can be analysed by any qualitative analysis method as long as researchers adhere to the principles of the particular approach.

References

Aquino, M.R.J.V., Olander, E.K. and Bryar, R.M. (2018). A focus group study of women's views and experiences of maternity care as delivered collaboratively by midwives and health visitors in England. *BMC Pregnancy and Childbirth*, **18** (1). doi:10.1186/s12884-018-2127-0.

Arnold, R., van Teijlingen, E., Ryan, K. and Holloway, I. (2015) Understanding Afghan healthcare providers: a qualitative study of the culture of care in a Kabul hospital. *British Journal of Obstetrics and Gynaecology*, **122** (2), 260–267.

Asbury, J. (1995) Overview of focus group research. *Qualitative Health Research*, **5** (4), 414–420.

Barbour, R. (2018) *Doing focus Groups*, 2nd edn, Sage, London.

Barnett, K.N., Weller D., Smith, S. *et al.* (2017) Understanding of a negative bowel screening result and potential impact on future symptom appraisal and help- seeking behaviour: a focus group study. *Health Expectations*, **20** (16), 582–584.

Boateng, B. and Nelson, M. (2016) focus groups with parents and adolescents with heart transplants: challenges and opportunities. *Journal of Pediatric Nursing*, **42** (3), 120–154.

Bradbury-Jones, C., Sambrook, S. and Irvine, F. (2009) The phenomenological focus group: an oxymoron? *Journal of Advanced Nursing*, **65** (3), 663–671.

Carey, M.A. and Smith, M.W. (1994) Capturing the group effect in focus groups. *Qualitative Health Research*, **4** (1), 123–127.

Finch, H., Lewis, J. and Turley, C. (2014) Focus groups, in *Qualitative Research Practice* (eds. J. Ritchie, J. Lewis, C. McNaughton Nicholls and R. Ormiston), 2nd edn, Sage, London.

Greenbaum, T.L. (1998) *The Handbook for Focus Group Research*, 2nd edn, Lexington Books/DC Heath and Co., Lexington, MA.

Hvidt, E.A., Søndergaard, J., Hansen, D.G. *et al.* (2017). 'We are the barriers': Danish general practitioners' interpretations of why the existential and spiritual dimensions are neglected in patient care. *Communication & Medicine*, **14** (2), 106–120.

Jones, J. (2015) The contested terrain of focus groups, lived experience, and qualitative research traditions. *Journal of Obstetric Gynecologic & Neonatal Nursing*, **44**, 565–566.

Kitzinger, J. (2005) Focus group research: using group dynamics to explore perceptions, experiences and understandings, in *Qualitative Research in Health Care* (ed. I. Holloway), Open University Press, Maidenhead, pp. 56–70.

Krueger, R.A. and Casey M.A. (2015) *Focus Groups: A Practical Guide for Applied Research*, 5th edn, Sage, Thousand Oaks, CA.

Merton, R.K. and Kendall, P.L. (1946) The focused interview. *American Journal of Sociology*, **51**, 541–557.

Merton, R.K. and King, R. (1990) *The Focused Interview: A Manual of Problems and Procedures*, Free Press, New York, NY.

Merton, R.K., Fiske, M. and Kendall, P.L. (1956) *The Focused Interview*, Columbia University Press, New York, NY.

Morgan, D.L. (2010) Reconsidering the role of interaction in analyzing and reporting focus group discussions. *Qualitative Health Research*, **20** (5), 718–722.

Morgan, D. (2019) *Basic and Advanced Focus Groups*, Sage, Thousand Oaks, CA.

Schipper, K., Abma, T.A., Koops, C. *et al.* (2014) Sweet and sour after renal transplantation: a qualitative study about the positive and negative consequences of renal transplantation. *British Journal of Health Psychology*, **19** (3) 580–591.

Sim, J. (1998) Collecting and analysing qualitative data: issues raised by focus groups. *Journal of Advanced Nursing*, **28** (2), 345–352.

Stewart, D.W. and Shamdasani, P.N. (2014) *Focus Groups: Theory and Practice*, 3rd edn, Sage, Thousand Oaks, CA.

Streubert Speziale, H.J. and Rinaldi Carpenter, D.R. (2011) *Qualitative Research in Nursing: Advancing the Humanistic Imperative*, 5th edn, Lippincott, Williams & Wilkins, Philadelphia, PA.

Tausch, A.P. and Menold, N. (2016) Methodological aspects of focus groups in health research: results of qualitative interviews with focus group moderators. *Global Qualitative Nursing Research*, **3**, 1–12.

Usher-Smith, J.A., Silarova, B., Ward, A. *et al.* (2017) Incorporating cancer risk information to promote behaviour change for cancer prevention into general practice: a qualitative study using focus groups with healthcare professionals. *British Journal of General Practice*, **67** (656), e218–e226. doi:10.3399/bjgp17X689401.

Webb, C. and Kevern, J. (2001) Focus groups as a research method: a critique of some aspects of their use in nursing research. *Journal of Advanced Nursing*, **33** (6), 798–805.

Wirtz, A.L., Cooney, E.E., Chaudry, A. and Reisner, S.L. (2019) Computer-mediated communication to facilitate synchronous online discussions: feasibility study for qualitative HIV research among transgender women across the United States. *Journal of Medical Internet Research*, **21** (3), e12569.

Further Reading

Hennink, M.M. (2014) *Focus Group Discussions: Understanding Qualitative Research*, Oxford University Press, Oxford.

Morgan, D.L. (2019) *Basic and Advanced Focus Groups*. Sage, Thousand Oaks, CA.

Tausch, A.P. and Menold, N. (2017) Methodological aspects of focus groups in health research: results of qualitative interviews with focus group moderators. *Global Qualitative Nursing Research*, **3**. doi:10.1177/2333393616630466.

Chapter 9

Sampling Strategies

Before collecting data from interviews, observation or other sources, researchers decide on their sampling strategies. This action involves questions as to *where, what, whom* and *how* to sample. Sampling is a complex process which is informed by the research question, practical and theoretical considerations, and of course it is guided by the phenomenon under investigation as well as by ethical principles.

In qualitative research, purposeful or purposive sampling is the main procedure. This means that the sample is carefully selected to achieve the research aim, hence it is often called criterion-based sampling (Creswell and Poth, 2017) – certain criteria are applied, and the sample is chosen accordingly. Much qualitative research also includes theoretical sampling – note that it is a 'must' in grounded theory, that is sampling in which researchers follow up questions, concepts or problems which emerge during the process of the inquiry. Ritchie *et al.* (2014: 115) state that 'the key criteria for selection in the theoretical sample are theoretical purpose and theoretical relevance'. (See also later in this chapter.) Gentles *et al.* (2015) give a useful overview of sampling in a variety of qualitative approaches.

Sampling decisions

Researchers generally make their initial sampling decisions at an early stage in the project. Qualitative approaches demand different sampling techniques from the randomly selected and probabilistic sampling used by quantitative researchers. It is, however, just as important for qualitative researchers to make their sampling decisions on a systematic basis and on rational grounds. A sample in qualitative research consists of sampling units of people, time or setting. Professional researchers (nurses, physiotherapists, midwives, occupational therapists and others) have to select the individuals or group members (*whom* to sample), the time and context (*what* to sample) and the place (*where* to sample), because they cannot investigate everything and have a specific aim for their research. Hammersley and Atkinson (2019) also stress the importance of context.

Qualitative Research in Nursing and Healthcare, Fifth Edition.
Immy Holloway and Kathleen Galvin.
© 2024 John Wiley & Sons Ltd. Published 2024 by John Wiley & Sons Ltd.

> **KEY POINT**
>
> People and places must be available and accessible for selection.

The sampling strategies adopted can make a difference to the whole study. The rules of qualitative sampling are focused on accessing those who know about the phenomenon under study and who can talk about it, and/or contexts where the phenomenon is likely to be visible. This complex requirement needs pre-planning with some flexibility and therefore sampling strategies are less rigid than those of quantitative methods, but sampling needs to be explicit, appropriate and adequate, as Morse and Field (1996) stated in their early text and can lead to saturation, especially in grounded theory studies (Morse, 2012). Appropriateness means that the method of sampling fits the aim of the study and helps the understanding of the research problem. A sampling strategy is adequate if it generates adequate and relevant and rich information and sufficient quality data. Saturation or redundancy has been reached when no new concepts turn up after thorough exploration (this term has its origin in GT. See also later in this chapter).

> **KEY POINT**
>
> The sample must be adequate to enable the researcher to examine the topic or phenomenon in depth.

Sampling takes place after the research focus has been decided. Although qualitative researchers start selecting participants at this stage, they can continue the selection throughout the process if more are needed because of the changing focus or extension of ideas as the study progresses, especially in grounded theory and ethnography. In most cases, it is not necessary to specify the overall sample and give an exact number of informants from the beginning of the study, although an initial sample should be given. Indeed, Cleary *et al.* (2014: 473) state in an editorial for the *Journal of Advanced Nursing* that the sample is 'commonly sequential rather than pre-determined'. This sampling strategy differs from quantitative research where respondents are chosen before the project begins. A qualitative proposal could state, for instance, that the initial sample should consist of *x* (number of) informants. Grounded theory and ethnography favour this type of sampling to which they can add at a later stage, depending on emerging concepts, while phenomenologists choose a sample from the start, often employing maximum variation, without adding to the sample at a later stage. (Ethics committees do not always accommodate the idea of unspecified or theoretical sampling and wish to know the exact number and clear description of the sample.) One way to approach this requirement is to specify the likely size, range (minimum number and maximum number of participants) and potential variations in sampling for the study, with a rationale.

Sampling is the purposeful selection of an element of the whole population to gain knowledge and information. The question is: *Whom* do the researchers choose and *how* do they choose (of course, there is also other sampling such as time, location and so on which is not discussed fully here). In qualitative inquiry, it differs in several significant ways from the sampling strategies which quantitative researchers carry out; probability sampling, for instance, is inappropriate in qualitative research. Sampling is an important part of the research procedures and has to be suitable for the specific research topic and question. As in other forms of inquiry, researchers have a sampling frame that includes a target population and its subset, the study population from which the sample is taken (Hunt and Lathlean, 2015). The accessible population that has the particular experience or knowledge of the phenomenon which the researcher is seeking to explore is the target population. The study population consists of the individuals to whom the researcher can gain access and who have the appropriate knowledge and experience, while the sampling frame is the population from which the sample is chosen. The terms mentioned above however are not often discussed in qualitative research, although they hold for any type of research.

The researchers do not only describe the sampling strategies and justify the selection of the sample but also explain how they gained access to the participants in the research.

Purposeful (or purposive) sampling

The sampling strategies of the qualitative researcher are guided by principles of ethics and the opportunity of gaining access to people whom they can observe and interview in-depth, and from whom they can obtain rich data. The selection of participants, settings or units of time is criterion based. When choosing participants, age or gender can be a criterion, and in research with patients, the type of condition is also important, as well as other criteria chosen by the researcher. Sampling units are selected for a specific purpose on which the researcher decides. For instance, the researcher chooses a sample on the basis of group membership, on the basis of the experiences that participants have had or the type of treatment and care that they were given.

The specific group is specified in advance but might change in the course of the research. Purposeful or purposive sampling is based on the judgement of the researcher. Apart from people, purposeful sampling can also include the site or setting of the research or indeed the time of day or night when the research takes place (of course, most sampling strategies, even random or theoretical sampling, are purposive).

People generally form the main sampling units. The appropriate informant is chosen by the researcher or may be self-selected. Sometimes researchers can easily identify individuals or groups with special knowledge of a topic, occasionally they advertise or ask for informants who have insight into a particular situation or are experts in an area of knowledge. These voluntary participants selected for the research are often those that are most articulate because the researchers find it easier to communicate with them and elicit rich data, but this might lead to a neglect of certain individuals that are powerless or inarticulate and who should be included; indeed, they might be very important as their voices are often marginalised.

Individuals are sampled for the information they can provide about a specific phenomenon, be it a condition, such as an illness, a treatment (for instance a particular medicine, manipulation, counselling), a type of care, professional decision making and so on. They could be nurses who have cared for people undergoing treatment, patients who have had day surgery or midwifery students who are interviewed about their clinical experience and so on. Identification of a particular population provides boundaries between those who are included in the study and those who stay outside it (inclusion and exclusion criteria). The members of the sample share certain characteristics. The sample is thus chosen on the basis of personal knowledge of the person selected about the phenomenon under study.

Useful informants would be people who have had experiences about which the researcher wants to gain information. For example, individuals who have diabetes might share experiences and the meanings that these have for them with the health researcher.

Informants with special knowledge or experience might consist of newcomers, people who are changing status or those who have been in the setting for a long time. Individuals who are willing to talk about their experiences and perceptions are often those persons who have a special approach to their work. Some have power or status; others are naïve, frustrated, hostile or attention-seeking, although researchers must remember that the latter are not always the best informants because they may have a mainly negative perception of the organisation or institution under discussion – 'an axe to grind'. Ethically, it is important that the persons in the sample are not jeopardised by 'confessing' to their practices (unless illegal) and uncovering their thoughts.

As in all research, the researcher needs to clarify the rationale for inclusion and exclusion of particular people or other sampling units.

> **Example 9.1** Purposeful or Criterion-Based Sampling
>
> In research which has relevance internationally, Cheraghi *et al.* (2014) investigated the perceptions and expectations of the role of nurses with doctorates. They chose a purposive sampling strategy. It included 43 clinical nurses, some of whom were clinical and educational supervisors and senior managers. The sample was chosen from five different teaching hospitals in an urban area of Iran. This variety of settings and nurses (a maximum variation sample) required a larger sample than is usual in qualitative research. The analysis of data provided interesting comprehensive findings. Obviously, some advantages were seen for the nurses with a doctorate qualification, such as research skills, and among other factors, their role was reduced and constrained by the dominance of physicians in the system. The majority of the participants knew little about the doctoral preparation, although they expected nurses with a doctoral degree to demonstrate their knowledge and skills. Some were disappointed because those nurses with a doctorate did not seem to live up to the expectations because of constraints; high expectations included improvements in practice and meeting complex challenges. The main themes that arose thus were advantages of the doctoral degree, clarification of doctorally prepared nurses' role in clinical practice and unmet expectations of doctorally prepared nurses.

A variety of sampling types

There are various forms of sampling. We shall discuss only the most often used and important types. An overview of a whole range can be found in Ritchie *et al.* (2014) as well as in Creswell and Poth (2017), but many sampling types overlap. The most common strategies are as follows:

- Homogeneous sampling
- Heterogeneous sampling
- Total population sampling
- Chain referral sampling (snowball sampling)
- Convenience or opportunistic sampling
- Maximum variation sampling
- Theoretical sampling

Homogeneous sampling

This involves individuals who belong to the same subculture or have similar characteristics. Nurses often use homogeneous sample units when they wish to observe or interview a particular group, for instance specialist nurses or conditions that are common among a group of either men or women. Midwives may wish to examine the perspectives of community midwives on their role in the community. In these examples, a homogeneous group is being studied. The sample can be homogeneous with respect to a certain variable only – for instance, specific occupation, length of experience, type of experience, age or gender. The important variables would be established before the sampling starts.

Example 9.2 Homogeneous Sampling

Leahy *et al*. (2014) explored the experience of stroke among 12 Irish women. They chose a homogeneous sample who were all working in paid employment and had families.

Heterogeneous sampling

A heterogeneous sample contains individuals or groups of individuals who differ from each other in a major aspect. For instance, nurses may wish to explore the perceptions of nurses, social workers and doctors who care for patients with HIV. The three groups form a heterogeneous sample. Heterogeneous sampling is also called maximum variation sampling, because it involves a search for individuals with widely differing experiences and for variations in settings. Patton (2015) discusses types of sampling in detail in his text.

Example 9.3 Heterogeneous Sampling

Researchers might wish to explore the perspectives of people with a chronic condition and the strategies with which they manage their illness. They wish to select a large variety of participants, hence they observe and interview women and men in a broad age range with different jobs and from a variety of backgrounds. The condition is the main factor which is common to them all. This would maximise the contrast between different types of participants.

The sample might consist of people from a naturally occurring population – such as members of a local carers' group, a specific ward, a community of patients. Some sampling is based on early findings with a group and cannot be determined prior to the study. For instance, a midwife could sample women who have just given birth to their first child and find that it would be interesting to select older and younger primiparae because they might have different ideas about childbirth. Sometimes married couples are chosen as samples or people who live together. Occasionally, the sample consists of focus groups, for instance self-help groups, or groups with similar conditions or experiences. In this instance, three to six focus groups would be enough (see chapter on focus groups).

Total population sampling

A sample is called a total population sample when all participants selected come from a particular group; it is used infrequently in qualitative research. For instance, all the nurses with specific knowledge or a skill, such as those with training and experience in counselling, might be interviewed because the researcher focuses on this skill, and there might be few available with the particular expertise. There are some illness conditions where those who suffer from them are very small in number, and the researcher might interview all of these. All midwives in one midwifery unit might be observed, because the specific setting in which they work or the special techniques they adopt are seen as important. However, not many qualitative studies carry out total population sampling.

Chain referral or snowball sampling

A variation of purposive sampling is chain referral or *snowball* sampling (the former is a term originally coined by Biernacki and Waldorf (1981)). A previously chosen informant is asked to identify other potential participants with knowledge of a particular area or topic, and these in turn nominate other individuals for the research. Researchers use snowball sampling in studies where they cannot identify useful informants, where informants are not easily accessible or where anonymity is desirable, for instance in studies about drug or alcohol use or where patients are reluctant to be identified. Penrod *et al.* (2003) suggest that chain referral sampling is useful in situations where people are vulnerable and when they are not easily accessible: this might include groups that are labelled negatively by society (for instance, those that suffer from sexually transmitted diseases), those with whom researchers discuss sensitive topics (such as sexual behaviour) or those individuals who fear being exposed or criminalised (i.e. substance use). Of course, it is all the more important for researchers to follow ethical principles.

Convenience or opportunistic sampling

The terms *convenience* or *opportunistic* sampling are self-explanatory. The researcher uses opportunities to ask people who might be useful for the study and easy to access. To some extent, of course, most sampling is opportunistic and arranged for the convenience of the researcher. Researchers usually adopt this sampling strategy when recruiting people is difficult, although this is not the best way of sampling.

The researcher chooses individuals whose ideas or experiences will help achieve the aim of the research; occasionally variations in the sample have no specific influence on the phenomenon to be explored, and in this case a convenience sample can be selected. For example, a group of people in a hospital near to the researcher's base might be convenient to interview, or indeed all the occupational therapists in one hospital might be observed.

Maximum variation sampling

Maximum variation sampling entails selecting a purposive sample of a diversity of people and/or their situations. It may include, for instance both genders, young and old, whether, for example, a person is mobile or housebound or in residential care. The researcher intends to access a range of perspectives from many different people who have something in common (the phenomenon or condition of interest), but that are also diverse. This means that the sampling criteria need to be carefully thought through and coherent with the research question. This type of sampling is sometimes used in phenomenological research and is becoming more common in a range of qualitative research studies.

Example 9.4 Maximum Variation Sampling

McFarland *et al.* (2014) selected a purposive sample of people whom they interviewed for information about their perspectives on the prevention of venous thromboembolism (VTE). They wished to gain varied perspectives on the focus of the research and 'to reflect the diversity within a given population'. The sample comprised a variety of people with expertise in VTE from a number of hospitals and other organisations. The researchers chose, for instance, a consultant haematologist, a consultant VTE lead, a number of nurses with different tasks in the VTE field, a pharmacist and other members of these organisations who had a special interest in VTE.

Theoretical sampling

Glaser and Strauss (1967) advocate *theoretical sampling* in the process of collecting data. Theoretical sampling develops as the study proceeds, and it cannot be planned beforehand. Researchers select their sample on the basis of concepts and theoretical issues that arise during the research. The theoretical ideas control the collection of data; therefore, researchers have to justify the inclusion of particular sampling units. At the point of data saturation, when no new ideas arise that are of value to the developing theory, sampling can stop. Coyne (1997) discusses qualitative sampling in depth and differentiates between purposive and theoretical sampling, although she believes that theoretical sampling could be called 'analysis-driven purposeful sampling'. Sandelowski (1995) also maintains that all sampling in qualitative research is purposeful; it is intended to achieve a specific aim. She claims that theoretical sampling is merely a variation of purposive sampling. (See Chapter 11 for examples and further explanations of theoretical sampling.)

Other types of sample selection

Other methods of purposeful or criterion-based sampling sometimes overlap with those above and can be examples of purposive sampling (for a variety of these, see Schensul *et al.* (1999: 236)):

• Extreme case selection
• Typical case selection

- Unique case selection
- Deviant case selection

In *extreme case selection*, the researcher identifies certain characteristics for the setting or population. Extremes of these characteristics are sought and arranged on a continuum. The cases that belong at the two ends of this continuum become the extreme cases. For instance, nurses may study a very large or a very small ward. These can be compared with cases that are the norm for the hospital population.

In *typical case selection*, researchers create a profile of characteristics for an average case and find instances of this. They might exclude the very young or old, the almost healthy, the most vulnerable or any other participants at the end of a continuum. They would be those that are typical or normal for the investigation of a particular phenomenon.

When choosing *unique cases*, researchers study those that differ from others by a single characteristic or dimension such as people who share a particular condition but come from an unusual community, such as a sect or ethnic group. This type of sample consists of the uncommon and unique cases which are not normal or typical.

Deviant case selection is similar to the above and to extreme case selection.

However, only those people are included who think in a very different way from other people whose ideas have been researched before, or those who have a different experience from others, although they have had the same condition, treatment or care.

There are other terms for and types of sampling but the preceding are the most common. Kuzel (1999) lists five important elements of sampling which may occur in qualitative research:

1 Flexible sampling which develops during the study.
2 Sequential selection of sampling units.
3 Sampling guided by theoretical development which becomes progressively more focused.
4 Continuing sampling until no new relevant data arise (sampling to saturation).
5 Searching for negative or deviant cases.

When considering sampling, one must be aware that many sampling types overlap.

KEY POINT

Regardless of the type of sample and the overlap of sampling types, all sampling in qualitative research is criterion based.

Inclusion and exclusion criteria

When describing their sampling strategies, researchers describe inclusion and exclusion criteria. Inclusion criteria state which particular people are included in the research, while participants who are excluded – although meeting some of the inclusion criteria – might be too vulnerable to be interviewed or have certain traits that might make the research problematic. For instance, in Britain or the United States, people who do not understand the English language might have to be excluded for practical or access reasons (although, of course, they might also be the target population in some studies). Because of the support and resources required, undergraduates are advised to exclude from their sample vulnerable people, for example children, or those with enduring mental health problems. In a study of the birth process, women with normal birth experience might be included while those who underwent caesarean section or those with still-born babies might be excluded for ethical reasons. The exclusion and inclusion criteria depend, of course, on the aim of the particular study. One of the most important inclusion criteria is voluntary participation.

Sampling parameters

The investigators do not only decide on the participants in their study but also on the time and location of the research as stated earlier. The criteria for selecting must be clearly identified.

The sample might consist of people, context and time. In an ethnographic study for instance, a particular subculture might be researched in different settings and situations. The people in the study are chosen for their experience and knowledge of the phenomenon under study. A particular phenomenon might be researched in a range of contexts in which it occurs. Different times of the day, year or stages in the process of care might also be a significant factor in the research.

The criteria for site selection, location and size also depend on the aim of the research. The setting can be small or large depending on the type of study; for instance, it might be a ward, a general practice, the community or a hospital. For a multi-centre study, it might be particular types of hospitals or a number of clinics. The research might also take place during a particular, important or critical time of the day.

Example 9.5 Setting and Site

A medical researcher is determined to examine the role of the gastroenterologist. She chooses a variety of hospitals in the North and South of England to explore this role with the specialist participants. These hospitals are the setting for her research.

> **Example 9.6** Time
>
> A nurse has observed a trend of many falls in a ward for elderly people. He thinks that they take place mainly at night. The decision is to observe day-time and night-time activities and events and ask the ward nurses about their perceptions about events in the hours of night and day.

Sample size

The sample may be small or large, depending on the type of research question, material and time resources as well as on the number of researchers. Generally, qualitative sampling consists of small sample units studied in depth. Sample size differs greatly in qualitative studies; a large sample is rarely necessary in qualitative research. Todres *et al.* (2005; also, Todres and Galvin, 2006), for instance, selected just one person for their phenomenological research which arose from collaboration between the researchers and the partner and carer of an individual with Alzheimer's. However, researchers must be warned that some funding agencies and even some members of ethics committees do not have the appropriate specialised knowledge of sampling and can sometimes reject the small sample that qualitative research entails. Grounded theory studies are generally larger (generally around 20, sometimes more), while ethnographies often consist of many participants as the researcher is exploring a culture. The size depends on the aim of the study, its focus and the type of sample. Obviously, researchers need more participants for a maximum variation sample, while a deviant case sample need not include many people.

> **KEY POINT**
>
> The sample in qualitative research depends on many factors. It need not be large but should uncover in-depth data related to the focus of the inquiry.

Although there are no rigid rules; as far as people in the setting is concerned, 6–8 data units are seen as sufficient when the sample consists of a homogeneous group, while between 14 and 20 might be needed for a heterogeneous sample. Most often, the sample consists of between 4 and 40 informants, although certain research projects contain as many as 200 participants and as few as 2. Qualitative studies that include a large sample do exist but are rare. Sample size, however, does not necessarily determine the importance of the study or the quality of the data. Morse also adds that larger sample sizes are possible through technologies such as for instance, telephones, recordings and cell phones.

There is rarely justification for a very large sample in qualitative research. Students or experienced researchers often choose these pragmatically to appease funding bodies, which are used to large samples, or research committees which do not always know details of qualitative research. Often, qualitative researchers select larger samples because they are trained in quantitative research where generalisation is demanded, or because they are anxious that an external examiner might query the sample size. A large sample, however, might be unnecessary and result in less depth and richness as the researcher's intention is usually to research a specific setting and has a purposive sample. An overlarge sample might not capture the meanings participants ascribe to their experience, and it could result in the loss of the unique and specific. In some cases, particularly in phenomenology, even a sample of one can be meaningful and yield useful insights (Todres *et al.*, 2005; Todres and Galvin, 2006).

Morse (2020) summarises what the researchers should take into account:

1 The complexity of questions
2 The scope of the research
3 The flexibility of the data collection
4 The amount of strategies
5 The variation in participants
6 The methods, aims and goals
7 The nature of the participants

She states that one cannot predict this in the initial proposal. We would add the availability of the participants as a factor.

Saturation

Saturation indicates that everything of importance to the agenda of a research project will emerge in the data and concepts obtained; Lincoln and Guba (1985) call this 'informational redundancy'. *Data saturation* means sampling to redundancy. *Theoretical saturation* denotes that no new concepts or dimensions for categories can be identified which are important for the study. It does not mean that nothing new can be found at all. Indeed, Morse (1995) specifically states that frequency, quantity and repetition of ideas in the data do not signify saturation or data adequacy. Unfortunately, no specific rules or guidelines exist pertaining to saturation, so researchers have to decide for themselves when this has happened.

Many approaches aim at data or theoretical saturation but fail to achieve it (O'Reilly and Parker, 2013). Bowen (2008) also deplores that researchers often state that saturation has been achieved but do not clarify what it means in the context of their own specific study. Often there are time constraints and other barriers to sample saturation; hence, it is not always appropriate to confirm saturation.

Morse (2012) maintains that careful choice of sampling and the cohesiveness of the sample can help to achieve saturation.

Giving a label to the participants

It is difficult for researchers to know what term to use for the people they interview and observe, especially as this name makes explicit the stance of the researchers and their relationship to those being studied. We favour the terms 'participant' or 'informant'. In surveys, by both structured interviews and written questionnaires, the most frequent term has been 'respondents', and, indeed, many qualitative researchers and research texts still use it, but it seems less frequent now in qualitative research texts and reports.

Morse (1991) developed a debate about terms almost two decades ago, and her thoughts on sampling are still valid. She claims that 'respondent' implies a passive response to a stimulus – the researcher's question. It sounds mechanistic. Medical and business researchers still use this term often in qualitative research. Biomedical researchers refer to 'subjects', again a word that expresses passivity of the people involved in a study. Interestingly, it is used in legal documents and sometimes in ethical guidelines (see Chapter 4). West and Butler (2003) quote Margaret Mead who, decades ago, criticised the word 'subject' and maintains that research *with* informants would yield better data. In qualitative research, this word would be inappropriate. 'Interviewee' sounds clumsy and boring. The American Psychological Association now also uses the term 'participants' when discussing human beings involved in research (APA, 2018).

Anthropologists refer to 'informants', those members of a culture or group who voluntarily 'inform' the researcher about their world and play an active part in the research. Hammersley and Atkinson (2019) do use this term in their texts. Morse (2012) usually chooses this term, although she acknowledges the suggestion by some journal editors that it might be seen to have links to the word 'informant' as used by the police. Most ethnographers, however, still use the term and do not perceive it as negative. Generally, qualitative researchers prefer the term 'participant'; this expresses the collaboration between the researcher and the researched (DePoy and Gitlin, 2015) and the equality of their relationship, but the term could be misleading as the researcher, too, is a participant in the research. Van den Hoonaard (2008) debates the term 'human subject', its alternatives and ethical implications in his article; he too prefers the term 'participant' or 'informant' to the word 'subject' as it is more appropriate for social and interactive individuals, although biomedical researchers still talk of 'human subjects'.

In the end, however, the nurses, midwives, doctors and allied health professionals must choose for themselves which term suits their research. In Morse's words, 'Subjects, respondents, informants, participants – choose your own term, but choose a term that fits' (1991: 406). We suggest that students use the terms 'participant' or informant in ethnographic studies, but never the word 'subject'.

Summary

The following are the important features of qualitative sampling:
- Sampling is purposeful and criterion-based, chosen specifically for the study.
- Sampling units can consist of people, time, setting, processes or concepts (the latter is called theoretical sampling).
- The sample of individuals in qualitative research is sometimes small but yields rich data.
- Sampling is not always wholly determined prior to the study but may proceed throughout (for instance, in grounded theory).
- The individuals in the sample are usually called *participants* or *informants* (in qualitative research they should never be called 'subjects', which infers passivity).

References

American Psychological Association (2018) Ethics committee: rules and procedures. Available at https://www.apa.org/ethics/committee-rules-procedures-2018.pdf.

Biernacki, P. and Waldorf, D. (1981) Snowball sampling: problems and techniques of chain referral sampling. *Sociological Methods and Research*, **10** (2), 141–163.

Bowen, G.A. (2008) Naturalistic inquiry and the saturation concept: a research note. *Qualitative Research*, **8** (1), 137–152.

Cheraghi, M., Jasper, M. and Vaismoradi, M. (2014) Clinical nurses' perceptions and expectations of the role of doctorally prepared nurses: a qualitative study in Iran. *Nurse Education in Practice*, **14** (1), 18–23.

Cleary, M. Horsfall, J. and Hayter, M. (2014) Data collection and sampling in qualitative research: does size matter? *Journal of Advanced Nursing*, **70** (3), 473–475.

Coyne, I.T. (1997) Sampling in qualitative research: purposeful and theoretical sampling: merging or clear boundaries? *Journal of Advanced Nursing*, **26**, 623–630.

Creswell, J.W. and Poth C.N. (2017) *Qualitative Inquiry and Research Design: Choosing Among Five Approaches*, 4th edn, Sage, Thousand Oaks, CA.

DePoy, E. and Gitlin, L.N. (2015) *Introduction to Research: Multiple Strategies for Health and Human Services*, 5th edn, Elsevier, St. Louis, MO.

Gentles, S.J., Charles, C., Ploeg, J. and McKibbon, K. (2015). Sampling in qualitative research: insights from an overview of the methods literature. *The Qualitative Report*, **20** (11), 1772–1789. Available at http://nsuworks.nova.edu/tqr/vol20/iss11/5.

Glaser, B. and Strauss, A. (1967) *The Discovery of Grounded Theory*, Aldine, Chicago, IL.

Hammersley, M. and Atkinson, P. (2019) *Ethnography: Principles in Practice*, Routledge, Abingdon, Oxon.

Hunt, K. and Lathlean, J. (2015) Sampling, in *The Research Process in Nursing* (eds. K. Gerrish and A. Lacey), 7th edn, Wiley Blackwell, Oxford, pp. 173–184.

Kuzel, A.J. (1999) Sampling in qualitative inquiry, in *Doing Qualitative Research* (eds. B.F. Crabtree and W.L. Miller), 2nd edn, Sage, Thousand Oaks, CA, pp. 33–45.

Leahy, D., Desmond, D., Coughlan, T. *et al.* (2014) Stroke in young women: an interpretative phenomenological analysis. *Journal of Health Psychology*, **21** (5), 669–678.

Lincoln, Y.S. and Guba, E.G. (1985) *Naturalistic Inquiry*, Sage, Beverly Hills, CA.

McFarland, L., Murray, E., Harrison, S. *et al.* (2014) Current practice of venous thromboembolism prevention in acute trusts: a qualitative study. *BMJ Open*, **4** (6), e005074.

Morse, J.M. (1991) Subjects, respondents, informants and participants [Editorial]. *Qualitative Health Research*, **1**, 403–436.

Morse, J.M. (1995) The significance of saturation [Editorial]. *Qualitative Health Research*, **5** (2), 147–149.

Morse, J.M. (2012) *Qualitative Health Research*, Left Coast Press, Walnut Creek, CA.

Morse, J.M. (2020) The changing face of qualitative inquiry. *International Journal Qualitative Methods*. doi:10.1177/1609406920909938 (originally a conference keynote address).

Morse, J.M. and Field, P.A. (1996) *Nursing Research: The Application of Qualitative Approaches*, Macmillan, Basingstoke.

O'Reilly, M. and Parker, N. (2013) 'Unsatisfactory saturation': a critical exploration of the notion of saturated sample sizes in qualitative research. *Qualitative Research*, **13** (2), 190–197.

Patton, M. (2015) *Qualitative Evaluation and Research Methods*, 5th edn, Sage, Thousand Oaks, CA.

Penrod, J., Preston, D.B., Cain, R.E. and Starks, M.T. (2003) The discussion of chain referral as a method of sampling hard-to-reach populations. *Journal of Transcultural Nursing*, **14** (2), 100–107.

Ritchie, J., Lewis, J., Elam, G. *et al.* (2014) Designing and selecting samples, in *Qualitative Research Practice: A Guide for Social Science Students and Researchers* (eds. J. Ritchie, J. Lewis, C. MacNaughton Nicholls and R. Ormston), Sage, London, pp. 111–135.

Sandelowski, M. (1995) Focus on qualitative methods: sample size in qualitative research. *Research in Nursing and Health*, **18**, 179–183.

Schensul, S.L., Schensul, J.J. and LeCompte, M.D. (1999) *Essential Ethnographic Methods 2: Observations, Interviews and Questionnaires*, Altamira Press, Walnut Creek, CA.

Todres, L. and Galvin, K. (2006) Caring for a partner with Alzheimer's disease: intimacy, loss and the life that is possible. *International Journal of Qualitative Studies on Health and Well-being*, **1**, 50–61.

Todres, L., Galvin, K. and Richardson, M. (2005) The intimate mediator: a carer's experience of Alzheimer's disease. *Journal of Clinical Nursing*, **12** (3), 422–430.

Van den Hoonaard, W.C. (2008) Re-imagining the subject: conceptual and ethical considerations on the participant in qualitative research. *Ciência and Saúde Coletiva*, **13** (2), 371–379.

West, E. and Butler, J. (2003) An applied and qualitative LREC reflects on its practice. *Bulletin of Medical Ethics*, **185**, 13–20.

Further Reading

Campbell, S., Greenwood, M., Prior, S. *et al.* (2020) Purposive sampling: complex or simple? Research case examples. *Journal of Research in Nursing*, **25** (8), 652–661. (This describes a variety of sampling types with examples.)

Emmel, N. (2013) *Sampling and Choosing Cases in Qualitative Research: A Realist Approach*, Sage, London.

Part Three

Approaches in Qualitative Research

Chapter 10

Ethnography

Ethnography is the description and representation of a culture, group or community. It is, however, an overall term for a number of approaches. Sometimes researchers use the term as synonymous with qualitative research in general (for instance, Hackett and Hayre, 2021) while at other times its meaning is more specific. In this chapter, we adopt the original meaning of the term, as a method within the social anthropological tradition and includes forms of qualitative research. In its early days, it could be qualitative and quantitative, although ethnographers in the healthcare field adopt now mostly qualitative procedures, and we shall focus on these.

As one of the oldest forms of research, it has been used since ancient times in its simplest form; for instance, in the descriptions of Greeks and Romans who wrote about the cultures they encountered in their travels and wars. Deriving from the Greek, the term ethnography means a description of the people – 'writing of culture'. Ethnographers focus on phenomena and problems in the context of culture and cultural groups. Ethnographic data collection takes place mainly through observation and interviews (see chapters on observation and interviewing).

Researchers stress the importance of studying human behaviour in the context of culture in order to gain understanding of cultural rules, norms and routines. Ethnography refers to both a *process* – the methods and strategies of research– and a *product* – the written story – as the outcome of the research. People 'do' ethnography: They study a culture, observe its members' behaviours and listen to them. They 'produce' *an ethnography*, a written text (or sometimes a performed piece of work), the ethnographic account, a portrait of the group they study.

KEY POINT

Ethnography differs from other qualitative approaches by its focus on culture or cultures

---

Qualitative Research in Nursing and Healthcare, Fifth Edition.
Immy Holloway and Kathleen Galvin.
© 2024 John Wiley & Sons Ltd. Published 2024 by John Wiley & Sons Ltd.

The development of ethnography

Modern ethnography has its roots in social anthropology and emerged in the 1920s and 1930s when famous anthropologists, such as Malinowski (1922) and Mead (1935), explored a variety of non-Western cultures and the life ways of the people within them. After the First and Second World Wars, when tribal groups in the traditional sense were disappearing, researchers wished to preserve aspects of disappearing cultures by studying them. As Gobo (2017) claims, in some form, ethnography as a method is around a century old but its origins are much older.

In the beginning, these anthropologists explored only 'primitive' cultures (a term that demonstrates the patronising stance of many early anthropologists). When cultures became more linked with each other and Western anthropologists could not find homogeneous, isolated cultures abroad, they turned to research their own cultures, acting as 'cultural strangers'; that is trying to see them from outside while still being an insider. The ethnographers and sociologists, who research their own society, take a new perspective on that which is familiar. It is important, however, that they do not take assumptions about their own cultural group for granted.

The Chicago School of Sociology had an influence on later ethnographic methods; its members examined marginal cultural and 'socially strange' subcultures such as the slums, ghettos and gangs of the city. A good early example is the study by Whyte (1943), who investigated the urban gang subculture in an American city – research which became a model for other sociologists.

The cultural context

Ethnography differs from other approaches by the emphasis on culture. Culture can be defined as the way of life of a group – the learnt behaviour that is socially constructed and transmitted. The life experiences of members of a cultural group include a shared communication system. This consists of signs such as gestures, mime and language as well as cultural artefacts – all messages that the members of a culture recognise, and whose meaning they understand. Individuals in a culture or subculture hold values and ideas acquired through learning from other members of the group. The researchers' responsibility is to describe the patterns of beliefs and behaviour and the unique processes in the subculture or culture they study. It must be stressed, however, that the values and beliefs of cultural members depend on their location in the culture or subculture in which they live, on their gender, age or ethnic group. Indeed, sometimes conflicting value systems may exist.

KEY POINT

Cultures are not uniform, monolithic or unchanging. They include subgroups which, although sharing many values, have different ideas depending on their social location.

Social anthropologists aim to observe and study the modes of life in a culture through the method of ethnography. They analyse, compare and examine groups and their rules of behaviour. The relationship of individuals to the group and to each other is also explored. The study of change helps ethnographers understand cultures. In areas where two cultural groups meet, they might focus on the conflict between groups if this is seen as important. In healthcare, for instance, researchers could study the interaction of nurses or midwives with doctors.

Applying ethnographic methods – especially observation – helps health professionals to contextualise the behaviour, beliefs and feelings of their clients or colleagues. Through ethnography, researchers become culturally sensitive and can identify the cultural influences on the individuals and groups they study. The goals of ethnographers in the health arena, however, differ from those of researchers in a subject discipline such as anthropology or sociology. They often intend to improve practice. Health professionals for instance, generally see the production of knowledge only as a first step; on the basis of this, they seek to enhance care for their clients.

Health researchers often examine subcultures and situations with which they are familiar.

Example 10.1 Descriptive Qualitative Ethnography

Meng *et al.* (2019) carried out research in China which examined nursing practice in stroke rehabilitation from the perspective of multi-disciplinary healthcare providers. They interviewed and observed three healthcare organisations and found distinctive multiple patterns. They developed a descriptive ethnography.

From clinical practice

The importance of clinical practice is described by an ethnography about nurses working with homeless people in Canada. Researchers (Paradis-Gagne and Pariseau-Legault, 2020) found four main themes in their inquiry but focus on stigma and disaffection in this article. They found that nurses had to find acceptance in the setting to gain trust and make relationships. It also meant that they themselves might be affected by stigma.

From education

Our colleagues Scammell and Olumide (2012) conducted ethnographic research in a nurse education department in England. They aimed to explore constructions of difference within mentorship relations which involve internationally recruited nurse mentors and white British nursing students. The study involved interviews with 10 internationally recruited nurses, 25 nursing students, 2 university lecturers and 5 placement-based staff development nurses. Encounters were observed and documentary analysis was also included. The study showed that many participants saw difference as a problem, separating 'them' from 'us'. The reality of racism and 'whiteness as a source of power' was however ignored or denied, indicating a failure of pre-registration nurse education. The implications of the study were that an understanding of 'unwitting' racism is necessary before institutional racism can be eliminated.

Ethnographic methods

Researchers distinguish between several types of ethnography, some of which overlap. Approaches to ethnography might arise from different ideological or procedural bases, but they are similar in data collection and management.

The main ways of using the ethnographic approach are through the following:

- Descriptive or conventional ethnography
- Critical ethnography
- Auto-ethnography

Descriptive or conventional ethnography focuses on description, and, through analysis, uncovers patterns, typologies and categories.

Critical ethnography is based in critical theory and, as discussed decades ago by Thomas (1993) and later by Madison (2019), it involves the study of macrosocial factors such as power and control. It examines common-sense assumptions and hidden agendas and is therefore more political. Thomas (p. 4) states the difference: 'Conventional ethnographers study culture for the purpose of describing it; critical ethnographers do so to change it'. Critical ethnography can be important for health researchers, particularly nurses, physiotherapists and midwives, because they are concerned with the empowerment and emancipation of people.

Example 10.2 Critical Ethnography

Newnham *et al.* (2021) discuss three critical ethnographic research projects about methodological understanding in maternity care. They use some key traits of critical ethnography discussed by Thomas and others, identification of consequences and potential harm, collaboration between researchers and participants and equity between them. They discuss power, control and oppression in a cultural context of the three separate studies, and show opportunities in maternity care research to be flexible, creative but also rigorous.

Auto-ethnography implies that researchers focus their studies on themselves, their own thoughts and feelings rather than centre their research on others. All qualitative research has a reflexive element which takes into account their own location, thoughts and feelings. Anderson (2006), however, differentiates between evocative and analytic auto-ethnography. The former focuses on the researchers' feelings, while the latter is designed to discuss social phenomena reaching beyond the researcher's own experience though taking it as a resource.

Example 10.3 An Auto-Ethnography

An academic (Fox, 2020) who uses the mental health services, explores their own experiences in these services. It was found that a commitment of policymakers to involve users existed, but the research states that it is still underdeveloped and not consistent. The service, according to Fox, needs systematic change.

Another example of auto-ethnography is the approach by *Walker et al.* (2020) who examined the experience of a medical student with dyspraxia. This in-depth account of experiences illuminates how auto-ethnography be of help and support.

Ethnography in healthcare

Ethnographic methods were first used in healthcare, specifically in nursing in the United States. One of the best-known nursing ethnographers is Janice Morse, who has written several well-known texts and is probably the best-known qualitative researcher in the nursing arena and has qualifications in anthropology. Leininger (1985), the nurse anthropologist, used the term 'ethnonursing' for the use of ethnography in nursing. She developed this as a modification and extension of ethnography. Ethnonursing deals with studies of a culture like other ethnographic methods, but it is also about nursing care and specifically generates nursing knowledge. Nurse ethnographers differ from other anthropologists in that they only live with informants in their working day and spend their private lives away from the location where the research takes place. Nurses, of course, are familiar with the language used in the setting, while early anthropologists rarely knew the language of the culture they examined from the beginning of the research, and even modern anthropologists are not always familiar with the setting, the terminology and the people they study. Robinson (2013) adds that the theory of culture care diversity is rooted in the belief that care is at the heart of nursing practice (and – one would have to add – in other health professionals' clinical practice too).

Ethnography in the healthcare arena is applied research. In nursing and midwifery as well as medicine and allied health professions, the method is used as a way of examining behaviours and perceptions in clinical settings, generally in order to improve care and clinical practice.

The ethnographic approach can also be a useful way of studying health promotion issues as it provides the social context and explores the social conditions in which participants live and by which they are influenced (Cook, 2005). In particular, critical ethnography offers an understanding of the differences and inequalities in the health of people.

Ethnographies in this field incorporate studies of healthcare processes, settings and systems. They are typified by observations of wards or investigations of patient perspectives or specific groups whose members have experienced a condition or illness. Socialisation studies are also important in the field of professional practice. They often examine the negotiation and interaction in the subculture of clinical practice or ward and classroom settings. Robinson also argues that ethnography is based in human sciences; it also explores the meaning of action and interaction and hence is particularly useful in the health and teaching professions. She claims in particular that there is a natural fit between nursing and ethnography and finds it surprising that nurses do not use ethnography as often as grounded theory and phenomenology, and believes that the reason for this is a misunderstanding of the term 'culture'.

As Thomson (2011) argues, ethnographic methods are useful not only in investigating patient or hospital cultures but also in developing an insider perspective on health professionals' lives, work and education. Schensul *et al.* (1999) give useful advice to ethnographers that might be adopted by health researchers too. They can take a number of steps:

- They describe a problem in the group under study.
- Through this, they understand the causes of the problem and may prevent it.
- They help the cultural members to identify and report their needs.
- They give information to affect change in (clinical or professional) practice.

Ethnographers do not always investigate their own cultural members. In modern Britain, health professionals care for patients from a variety of ethnic groups and need to be knowledgeable about their cultures. Culture becomes part of all aspects of healthcare because both professionals and clients are products of their group in a particular social context. Savage (2006) gives examples from the area of healthcare such as research carried out in hospice settings, studies on rules and rituals, pain and illness experience.

There are many ethnographic studies in healthcare. We cite just one of them.

Example 10.4 Involvement of Health Professionals and Patients

In the United States, Coughlin (2013) examined major events during hospitalisation by exploring patients' perceptions of the care they received and the perspectives of nurses on the care that had been given. The findings indicated that the perception and focus of patients differed from those of the nurse participants. The implications for clinical practice demonstrated the importance of gaining patients' views on the experience in order for nurses to enhance their care.

The main features of ethnography

The main features of ethnography are the following:
• Data collection mainly through observation and interviews
• The use of 'thick' description
• Selection of key informants and settings
• The emic–etic dimension

Data collection through observation and interviews

Researchers collect data by standard methods, mainly through observation and interviewing, but they also rely on documents such as letters, diaries and digitally recorded oral histories of people in a particular group or connected with it. (See also the chapters on observation and interviewing.)

As in other qualitative approaches, the researcher is the major research instrument (a term that is useful but not humanising). Direct participant observation is the main way of collecting data from the culture under study, and observers try to become part of the culture, taking note of everything they see and hear as well as interviewing members of the culture to gain their interpretations. Huby *et al.* (2007) make the point that data can be collected both formally and informally, which is one of the advantages of being immersed in setting.

Health researchers commonly observe behaviour in clinical or educational settings. The decisions about inclusion and exclusion depend on the research topic, the emerging data and the experiences of the researchers. The participants and their actions as well as the ways in which they interact with each other are observed. Special events and crises, the site itself and the use of space and time can also be examined. Observers study the rules of a culture or subculture and the change that occurs over time in the setting. It does not suffice, however, to use the fieldnotes for description only and add a description of the interview data. The participants' accounts are transformed and translated by the researcher into more abstract and theoretical concepts as in most qualitative research reports.

Observations might become starting points for in-depth interviews. The researchers may not understand what they see, and ask the members of the group or culture to explain it to them. Participants share their interpretations of events, rules and roles with the interviewer. Some of the interviews are formal and structured, but often researchers ask questions on the spur of the moment and have informal conversations with members. Often, they uncover discrepancies between words and actions ('words and deeds') – what people do and what they say – a problem originally discussed by Deutscher (1970). On the other hand, there may be congruence between the spoken work and behaviour. If any discrepancies exist, they must be explained and interpreted.

Ethnographers take part in the life of people; they listen to their informants' words and the interpretation of their actions. In essence, this involves a partnership between the investigator and the informants.

The use of 'thick description'

One of the major characteristics is *thick description*, a term used by the anthropologist Geertz (1973) who borrowed it from the philosopher Ryle. It is description that makes explicit the detailed patterns of cultural and social relationships and puts them in context. Ethnographic interpretation cannot be separated from time, place and events. It is based on the meaning that actions and events have for the members of a culture within the cultural context. Description and analysis have to be rooted in reality; researchers think and reflect about social events and conduct. Thick description must be theoretical and analytical in the sense that researchers concern themselves with the abstract and general patterns and traits of social life in a culture. Denzin (1989) claims that thick description aims to give readers a sense of the emotions, thoughts and perceptions that research participants experience. It deals with the meaning and interpretations of people in a culture.

Thick description can be contrasted with 'thin description', which is superficial and does not explore the underlying meanings of cultural members. Any study where thin description prevails is not a good ethnography.

Selection of key informants and settings

As in other types of qualitative research, ethnographers generally use sampling that is purposive (criterion based) and non-probabilistic. This means ethnographers adopt certain criteria to choose a specific group and setting to be studied, be it a ward, a group of specialists or patients with a specific condition. Some researchers use samples from such subcultures as groups of recovering alcoholics and patients with myocardial infarction, or from professional education such as an investigation of mentoring. The criteria for sampling must be justified in the study and be explicit. Researchers should choose key informants carefully to make sure that they are suitable and representative of the group under study. Key actors often participate by informally talking about the cultural conduct or customs of the group. They become active collaborators in the research rather than passive respondents.

The sample is taken from a particular cultural or subcultural group. Ethnographers have to search for individuals within a culture who can give them specific detailed information about the culture. Key informants hold special and expert knowledge about the history and subculture of a group, about interaction processes in it and cultural rules, rituals and language. Thomson (2011) states that they must have been in the setting for some time.

These key actors help the researcher to become accepted in the culture and subculture. Researchers can validate their own ideas or perceptions with those of key informants by going back to them at the end of the study and asking them to check the script and interpretation; this is called member check (see also Chapter 18).

The bond between researcher and key informant strengthens when the two spend time with each other. Through informal conversations, researchers can learn about the customs and conduct of the group they study, because key informants have access to areas which researchers cannot reach in time and location. For instance, a midwife might wish to gain information about midwifery in wartime, or a doctor to discover the problems of working in the nineteenth century, and have no access themselves to the past or the location. These researchers use informants who have this special knowledge, in these instances midwives who practised during the war or physiotherapists who have worked extensively abroad, or they consult documents from former times.

Key informants may be other health professionals or patients. Patients are most often the cultural group being studied. They tell the health carers of their condition in the context of their group, and of the expectations and health beliefs that form part of it. Spradley (1979) advises ethnographers to elicit also the 'tacit' knowledge of cultural members – the concepts and assumptions that they have but of which they are unaware.

Fetterman (2020) warns against prior assumptions which key informants might have. If they are highly knowledgeable, they might impose their own ideas on the study and the researcher; therefore, the latter must try to compare these tales with the observed reality. There might be the additional danger that key actors might only tell what researchers wish to hear. This danger is particularly strong in the health system. Clients are aware of labelling processes and often want to please those who care for them or deal with them in a professional relationship. However, the lengthy contact of interviewer and informants and 'prolonged engagement' in the setting help to overcome this.

The emic–etic dimension

Ethnographers use the constructs of the informants and also apply their own scientific conceptual framework, the so-called *emic* and *etic* perspectives (Harris, 1976). First, the researcher needs an understanding of the emic perspective, the insider's or native's perceptions. Insiders' accounts of reality help to uncover knowledge of the reasons why people act as they do. A researcher who uses the emic perspective gives explanations of events from the cultural member's point of view. This perspective is essential in a study, particularly in the beginning, as it prevents the imposition of the values and beliefs of researchers from their own culture to that of another. The outsider's perspective, the etic view, has been prevalent for too long in healthcare and health research. Outsiders, such as health professionals or professional researchers, used to identify the problems of patients and described them rather than listening to the members' own ideas. Now, those who experience an illness are allowed to speak for themselves as they are 'experts' not only on their condition but also on their own feelings and perceptions; as Harris (1976: 36) states, 'The way to get inside of people's heads is to talk with them, to ask questions about what they think and feel'.

The emic perspective corresponds to the reality and definition of informants. The researchers who are examining a culture or subculture gain knowledge of the existing rules and patterns from its members; the emic perspective is thus culturally specific. For health researchers who explore their own culture and that of their patients, the 'native' view is not difficult to obtain because they are already closely involved in the culture. This prior involvement can be dangerous, because health professionals, by being part of the culture they examine, lose awareness of their role as researchers and sometimes rely on assumptions which do not necessarily have a basis in reality. Therefore, reflection on prior assumptions is important. For instance, a researcher might have a similar illness as the participants and might assume that they experience the same emotions. It is important to keep an open mind.

Example 10.5 On Making Assumptions

In her ethnographic study on the adjustment experiences of international students, Brown (2009), one of our colleagues, expected to find that one of the biggest stressors in the new cultural environment would be anxiety over language use as this had been one of the preoccupations of the international students she usually worked with. However, interviews revealed that what preoccupied students the most was food, in particular the difficulty in adapting to a new food culture and missing the food associated with home. This finding took Lorraine to the literature on the eating habits of migrants (none existing on international students directly), which revealed that behaviour around food was the last to adapt to living in a new culture.

Of course, the etic view is important too. Etic meanings focus on the ideas of ethnographers themselves, their abstract and theoretical view where they distance themselves from the cultural setting and try to make sense of it. Harris (1976) explains that etics are scientific accounts by the researcher, based on that which is directly observable. The researchers place individuals' ideas within a framework and interpret it by adopting a social science perspective on the setting. Emic and etic perspectives provide a partnership between researchers and participants. Not only do outsiders recognise patterns and ideas of which the people in the setting are not aware, but they also translate the insights and words of the participants into the language of science.

The meaning of the participants differs from scientific interpretations. Researchers move back and forth, from the reality of informants to scientific interpretation, but they must find a balance between involvement in the culture they study and scientific reflections and ideas about the beliefs and practices within that culture. This can be described as 'iteration', where researchers revise ideas and build upon previous stages (Fetterman, 2020) (see also Chapter 1).

Fieldwork

The term fieldwork is used by ethnographers and other qualitative researchers to describe data collection outside laboratories. The major traits of ethnography have their basis in 'first-hand experience' of the group or community, and this usually, although not only, involves participant observation and interviewing (Atkinson *et al.*, 2007). Ethnographers gain most of their data through fieldwork. They become familiar with the community or group with which they want to carry out research. Fieldwork in qualitative research means working in the natural setting of the informants, observing them and talking to them over prolonged periods of time. This is necessary so that informants get used to the researcher and behave naturally rather than putting on a performance. The observation of a variety of contexts is important. Spradley (1980: 78) provides a list in order to guide researchers when they observe a situation, although these guidelines cannot be seen as complete or all inclusive (see Chapter 7). The physical location of the researcher in the setting is necessary for observation in fieldwork.

The initial phase in the field consists of a time for exploration. Health researchers learn about an area of study and become familiar with it. This is not difficult, because they are already part of the community and well aware of patient and professional cultures. Acceptance need not be earned because health professionals have been part of these cultures, while anthropologists in foreign cultures must achieve entry through learning the ways of the group from the beginning. Fieldwork aims to uncover patterns and regularities in a culture which the people living in that community can recognise. There are several steps in fieldwork. In the first stage the researchers gain access to observe and study the culture in which they are interested and write notes on their observations. In the second stage, researchers start focusing on particular issues. They question the informants on the initial observations. In the third stage researchers realise that saturation has occurred, and they start the process of disengagement.

The best method of data collection in ethnographic research is participant observation, the most complete immersion in a culture. For instance, a nurse who intends to explore the work of a nursing development unit would either be a member of this unit or take part in it in order to observe the practices and reactions of the individuals within.

The ethnographic interview usually follows from observation of the group under study. Its role is to capture the experiences of informants, particularly key informants who have expert knowledge of the culture. Robinson (2013) suggests that researchers use it to gain in-depth information to 'discover cultural knowledge and beliefs' (p. 17), and to examine how this knowledge is structured.

According to Robinson, interviews can be formal or informal. We found that informal interviews often generate richer data. Thomson (2011) adds that interviewing in ethnography differs from other types of interviews if it is carried out after observation: The researchers have already developed a relationship with the participants and can explore the meaning of the behaviour and language they observed. Of course, not all ethnographic studies in health and care take place in the researchers' own countries and cultures; some are carried out in settings where they are outsiders, 'cultural strangers'.

Example 10.6 Outsider Research

Arnold *et al.* (2015), a midwifery researcher, carried out research in a maternity hospital in Kabul. The aim of the study is to describe the culture of care and to examine the perspectives of midwives, doctors and cleaners on their role and care within that hospital. In a country striving to reduce its high rate of maternal mortality, the provision of quality of care for women in Kabul's maternity hospitals is vital. The ethnographic research explores the culture of care in this hospital to identify the barriers and facilitators to healthcare. The thematic analysis of the fieldnotes and interviews demonstrated the 'centrality of the family and family obligations' in Afghan society. Another theme is 'the struggle for survival' within the hospital system, which is a motivator for the work which participants do.

The ethnographic record: field and analytic notes

Researchers collect data by standard methods, mainly through observing and interviewing, but also rely on documents such as letters, diaries and the oral history of people in the culture they study. From the beginning of their research, ethnographers record what goes on 'in the field' – the setting and situation they are studying. This includes noting down fleeting impressions as well as accurate and detailed descriptions of events and behaviour in context. While writing notes and describing what occurs in the situation, ethnographers become reflective and analytic.

Spradley (1979) lists four different types of fieldnotes in ethnography:
- The condensed account
- The expanded account
- The fieldwork journal
- Analysis and interpretation notes

Condensed accounts are short descriptions made in the field during data collection, while expanded accounts extend the descriptions and fill in detail.

Ethnographers extend the short account as soon as possible after observation or interview if they were unable to record during data collection. In the field, journal ethnographers note their own biases, reactions and problems during fieldwork.

Researchers use additional ways to record events and behaviour such as digital audio recordings, films or photos, flowcharts and diagrams.

Fieldwork proceeds in progressive stages. Initially researchers gain the broad picture of the group and the setting. They observe behaviour and listen to the language that is used in the community they study. For nurses and midwives in a clinical setting, this is not difficult because patients, colleagues and other health professionals trust them to record accurately and honestly. After initial observation, researchers focus on particular issues that seem important to them. Finally, writing becomes detailed analysis and interpretation of the culture under study.

KEY POINT

The final outcome of ethnography is a portrait of a culture or subculture.

Micro- and macro-ethnographies

Micro-ethnographies (also called focused ethnographies) investigate subcultures or settings such as a single ward or a group of specialist nurses. Fetterman (2020) claims that micro-studies consist of research in small units, or focus on activities within small social settings. Much health research is indeed micro-ethnographic. Ethnographers might select a setting such as a pain clinic, an operating theatre, a labour ward or a GP practice; one colleague for instance studied time in hospital, another focused on handovers. Most student researchers choose micro-ethnographic studies like these as they make fewer demands on their time than macro-ethnography. It also seems more immediately relevant to the world of the health professional, while policy makers would find macro-ethnography more useful.

There is a continuum between large- and small-scale studies, macro- and micro-ethnographies. A macro-ethnography examines a larger culture with its institutions, communities and value systems. This might be a hospital, or the nursing, midwifery or physiotherapy subculture. A large-scale study means a long period of time in the setting and often involves the work of several research-ers. Both types of ethnography demand a detailed picture of the community under study as well as strategies for data collection and analysis. The type of project depends, of course, on the focus of the investigation and the researcher's own interests.

Ethnographic research can be useful during changes in a culture. In a chang-ing healthcare system, health professionals sometimes study developments not only in larger settings such as hospitals or communities but also in the smaller world of wards and operating theatres. Change – the transition from one stage or one ideology to another (often due to changes in government) – can provide a useful focus for health or health policy research. Maternity wards, GP surgeries and other small units but also bigger sites and settings can be appropriate settings for ethnography. Allen (2015) provides illustrations applied to the work of nurses.

(Most of the examples in this chapter are micro-ethnographic studies. Macro-ethnographies often contain both quantitative and qualitative data.)

Doing and writing ethnography

When writing up, researchers take all the stages of the process into account. Ethnography is analytic as well as descriptive and interpretative. Ethnographers describe what they see and hear while studying a culture; they identify its main features and uncover relationships between them through analysis; they interpret the findings by asking for meaning and inferring it from the data. They take into account the social context in which the study takes place.

Description

As mentioned earlier, ethnography uses description. We must warn, however, that it is never as simple as it seems. Writers select specific situations for observation, disregard some events and interactions in favour of others and focus on particular issues that they perceive as relevant and significant. Not everything observed or heard is described but only that which is relevant for the study at hand. This involves analysis and interpretation.

Researchers describe by writing a story, which is a report of the actions, interactions and events within a cultural group. The reader should get a sense of the setting or a feel for it and understand what is going on there. The description is enhanced by the portrayal of critical events and ordinary life, as well as rituals and roles. Wolcott (1994) demands that during description the writer follow an analytical structure that gives a framework to the account.

Analysis

There are a number of ways in which qualitative ethnographic data can be analysed, see for instance Gobo (2017), Hammersley and Atkinson (2019).

Or the older nursing text by Roper and Shapira (2000). There are also recommended early foundational books such as Spradley (1979, 1980), and these include analytic procedures. Analysis entails working with the data. To provide a simple overview, the researchers process the data by coding/labelling and transform the raw data through finding themes and by making linkages between ideas. This process will generate recognisable patterns. Analysis cannot proceed without interpretation but is more scientific and systematic; it brings order to disorderly data, and the researchers must show how they arrived at the structures and linkages. The informants' perspectives might be different, depending on their location in the hierarchy or their background and career, and this has to be taken into account and the question 'who says what?' is important. At the findings stage, other people's research connected with the emergent themes becomes part of the analytic process through comparison and integration in the study. It is important that the analysis accurately reflects the data. Whatever the analyst finds has to be related back to the data in order to see whether there is a fit between them and the analytic categories and themes.

Steps in the analysis

As in other qualitative research, data analysis takes place from the beginning of the observation and interviews. The focus becomes progressively clearer. In the data analysis, the researcher revisits the aim and the initial research question. Analysis takes more time than data collection. In any type of ethnography, mere description of behaviour and events is not enough as the aim of ethnography is analytic description of a culture or subculture. Ethnographers often start with domain analysis, that is the area which they study and where they note specific events, incidents and activities.

The process of analysis involves several steps though ethnographers might explain this in different ways (see, for instance, the table in LeCompte and Schensul, 1999: 82–83):

1 Ordering and organising the collected material.
2 Breaking the material into manageable – and meaningful – sections.
3 Building, comparing and contrasting categories.
4 Searching for relationships and grouping categories together.
5 Recognising and describing patterns, themes and typologies.
6 Interpreting and searching for meaning.

These processes must not be seen necessarily as linear or sequential, and each step or stage can be revisited or repeated. There is also overlap between these activities. Spradley (1979: 92) claims that analysis involves the 'systematic examination of something to determine its parts, the relationship among parts, and their relationship to the whole'. Agar (1980) stresses the non-linear nature of the process: researchers collect data through which they learn about a culture, they try to make sense of what they saw and heard, and then they collect new data on the basis of their analysis and interpretation.

Researchers listen to their recordings, read the transcripts and fieldnotes from observation and note down significant elements. Of course, they re-read and listen many times, and sometimes recognise differences between the first and the second reading and listening.

The data are scanned and organised from the very beginning of the study. If gaps and inadequacies occur, they can be filled by collecting more data or refocusing on the initial aims of the study. While this work goes on, researchers choose to focus on particular aspects which they examine more closely than others. While re-reading the data, thoughts and observations are being recorded, and a search for regularities can begin. The material is organised and broken down into manageable chunks. These pieces (of sentences, groups of words or paragraphs) are each given a meaningful label. This initial coding of data generates categories. The 'coding for descriptive labels' (Roper and Shapira, 2000) reduces or collapses the mass of data obtained. (Indeed, these processes are similar to those in other qualitative approaches.)

For instance, the first interview – or the first detailed description of observation – is scanned and marked off into chunks, which are given labels. The second and third interview transcripts are then coded and compared with the first. Commonalities and similar codes are sorted and grouped together. This happens for each interview (or observation). Thematically, similar sets are placed together and grouped into categories. The researcher then tries to find the ideas that link the categories, and describes and summarises them. From this stage onwards diagrams are helpful because they present the links and patterns graphically.

The researcher compares the emerging categories and reduces them to (or collapses into) themes (major categories, constructs) and tries to find regularities. Broad patterns of thought and behaviour emerge. The patterns and regularities have their basis in the actual observations and interviews; they will be connected with the personal experiences of the researcher.

At that stage a dialogue starts with categories and themes drawn from the relevant and related literature. Ethnographic texts describe this 'taxonomic analysis' – analysis by classification or grouping of categories into an organised system which points to the relationship between these categories. They also might uncover a typology of participants, for instance, a midwife might recognise in the research on a maternity unit three 'types' of professional – the 'dependent', the 'independent' and the 'controlling' professional. In a further example, a doctor might classify patients into passive and active individuals. These kinds of grouping common in ethnographic research generate a typology.

However, this does not present all the processes of ethnographic research. It also means searching for contrasts between categories, stating their dimensions and looking for conditions under which certain actions occur (see also Gobo, 2017).

Interpretation

Researchers take the last step, that of interpretation, during and after the analysis, making inferences, providing meaning and giving possible explanations for the phenomena. While describing and analysing, they interpret the findings, that is they gain insight and give meaning to them. Interpretation involves some speculation, theorising and explaining, although it must be directly grounded in the data. It links the emerging ideas derived from the analysis to established theories through comparing and contrasting others' work with the researcher's own.

Eventually the story is put together from the descriptions, analyses and interpretations. LeCompte *et al.* (1997) compare this to assembling a jigsaw puzzle where a frame is quickly outlined and small puzzle pieces are collected together and placed in position within the frame. The difference is that one knows about the final picture of a jigsaw and has something to work towards, while in qualitative ethnographic research the eventual portrait may include radical changes.

Pitfalls and problems

There are a number of problems with ethnographic research in the health arena. First, it is difficult as an insider to become a 'cultural stranger' questioning the assumptions of the familiar culture whose rules and norms have been internalised. Vigilance and advice from outsiders are very important. Second, because health professionals often have a background in the natural sciences and are taught to adopt a systematic approach to their clinical work, they sometimes may find it difficult to bear ambiguity. Here, it is better to admit to uncertainty than to make unwarranted claims about the research. The ethnographic outcome resembles a diagnosis: signs and symptoms are examined for meaning but should never become once-and-for-all interpretation. Findings can be re-interpreted at a later stage in the light of reflection or new evidence.

Our students often write up their research and make statements that seem to be applicable to a whole range of similar situations. The findings from ethnography cannot simply be generalised, however, and they are not automatically applicable to other settings though often theoretical ideas can be generalised. The researcher can compare with other specific situations similar to the case studied and can achieve typicality.

Novice researchers are often too descriptive and present raw data without analysis and interpretation, but even the quotes of the participants in the study are not raw data but purposefully selected by the researcher (see Chapter 17). Nevertheless, at the start of a research journey, it is advisable to give more descriptive detail, clear analysis and to be careful with interpretation. With experience, the balance might change. It is interesting that on revisiting the work at a later stage, many researchers start reinterpreting the data.

Summary

The main features of ethnography as a research method are as follows.
- Ethnographers describe, analyse and interpret the culture and the local, emic perspective of its members while making their own etic interpretations.
- Ethnographers immerse themselves in the culture or subculture they study.
- Data are acquired during fieldwork through participant observation and interviews with key informants as well as through documents or diaries.
- Researchers observe the rules and rituals in the culture and try to understand the meaning and interpretation that informants give to them.
- Fieldnotes are written throughout the fieldwork about events and behaviour in the setting.
- The main evaluative criterion is the way in which the study presents the culture as experienced by its members.

References

Agar, M.H. (1980) *The Professional Stranger: Informal Introduction to Ethnography*, Academic Press, New York, NY.

Allen, D. (2015) *The Invisible Work of Nurses: Hospitals, Organisations and Healthcare*, Routledge Oxon, Abingdon. Kindle Edition

Anderson, L. (2006) Analytic autoethnography. *Journal of Contemporary Ethnography*, **35** (4), 373–395.

Arnold, R., Van Teijlingen, E., Ryan, K.C. and Holloway, I. (2015) Understanding Afghan healthcare providers: a qualitative study of the culture of care in a Kabul maternity hospital. *BJOG: An International Journal of Obstetrics and Gynaecology*, **122** (2), 260–267.

Atkinson, P., Coffey, A., Delamont, S. *et al.* (eds.) (2007) Introduction to part one, in *Handbook of Ethnography* Sage, London, pp. 9–10.

Brown, L. (2009) The role of food in the adjustment journey of international students, in *The New Cultures of Food: Marketing Opportunities from Ethnic, Religious and Cultural Diversity* (eds. A. Lindgreen and M. Hingley), Gower, London, pp. 36–56.

Cook, K.E. (2005) Using critical ethnography to explore issues in health promotion. *Qualitative Health Research*, **15** (1), 129–138.

Coughlin, C. (2013) An ethnographic study of main events during hospitalization: perceptions of nurses and patients. *Journal of Clinical Nursing*, **22** (15–16), 2327–2337.

Denzin, N.K. (1989) *Interpretive Interactionism*, Sage, Newbury Park, CA.

Deutscher, I. (1970) Words and deeds: social science and social policy, in *Qualitative Methodology: Firsthand Involvement with the Social World* (ed. W.J. Filstead), Markham Publishing, Chicago, IL, pp. 27–51.

Fetterman, D.M. (2020) *Ethnography: Step by Step*, 4th edn, Sage, Thousand Oaks, CA.

Fox, J. (2020) Experiences of user involvement in mental health research: exploring perspectives from a service user researcher using autoethnography. Discussion paper, *Mental Health Review Journal*. Available at https://arro.anglia.ac.uk/id/eprint/705768/6/Fox_2020.pdf.

Geertz, C. (1973) *The Interpretation of Cultures*, Basic Books, New York, NY.

Gobo, G. (2017) *Doing Ethnography*, 2nd edn, Sage, Thousand Oaks, CA.

Hackett, P.M.W. and Hayre, C.N. (2021) *Handbook of Ethnography in Healthcare Research*, Abingdon, Oxon, Routledge.

Hammersley, M. and Atkinson, P. (2019) *Ethnography: Principles in Practice*, 4th edn, Routledge, Milton Park.

Harris, M. (1976) History and significance of the emic/etic distinction. *Annual Review of Anthropology*, **5**, 329–350.

Huby, G., Hart, E., McKevitt, C. and Sobo, E. (2007) Editorial: addressing the complexity of health care: the practical potential of ethnography. *Journal of Health Services Research Policy*, **12** (4), 193–194.

LeCompte, M.D. and Schensul, J.J. (1999) *Analyzing & Interpreting Ethnographic Data*, Altamira Press, Walnut Creek, CA.

LeCompte, M.D., Preissle, J. and Tesch, R. (1997) *Ethnography and Qualitative Design in Educational Research*, 2nd edn, Academic Press, Chicago, IL.

Leininger, M. (ed.) (1985) *Qualitative Research Methods in Nursing*, WB Saunders, Philadelphia, PA.

Madison, D.S. (2019) *Critical Ethnography: Method, Ethics and Performance*, 3rd edn, Sage, Thousand Oaks, CA.

Malinowski, B. (1922) *Argonauts of the Western Pacific: An Account of Native Enterprise and Adventure in the Archipelagoes of Melanesian New Guinea*, Dutton, New York, NY.

Mead, M. (1935) *Sex and Temperament in Three Primitive Societies*, Morrow, New York, NY.

Meng, X., Chen, X., Liu, Z. and Zhou, L. (2019) Nursing practice in stroke habilitation: perspectives from multidisciplinary health professionals. *Nursing and Health Sciences*, **22** (1), 28–37.

Newnham, E., Small, K. and Allen, J. (2021) Critical ethnography in maternity care: bridging creativity and rigour. Discussion paper. *Midwifery*, **99** (103014) doi:10.1016/j.midw.2021.103014.

Paradis-Gagné, E. and Pariseau-Legault, P. (2020) Critical ethnography of outreach nurses of the clinical issues associated with disaffiliation and stigma. *Journal of Advanced Nursing*, **77** (3), 1357–1367.

Robinson, S.G. (2013) The relevancy of ethnography to nursing. *Nursing Science Quarterly*, **26** (1), 14–19.

Roper, J.M. and Shapira, J. (2000) *Ethnography in Nursing Research*, Sage, Thousand Oaks, CA.

Savage, J. (2006) Ethnographic evidence: the value of applied ethnography in health care. *Journal of Research in Nursing*, **11** (5), 383–393.

Scammell, J. and Olumide, G. (2012) Racism and the mentor–student relationship: nurse education through a white lens. *Nurse Education Today*, **32** (5), 545–550.

Schensul, S.L., Schensul, J.J. and LeCompte, M.D. (1999) *Essential Ethnographic Methods: Observations, Interviews and Questionnaires*, Altamira Press, Walnut Creek, CA (from the Ethnographic Toolkit).

Spradley, J.P. (1979) *The Ethnographic Interview*, Harcourt Brace Johanovich College Publishers, Fort Worth, TX.

Spradley, J.P. (1980) *Participant Observation*, Harcourt Brace Johanovich College Publishers, Fort Worth, TX.

Thomas, J. (1993) *Doing Critical Ethnography*, Sage, Newbury Park, CA.

Thomson, D. (2011) Ethnography: a suitable approach for providing an inside perspective on the everyday lives of health professionals. *International Journal of Therapy and Rehabilitation*, **18** (1), 10–17

Walker, E.R., Shaw, S.C.K. and Leeds Anderson, J. (2020) Dyspraxia in medical education: a collaborative autoethnography. *The Qualitative Report*, **25** (11), 4072–4093.

Whyte, W.F. (1943) *Street Corner Society: The Social Structure of an Italian Slum*, University of Chicago Press, Chicago, IL.

Wolcott, H.F. (1994) *Transforming Qualitative Data: Description, Analysis, and Interpretation*, Sage, Thousand Oaks, CA.

Further Reading

Atkinson, P. (2020) *Writing Ethnographically*, Sage, London.

Stanley, L. (2018) *Feminist Sociology and Institutional Ethnography*, Xpress, Edinburgh.

Chapter 11

Grounded Theory Methodology

Many experienced researchers use grounded theory methodology (GTM), because it is a systematic research approach to collecting and analysing data. This generates a theory grounded in the data. It has been popular since the initial text by Glaser and Strauss was published (1967). (Although the book is called 'Grounded Theory', recent researchers often call it Grounded Theory Methodology and suggest that only the result should be called 'a grounded theory.)

Stern and Porr (2011) stated that it was initially used for nursing and healthcare research predominantly, before it became widespread in other disciplines. The finished product of this research is called a grounded theory – a development of theory directly based and grounded in the data collected by the researcher. Over the years, the original approach has evolved, not only through the main protagonists themselves but also by others researchers who adopted and adapted it during its application to their own inquiry. It has taken different directions, not only in underlying philosophies, the use of literature, and even in analytic strategies. In this chapter, we will describe the main features of GT or GTM (grounded theory method) and trace its development and changes over time.

The approach has its origin in sociology, and, in its early days, was developed through the collaboration of the sociologists Barney Glaser and Anselm Strauss who were trained respectively in quantitative and qualitative methods. Although GT can comprise both qualitative and quantitative procedures, it is most often allied to qualitative research. GT is not tied, however, to a specific discipline or even to a particular form of data collection – there are studies in psychology, healthcare, business management and other fields. GT, like other qualitative approaches, is often adopted by researchers where not much knowledge exists about the phenomenon they wish to study.

Data sources can be varied, such as interviews, observations or documents and visual and oral presentations or events. Health researchers particularly appreciate the systematic and organised way of the GT process. Caring is an interactive process, hence the focus in GT on interaction, communication and active engagement in social situations suits most health professionals.

Qualitative Research in Nursing and Healthcare, Fifth Edition.
Immy Holloway and Kathleen Galvin.
© 2024 John Wiley & Sons Ltd. Published 2024 by John Wiley & Sons Ltd.

History and origin

GT originated in the 1960s by Barney Glaser and Anselm Strauss, who worked together on research about health professionals' interaction with dying patients in 1965. From research, writing and teaching, the classic text *The Discovery of Grounded Theory* (Glaser and Strauss, 1967) emerged. Four other books on GT followed – *Field Research: Strategies for a Natural Sociology* (Schatzman and Strauss, 1973), *Theoretical Sensitivity* (Glaser, 1978), *Qualitative Analysis for Social Scientists* (Strauss, 1987) and *Basics of Qualitative Research* (Strauss and Corbin, 1990, 1998), which was an attempt by Strauss and Corbin (Corbin is a researcher with a nursing background) to modify earlier ideas on GT. The last book on which Strauss (who died in 1996) worked is a clear and practically useful book on GT; it describes an approach which has been tried and developed. In 2008, Corbin followed this up with a later book (Corbin and Strauss, 2008). Although at times called formulaic and prescriptive, the 1990 and 1998 editions have helped many health researchers find certain elements on GT such as theoretical sampling and saturation (these terms will be explained later). The early book edited by Chenitz and Swanson (1986) discussed GT in relation to nursing research. Strauss and Corbin (1997) edited a book in which they show how researchers have applied GT in practice. In the early nineties, Glaser (1992) criticised the approach taken by Strauss and Corbin and asserted that what they described was not true GT but 'conceptual description'. Since then, Glaser has written prolifically – including various readers on GT – and developed his own perspective in books and website. He founded his press (Sociology Press, Mill Valley, CA), established a 'Grounded Theory Institute' and now published the international journal *The Grounded Theory Review*. His books are too numerous to quote and his collaborators were many. The ideas of Glaser and Strauss diverged in later years. Recently Kathy Charmaz (2006, 2014) developed a constructivist GT from earlier work. An edited handbook by Bryant and Charmaz was last updated in 2019. See also *Developing Grounded Theory: Second Generation* (Morse et al., 2021).

A wealth of research exists in the field of healthcare and nursing. In this area, the GT approach has been popular from its inception; Benoliel (1996: 419–421) lists the GT research studies that have been carried out in nursing between 1980 and 1994 and gives a good overview of the history of GT. There are also chapters in Munhall (2012) and in many of Morse's publications in the United States. Melia in the 1980s and 1990s, and Cutcliffe (2000, 2005) in Britain are some of the better-known nurse researchers who have used and/or discussed GT approaches. Schreiber and Stern (2001) edited a GT text specifically for nurses, and even in the 2020s many articles and books are being written. It has also been used in medical education research (see, for instance, Watling and Lingard, 2012).

Symbolic interactionism

In their original book, Glaser and Strauss did not discuss a philosophical base for their approach in detail (Chamberlain-Salaun *et al.*, 2013), nor did they create a theoretical framework (one of the reasons for the popularity of GT which could be used in any discipline). However, when initially used, GT had a strong link to symbolic interactionism, focusing on the processes of interaction between people exploring human behaviour and social roles (although it must be said that Glaser sees SI as just one of the contributions to the approach). SI explains how individuals attempt to fit their lines of action to those of others (Blumer, 1971), take account of each others' acts, interpret them and reorganise their own behaviour. Mead (1934) established the philosophical framework, and Blumer contributed to GT the idea that human beings are active participants in their situation rather than passive respondents.

Mead, the main proponent of SI, sees the self as a social rather than a psychological phenomenon. Members of society affect the development of a person's social self by their expectations and relationships. Initially, individuals model their roles on the important people in their lives, 'significant others'; they learn to act according to others' expectations, thereby shaping their own behaviour. The observation of these interacting roles is a source of data in GT, and individual actions can only be understood in context.

SI focuses on actions and perceptions of individuals and their ideas and intentions. The Thomas theorem states that 'If men [*sic*] define situations as real, they are real in their consequences' (Thomas, 1928: 584), thereby claiming that individual definitions of reality shape perceptions and actions. In particular, researchers use GT to investigate the interactions, behaviours and experiences as well as individuals' perceptions and thoughts about them. Researchers also investigate social processes – for example *being diagnosed* or *helping dying patients*. The previous references are now quite old, but GT has lost none of its popularity with present day health researchers.

The main features of grounded theory

The main aim of GT is the *systematic* generation of theory from the data collected by researchers, but existing theories can also be modified or extended through GT. Researchers start with an area of interest, collect and analyse the data and allow relevant ideas to develop, without preconceived theories or preconceptions. Indeed, Glaser and Strauss (1967) advised that rigid preconceived assumptions prevent development of the research; imposing a framework might block the awareness of major concepts emerging from the data. The approach seeks *explanation* rather than being descriptive.

The theory generated through the research must be applicable to similar settings and contexts. GT researchers are able to adopt alternative perspectives rather than follow previously developed ideas. For this, they need flexibility and open minds, qualities related to the processes involved in healthcare.

The GT style of research uses constant comparison. The researcher compares each section of the data with every other throughout the study for similarities, differences and connections. Included in this process are the themes and categories identified in the literature. All the data are coded and categorised, and from this process, major concepts and constructs are formed. The researcher takes up a search for major themes that link ideas to find a core category for the study.

Strauss (1987) sees the processes of both induction and deduction as essential in GT. GT does not start with a hypothesis though researchers might have 'hunches'. After collecting the initial data, however, relationships are established and provisional hypotheses (or 'working propositions') conceived. These are checked out against new incoming data. Glaser (1992), however, stresses the inductive element and the 'emergence' of theory.

Grounded theorists accept their role as interpreters of the data and do not stop at merely reporting them or describing the participants' experiences. Researchers search for relationships between concepts, unlike some other forms of qualitative research which often generate major themes but, generally, do not develop theories. Much research which adopts the name of GT is descriptive or modified grounded theory method.

KEY POINT

Researchers who call their approach grounded theory should include its elements and develop a theory.

Grounded theory has been one of the most popular and commonly used qualitative research approaches in healthcare and especially nursing. It has a key advantage that may explain its extensive use. Grounded theory is particularly suited to the study of processes, trajectories or journeys through for instance, an illness condition, a care delivery system or organisational pathway. Because the key aim is to offer explanatory theory (explanations of what happens under what conditions), grounded in rich complex data, it is especially applicable to a diverse range of health research topics. In addition, the procedures are described very systematically and explicitly with attention to interpretive steps in the analysis which also makes it very attractive to health professionals, particularly nurses.

> **Example 11.1** A Grounded Theory in Healthcare
>
> Campbell and Nolan (2019) researched pregnant women's experience of taking part in yoga classes. They interviewed the participants three times at different points in time. Through their work, they developed a theory that 'yoga enhances women's self-efficacy for labour by building their confidence through a combination of techniques.'

Data collection, theoretical sampling and analysis

Data collection

Data are collected through observations in the field, interviews of participants, diaries and other documents such as letters or even newspapers. Researchers use interviews and observations more often than other data sources. Everything, even researchers' experience, can become sources of data; Glaser (1978) states that 'everything is data'. Data collection and analysis are linked from the beginning of the research, proceed in parallel and interact continuously. The analysis starts after the first few steps in the data collection have been taken; the emerging ideas guide and inform the collection of data and analysis. This process does not finish until the end of the research, because ideas, concepts and new questions continually arise which guide the researcher to new data sources and concepts. Researchers collect data from initial interviews, observations or documents and take their cues from the first emerging ideas to develop further interviews and observations. The collection of data becomes more focused and specific as the process develops (progressive focusing).

The researcher writes fieldnotes from the beginning of the data collection throughout the project. Certain occurrences in the setting, or ideas from the participants that seem of vital interest, are recorded either during or immediately after data collection. They remind the researcher of the events, actions and interactions and trigger thinking processes.

According to Glaser (1978), the following are necessary for GT:

- Theoretical sensitivity
- Theoretical sampling
- Data analysis: coding and categorising
- Constant comparison
- Literature as a source of data
- Integration of theory
- Theoretical memos and fieldnotes
- The core category

Theoretical sensitivity

Researchers must be theoretically sensitive (Glaser, 1978). Theoretical sensitivity means that researchers can differentiate between significant and less important data and have insight into their meanings. There are a variety of sources for theoretical sensitivity. It is built up over time, from reading and experience which guides the researcher to examine the data from all sides rather than stay fixed on the obvious. Birks and Mills (2015) maintain that the concept of theoretical sensitivity is difficult to understand, but reflection and insight into the meaning of the phenomenon under study is essential. They state that it has three main traits (p. 59):

1 It mirrors the researcher's personal and professional biography.
2 It can be increased by various instruments and strategies.
3 It is developed during the research journey.

Professional experience can be one source of awareness, and personal experiences, too, can help make the researcher sensitive. Mills and Birks (2015) also discuss theoretical sensitivity in the second edition of their book.

Example 11.2 Professional Experience

A study in rural Australia by Mulholland (2020) uncovered a grounded theory of interprofessional learning and paramedic care as not much was known about how paramedics and other health professionals interact and collaborate with each other. The researchers reported the importance of relationships, acknowledgement and cooperation but also that of occupational barriers. The authors' state: 'A successful collaboration produced a clinical environment where patient care was informed by contributions from all team members'. (To most of us it seems obvious, but it is known that some groups of professionals are sometimes seen as less important than others.)

Example 11.3 Personal Experience

A health professional suffered from a mild form of epilepsy. She decided to carry out research about the experience of epilepsy because she was an insider in this world. Her advisers, while acknowledging that she used her own experience as a source of knowledge, warned her of the possibility of personal biases and preconceptions which might leave her incapable to be flexible and able to set assumptions aside.

The literature sensitises in the sense that documents, research studies or autobiographies create awareness in the researcher of relevant and significant elements in the data. Strauss and Corbin (1998) – who call it just 'sensitivity' – believe that theoretical sensitivity increases when researchers interact with the data because they think about emerging ideas, ask further questions and see these ideas as provisional until they have been examined over time and are finally confirmed by the data.

Theoretical sampling

Sampling guided by ideas with significance for the emerging theory is called *theoretical sampling*. The developing theory directs this type of sampling. In the process of collecting data and analysing them, the researcher decides on the basis of emerging concepts, what data to collect next, and from whom, in order to advance the theory.

One of the main differences between this and other types of sampling is *time* and *continuance*. Unlike other sampling, which is planned beforehand, theoretical sampling in GT continues throughout the study and is not planned before the study starts as happens in some other qualitative research approaches.

At the start of the project, researchers do make initial sampling decisions. They decide on a setting and on particular individuals or groups of people able to give information on the topic under study. Once the research has started and initial data have been analysed and examined (one must remember that data collection and analysis interact) new concepts arise, and events and people are chosen who can further illuminate the problem. Researchers then set out to sample different situations, individuals, or a variety of settings, and focus on new ideas to extend the emerging theories. The selection of participants, settings, events or documents is a function of developing theories.

Theoretical sampling continues until *theoretical saturation*. Students do not always understand the meaning of the concept 'saturation', and believe it to be a stage when no new information or concepts are obtained through data collection and analysis. It occurs however, when no new data of importance for the developing theory and for the achievement of the aim of the research emerge. It is very difficult to reach saturation; indeed, one might ask if it can ever truly be established, but the attempt at saturation is necessary so that the researcher can account for all categories. Saturation takes place at a different stage in each research project and is difficult to recognise. Draucker *et al.* (2007) present a sampling guide to assist in both systematic decision-making and category development.

Example 11.4 Theoretical Sampling

A grounded theory was developed by Mcmillan *et al.* (2012). The researchers examined post-discharge issues of older people after a repair of their hip fracture. Their sampling was initially purposive and later focused on particular concepts for theoretical sampling. They initially contacted volunteer participants in their study. After developing the categories that emerged through constant comparative analysis, they used theoretical sampling as a strategy to strive for saturation by searching for the dimensions of the core category, *taking control*. Interviews were held with the first group of participants within 4 weeks of discharge, while those who had been at home longer formed a later participative group. The researchers also recruited participants who had been in an intermediate setting. All these settings added to the study of 'taking control' and its many forms and contexts.

Theoretical sampling, although originating in GT, is occasionally used in other types of qualitative analysis, but saturation cannot be applied to all cases in qualitative research (O'Reilly and Parker, 2013).

Data analysis: coding and categorising

Coding and categorising go on throughout the research. From the start of the study, analysts *code* the data. Coding in GT is the process by which concepts or themes are identified and named during the analysis. Data are transformed and reduced to build *categories* which are named and given a label. Through the emergence of these categories, theory can be evolved and integrated. Researchers form clusters of interrelating concepts, not merely descriptions of themes. Sometimes these codes consist of words and phrases used by the participants themselves to describe a phenomenon. They are called *in vivo* codes (Strauss, 1987). A new recruit to the profession might declare in an interview: 'I was thrown in at the deep end', for instance. The code might be 'thrown in at the deep end'. *In vivo* codes can give life and interest to the study and can be immediately recognised as reflecting the reality of the participants. In this process of analysis, the first step is concerned with open coding which starts as soon as the researcher receives the data. Open coding is the process of breaking down and conceptualising the data.

In GT, all the data are coded. Initial codes tend to be provisional and are modified or transformed over the period of analysis. At the beginning of a project or a study, line-by-line analysis is important, although it may be a long-drawn-out process for analysts. Codes are based directly on the data, and therefore the researcher avoids preconceived ideas. An example of an interview with a nurse tutor gives some idea of level 1 coding:

Well, I suppose most people get fed up with doing the same things year in, year out	Getting bored
I really felt like a change	Desire for change
Regular hours are important to me	Wish for regularity
I had not been promoted to the level to which I could function	Lack of promotion

The analyst groups concepts together and develops categories. At the start, a great number of labels are used, and after initial coding, analysts attempt to condense (or collapse) codes into groups of concepts with similar traits which are categories. Hutchinson (1993) called these level 2 codes. These categories tend to be more abstract than initial codes and are generally formulated by the investigator. These are examples of level 2 codes:

I had this fear that I was not going to survive	Fear of dying
Nobody, but nobody was there to help me and	Lack of support
I felt that I was completely alone	Feeling isolated
We all need somebody close to be with us when we are ill	Need for significant other

The broken-down data must be linked together again in a new form. The main features (properties) and dimensions of these categories are identified.

Level 3 constructs are major categories which, although generated from the data and based in them, are formulated by the researchers and rooted in their professional and academic knowledge. These constructs contain developing theoretical ideas and themes and through building these constructs, analysts reassemble the data. Categories are linked to subcategories. This process of reassembling the data is called *axial coding* by Strauss and Corbin though Glaser uses different terms. There is no reason, however, why researchers cannot use the categories that others have discovered. For instance, Melia (1987) borrows the term 'awareness context' from Glaser and Strauss, but usually health researchers develop their own useful categories. In developing the relationship between categories, researchers have to take the six c's into account (Glaser developed these and other theoretical coding families in 1978): causes, context, contingencies, covariances, consequences and conditions for each category.

1 *Causes* are reasons for or explanations for the occurrence of a category.
2 *Context* is the setting and factors surrounding the phenomenon.
3 *Covariance* occurs between the given category and others (i.e. a category changes with change in another).
4 The development of a category is affected by certain *conditions*.
5 *Contingency* means that the given category has an impact on another category.
6 *Consequences* are the outcomes or functions of a given category.

Glaser advises that most GT research fit into a causal model, a consequence model or a condition model. Even if the GT method is modified by researchers, it is useful to keep this in mind.

Although there is no initial hypothesis in GT, Strauss and Corbin (1998) (though not Glaser) suggest that during the course of the research, working propositions or hypotheses are generated. These must be based in and indicated by the data. The process of verification for the working hypotheses goes on throughout the research in the Straussian version of GT though it cannot be compared with that in quantitative research. Researchers also seek deviant or negative cases which do not support a particular working proposition. When these are found, the researcher must modify the proposition or find reasons why it is not applicable in this particular instance.

The process of coding and categorising stops only when

- No new information on a category can be found in spite of the attempt to collect more data from a variety of sources.
- The category has been described with all its properties, variations and processes.
- Links between categories are firmly established (Strauss and Corbin, 1998).

The core category

The researcher must discover the *core category*. In GT, the major category which links all others is called the core category or core variable. Like a thread the category should be woven into the whole of the study; it is part of the overall pattern. The linking of all categories around a core is called selective coding. This means that the researcher uncovers the essence of the study and integrates all the elements of the emergent theory.

The core category is the basic social–psychological process (BSP) involved in the research. The BSP is a process that occurs over time and explains changes in behaviour. It represents the ideas that are of major importance for the research and links the other categories (though the term BSP is not often used lately).

Strauss (1987) claims some major characteristics for the core category:

1 It must be the central element of the research related to other categories and explain variations.
2 It must recur often in the data and be part of a pattern.
3 It connects with other categories without a major effort by the researcher.
4 The core category develops in the process of identifying, describing and conceptualising.
5 The core category is usually fully developed only towards the end of the research.

Examples for core categories can be found in most grounded theory studies; examples of core categories are), 'Deciding to recover' (Newell, 2008), and 'Taking control' (McMillan *et al.*, 2012). Most GT research has a core category which expresses the essence of the study.

Constant comparison

Coding and categorising involve constant comparison. Initial interviews are analysed and codes and concepts developed. By comparing concepts and sub-categories, researchers are able to group them into major categories and label them. When they code and categorise incoming data, they compare new categories with those that have already been established. Thus, incoming data are checked for their 'fit' with existing categories. Each incident of a category is compared with every other incident for similarities and differences. The comparison involves the literature. Constant comparison is useful for finding the properties and dimensions of categories. It helps in looking at concepts critically as each concept is illuminated by the new, incoming data. Strauss and Corbin (1998: 4) stress that they do not offer prescriptions but 'essentially guidelines for suggested techniques'. However, it is useful if researchers are completely familiar with the main features of the GT approach, even if they modify it.

The three main approaches

Rather than using a modified grounded theory method – which is possible if it is made explicit – it would be more purist to follow an established approach. Researchers generally differentiate between three main approaches, all rooted in the first book by Glaser and Strauss in 1967. Rieger (2019) discusses *Straussian*, *Classic* (which Glaser and his followers call it. We shall use the term Glaserian in this text) and *Constructivist*. Deering and Williams (2020) add *Feminist* GT, but this could be encompassed in one of the previously cited approaches as long as researchers consider and explore the experiences of women and other oppressed groups. Each method has its own way of analysing the data and handling the literature (see later). Kenny and Fourie (2015) state that these have differing philosophical stances, coding strategies and use of literature. The latter is of particular importance. (The approaches will be further described in the section about pitfalls and problems. A novice researcher does not need these in detail, while a PhD student or an experienced researcher has to engage with them.)

Example 11.5 Straussian GT

A Straussian grounded theory was adopted by Johnsson and Nordgren (2019) in a study about decision-making by General Practitioners in Sweden. It included interviews and observations of sixteen doctors when making decisions based on conflicting demands and pressures from evidence-based medicine, patient-centeredness and ethics.

The researchers analysed the interviews about the participants' thoughts and the observations of their actions in parallel. They used constant comparisons by looking at incoming in relation to already collected data. Memos were written and working hypotheses developed.

The outcome of this research was a middle range theory, ethics was at the centre of the GPs' decision-making. They seemed to choose their tenets of action while being pressured by conflicting norms. The researchers attempted an understanding of ethical decision-making and the elements that influenced it.

Example 11.6 Glaserian or Classic GT

In a Danish study, Sorensen and Christensen (2018) explored behavioural patterns of adherence to respiratory muscle training in patients with chronic pulmonary disease. They uncovered three behavioural modes of adherence: *evading*, *misgiving* and *involving*. The research also showed patterns of intended and non-intended patterns of non-adherence.

Example 11.7 Constructivist GT

In two health service trusts of the United Kingdom, Andrews *et al.* (2020) researched the experience of nurses in self-care and self-compassion and the influence these factors had on the care of patients. They developed a constructivist grounded theory by interviewing and analysing the thoughts of general, mental health and general learning disability nurses. This theory demonstrated the need for permission to help nurses to self-care and self-compassion which might enable them to fulfil patients' needs.

Using the literature

The place of the literature in a GT study is problematic; experts have different perspectives on this. Informative lists of the differences between the approach of Strauss and Corbin and that of Glaser can be found in MacDonald (2001), Kenny and Fourie (2015) and Deering and Williams (2020).

Some purists believe that there should not be an initial literature review of the specific topic to be researched but an overview of the more general area Indeed Glaser and Strauss eventually developed diverging ideas on this. Deering and Williams argue that Glaser and his followers do not advocate an initial review – indeed we have heard this from him in various lectures. The reason for this is that researchers should not be directed to particular issues in their field, but their own data retain priority in the study. Others feel that an initial review sensitises the researcher to issues related to the topic and stimulates questions to be asked. Strauss and Corbin have argued that the researcher is not a 'blank sheet' without any prior knowledge and experience. They stress open-mindedness and advise not to follow previous assumptions. Charmaz and Thornberg (2020) add the element of reflexivity: Researchers need to take into account 'preconceived' ideas and reflect on them. Constructivist GT seems to take a position between the others.

One can give arguments for and against a long literature review before collection and analysis of data begins. Researchers must be able to justify their study, and therefore they need to find out the type and extent of knowledge that already exists in the field. They should not, however, generate a focus from other people's studies but rather from their own data which have priority.

Strauss and Corbin (1998) list a number of points about the use of the literature.

1 Concepts from the literature can be compared with those deriving from the study.
2 The literature can stimulate theoretical sensitivity. It can make researchers aware of existing ideas.
3 The literature can generate questions and problems.

4 Knowledge of existing theories can be useful in influencing the stance of the researcher.

5 The literature can be used as an added source of data although these do not have priority over the researchers' own data.

6 Researchers have to consider why the literature confirms or refutes their own ideas or data.

7 Even before the study starts, initial questions can help develop conceptual areas.

8 During the analysis process more questions can be generated, especially when the researchers' data and the findings of the literature show a discrepancy.

9 The literature can guide theoretical sampling. It can help decide where to go next. Ideas might arise which increase the chance of developing further the emerging theory.

10 The literature can be used to validate the researcher's categories. Concepts in the literature may confirm or refute the findings of the researcher.

Thornberg and Dunne (2019) advise that the literature should develop theoretical sensitivity in the researcher. The dialogue with the literature is critical in the process of theory development. Glaser speaks about several levels of literature and suggests that researchers initially read in the general area, while not studying the specifics related to their own research. The latter should not be carried out until fieldwork, coding and categorising is well under way; otherwise, researchers might rely on ideas by others rather than develop their own. We suggest that the grounded theorists trawl the literature initially to find the gap in knowledge where they can contribute to the field, without studying it in detail or being directed to specific ideas, otherwise they might lose the primacy of their own data and be constrained by others' writing. It is, however, now generally accepted that researchers need an initial review to give some boundaries to their research and to show where they fit in and fill the gap (see also later).

Most grounded theorists believe that the literature becomes a source for comparison. When categories have been found, researchers trawl and engage with the literature for confirmation or refutation of these categories. They try to discover what other researchers have found, and whether there are any links to existing theories. Researchers can also use the literature to compare their own theories with those previously developed.

KEY POINT

The dialogue and engagement with the literature is critical in the process of theory development.

Integration of theory

To be credible, the theory must have 'explanatory power', that is establish a causal relationship. This is different from descriptive qualitative research. In a good project, categories are connected with each other and tightly linked to the data. Researchers do not describe static situations but take into account and develop processes. We discuss later that Charmaz and Thornberg (2020) confirm the original statements by Glaser and Straus about quality in GT. They (2020) repeat the original authors' criteria for credibility: A detailed, lively description, showing the readers how research arrived at their conclusions, and comparisons to enhance the 'scope and generality of the theory'. We suggest that researchers read their article as they discuss these elements in detail and give examples. They add a useful checklist and guidelines for quality.

Glaser and Strauss (1967) state that two types of theory are produced: substantive and formal. Some also mention the term 'middle-range theory'. A term that Merton used many decades ago. Substantive theory emerges from the study of a particular context or setting – such as a ward, or patients with myocardial infarction, or professional education – hence this type of theory is very useful for health researchers. It has specificity and applies to the setting and situation studied; this means that it is limited. Formal theory, however, is generated from many different situations and settings, and it is conceptual. It might be a theory about vocational education, general experiences of suffering or being a mother, for instance. The 'career' of the dying patients in hospital, the stages through which patients proceed, which Glaser and Strauss investigated, is substantive theory. When this is linked to the concept of 'status passage', which can be applied to many different situations, it becomes formal theory. This type of theory has general applicability, that is it holds true not just for the setting of the specific study but also for other settings and situations, and it is not speculative but based in the data.

In a student project, it would be difficult to produce a formal theory with wide applications, but substantive theories can still be important and have general implications for the work of the health professional.

The theory developed is generalisable in the sense that it can be applied to other, similar situations. Other events and situations can be understood through the knowledge acquired in building the theory.

Theoretical memos and fieldnotes

While going through the process of research, the researcher writes fieldnotes and memos. When observing and interviewing, they produce fieldnotes throughout the process. Certain occurrences or sentences seem of vital interest and they are recorded either during or immediately after data collection and even during data analysis. They remind the researcher of events, actions and interactions and trigger thinking processes. There can be descriptions of the setting too to act as triggers for remembering.

Strauss and Corbin (1998: 110) define memos as 'records of analysis, thoughts, interpretations, questions and directions for further data collection', and they should be dated and detailed. Every GT researcher should write memos. They are meant to help in the development and formulation of theory. In theoretical memos, the researcher discusses tentative ideas and provisional categories, compares findings and jots down thoughts on the research. Initially, memos might contain notes to remind the researcher 'don't forget ...' or 'I intend to ...'. Later they encompass micro-codes, and later still, major emergent categories, hunches, implications and concepts from the literature; memos become ever more varied and theoretical over time. Ideas for follow-up, related issues and thoughts about deviant cases become part of these memos.

Strauss (1987) suggests that memos are the written version of an internal dialogue that goes on during the research. Diagrams in the memos can help to remind the researcher and structure the study. Memo writing continues throughout the whole of the research; it goes through stages and becomes more complex in the process. Memos and diagrams provide 'density' for the research and guide the researcher to base abstract ideas in the reality of the data. Eventually, memos become integrated in the writing.

KEY POINT

Grounded theory always involves an interaction of data collection and analysis, hence it is an error to collect all the data first and analyse them sequentially.

Pitfalls and problems

As in any research approach, there are some problems and pitfalls that novice researchers need to be aware of. Some of the issues identified historically remain just as problematic today. These include the problems of balancing openness with systematically reducing the data and funnelling the focus of the research; the extent to which the research process is sensitised by existing theory and literature; the complexity of theoretical saturation and the active search for contrary occurrences in the data as well as points of convergence in the analysis. These are all subjects of a controversy that has been debated by leading grounded theorists, which we will touch on in this and other chapters. This has given rise to several schools of GT. There are also many misunderstandings of grounded theory procedure and common mistakes evident in the GT studies literature.

For instance, Wilson and Hutchinson (1996) discuss some of the common mistakes made in GT. They list six of these:

1 Muddling method (or method slurring)
2 Generational erosion
3 Premature closure
4 Overly generic analysis
5 The importing of concepts
6 Methodological transgression

Some of these are discussed further in other chapters, as they are common to several approaches. There are also problems with building a GT. Many researchers, particularly students in dissertations, projects and even theses, give good conceptual descriptions but do not develop a theory or even theoretical ideas. The difference between conceptualisation and description is significant. It is not enough to describe the perspectives of the participants or discuss 'themes' to develop a truly 'grounded' theory. A grounded theory should offer theoretical explanation with illustration from empirical data, and a core category should be developed that makes sense of the findings in an explanatory way.

The term 'emerging categories' (or 'emerging theory') is problematic as they can only be achieved by hard work. This problem is linked to theoretical sampling. Often researchers use selective (or purposive) sampling procedures. Coyne (1997) differentiates clearly between purposeful and theoretical sampling. While the researcher decides on purposeful sampling beforehand according to certain criteria, dimensions and settings, for GT research this type of sampling is necessary but does not suffice. The decisions about theoretical sampling are not made on the basis of initial criteria but throughout on the basis of emerging concepts, because of the inductive nature of the research.

A number of computer programmes for qualitative research do exist. Becker argues that computers might prevent sensitivity to the data and the discovery of meanings. Computers distance researchers from the data. Although this need not be so, we realise that in health research, where emotional engagement and sensitivity is necessary, the use of computers could be problematic. Charmaz too maintains that in a study in which the researcher is deeply involved with the participants, computer analysis has an undesirable distancing effect.

Generalisability and replicability of GT research are often discussed. Of course, it is difficult to match the original situation and context. Each researcher has a personal approach and a relationship with the participants which cannot be exactly reproduced. However, if health professionals make procedures explicit and clearly describe the original conditions and setting, others can follow the same rules and procedures and discover the same general scheme. Strauss and Corbin (1998) maintain that the findings of a GT study become more generalisable if the study is systematic, relies on theoretical sampling and examination of special conditions and discrepancies. A range of similar theoretical concepts from a variety of sources can become cumulative.

Glaser's critique and further development

As discussed before, several versions of GT can be distinguished. The ideas of Strauss and Glaser, for instance, have diverged even during Strauss' life time. Glaser (1992) wrote a book in response to the book by Strauss and Corbin (1990), criticising the authors for distorting the procedures and meaning of GT. Glaser claims that their book does not truly describe GT. He accuses the authors of 'forced conceptual description' (p. 5). He exhorts researchers not to impose their research problem but start with an interest and a questioning mind so that they see their informants' perspectives with no preconceptions. Thus, the researcher does not start with a research question but with a research interest. Although agreeing that Strauss and Corbin have described a research method, Glaser denies that its roots have much in common with the original 1967 volume. The new method, he claims, results in conceptual descriptions rather than in the emergence of concepts and formation of the links between them that explain variations in behaviour.

The difference between the ideas in Strauss and Corbin's text and the original development lies in the way in which concepts are generated and relationships explained. Glaser states that GT should not be verificational but inductive, it does not move between inductive and deductive thinking (although the 1967 book does mention verification). Deduction is rarely used except for reasons of conceptual guidance; this differs from the ideas of Strauss and Corbin who include the element of verification by suggesting that researchers test working propositions or 'provisional hypotheses' during their research.

Glaser also argues that participant observation does not suffice for a truly GT; interviews which explain the meanings of the participants are always necessary (many researchers see interviews as an integral part of participant observation in any case). Other differences exist between the two camps. It is interesting that Glaser, who started out as a survey researcher, seems to have become more flexible and less structured over time, while Strauss develops a more prescriptive way of researching.

Glaser (1992) believes that any initial literature review on the specific topic would contaminate the data and denies the need for it because it might direct researchers to irrelevant ideas. This he had also stated in his earlier book (Glaser, 1978). However, he too suggests that the literature can be integrated in the developing concepts. Discrepancies between concepts developed from the researchers' original data and the data from the literature may be discovered and the reasons for them investigated. Theoretical sensitivity helps to generate ideas and relate them to theory.

Glaser also advises against recording and transcribing interviews as he believes it a waste of time and might neglect the essential message in an interview. We believe, however, that recording interviews can be important, due to the complexity of discursive data and its analysis, but not least it might help those who are forgetful or those who have difficulty writing fieldnotes while interviewing. Of course, listening to interviews after recording is of great importance. We would argue that the memory of researchers might not be accurate and lead to misinterpretation. Mills *et al.* (2006) suggest naming the branches of GT 'traditional' (Glaser, who himself calls it 'classic'), 'evolved' (Strauss and Corbin) and 'constructivist' (Charmaz uses this term).

Charmaz (2006) criticises some of the early ideas in the GT approach and argues that it has developed from a more prescriptive and positivist style of research to a flexible way of thinking. She claims that the methods have developed in a number of different ways depending on researchers' perspectives. She sees this as developmental and she welcomes the move towards a more constructivist GT. As Charmaz suggests (p. 187), the 'interpretation of the studied phenomenon is in itself a construction' and 'people ... construct the realities in which they participate'. This means that researcher, participants and readers co-construct the research. Reality emerges or is discovered in the context of interaction. Indeed, constructivists sometimes suggest that 'truth' and reality are socially constructed (many researchers would acknowledge the influence of context on research). Constructivist GT is hence more relativist and subjective.

Which approach for the health researcher?

The varied approaches within GT seem to be based on different epistemological and methodological perspectives, although we would claim strong similarity between them. The development of GT itself has illuminated its elements and aspects in different ways. Indeed, Dunne (2011) sees GT as an ever-evolving approach 'subject to multiple definitions and interpretations' (p. 113). Researchers can make up their own minds on which specific way to take when doing GT, as long as they are knowledgeable about it and can explain why they have adopted a particular stance or followed specific processes. In any case, many researchers adapt methods during the process of research or use elements which they find useful. For a study to be called a 'Grounded Theory', the major features of GT should be included; most importantly, the researcher must develop a theory, grounded in the data and with 'explanatory power'.

KEY POINT

Grounded theory aims at developing theory and explanations rather than being descriptive.

Summary

- The aim of the GT is the generation or (occasionally) modification of existing theory.
- Data usually are collected through non-standardised interviews and participant observation but also by access to other data sources.
- Data collection and analysis interact.
- Researchers code and categorise transcripts from interviews or fieldnotes.
- The dialogue with the literature is essential, particularly when discussing categories and findings.
- Throughout the analytic process, constant comparison and theoretical sampling takes place.
- Memos – theoretical notes – provide the researcher with developing theoretical ideas.
- The theory that is generated has 'explanatory power' and is grounded in the data.

References

Andrews, H., Tierney, S. and Seers, K. (2020) Needing permission: the experience of self-care and self-compassion in nursing: a constructivist grounded theory. *International Journal of Nursing Studies*. doi:10.1016/j.ijnurstu.2019.103436.

Benoliel, J.Q. (1996) Grounded theory and nursing knowledge. *Qualitative Health Research*, **6** (3), 406–428.

Birks, M. and Mills, J. (2015) *Grounded Theory: A Practical Guide*, 2nd edn, Sage, London.

Blumer, H. (1971) Sociological implications of the thoughts of G.H. Mead, in *School and Society* (eds. B.R. Cosin, I.R. Dale, G.M. Esland *et al.*), Open University Press, Milton Keynes, pp. 11–17.

Campbell, V. and Nolan, M. (2019) 'It definitely made a difference': a grounded theory study of yoga for pregnancy and women's self-efficacy for labour. *Midwifery*, **68**, 74–85.

Chamberlain-Salaun, J., Mills, J. and Usher, K. (2013) Linking symbolic interactionism and grounded theory methods in a research design: from Corbin and Strauss' assumptions to actions. *Sage Open*, **3** (3), 1–10.

Charmaz, K. (2006) *Constructing Grounded Theory: A Practical Guide through Qualitative Analysis*, Sage, London (second edition of this book in 2014).

Charmaz, K. and Thornberg, R. (2020) The pursuit of quality in grounded theory. *Qualitative Research in Psychology*. doi:10.1080/14780887.2020.1780357.

Chenitz, W.C. and Swanson, J.M. (eds.) (1986) *From Practice to Grounded Theory: Qualitative Research in Nursing*, Addison-Wesley, Menlo Park, CA.

Corbin, J. and Strauss, A.L. (2008) *Basics of Qualitative Research: Techniques and Procedures for Developing Grounded Theory*, 3rd edn, Sage, Los Angeles, CA.

Coyne, I.T. (1997) Sampling in qualitative research: purposeful and theoretical sampling: merging or clear boundaries? *Journal of Advanced Nursing*, **26**, 623–630.

Cutcliffe, J.R. (2000) Methodological issues in grounded theory. *Journal of Advanced Nursing*, **31**, 1476–1484.

Cutcliffe, J.R. (2005) Adapt or adopt: developing and transgressing the methodological boundaries of grounded theory. *Journal of Advanced Nursing,* **51** (4), 421–428.

Deering, K. and Williams, J. (2020) Approaches to reviewing the literature in grounded theory: a framework. *Nurse Researcher.* doi:10.7748/nr.2020.e1752.

Draucker, C.B., Martsolf, D.S., Ross, R. and Rusk, T.B. (2007) Theoretical sampling and category development in grounded theory. *Qualitative Health Research,* **17** (8), 1137–1138.

Dunne, C. (2011) The place of the literature in grounded theory methodology. *International Journal of Nursing Research,* **14** (2), 111–124.

Glaser, B.G. (1978) *Theoretical Sensitivity,* Sociology Press, Mill Valley, CA.

Glaser, B.G. (1992) *Basics of Grounded Theory Analysis,* Sociology Press, Mill Valley, CA.

Glaser, B.G. and Strauss, A.L. (1967) *The Discovery of Grounded Theory,* Aldine, Chicago, IL.

Hutchinson, S.A. (1993) Grounded theory: the method, in *Nursing Research: A Qualitative Perspective* (eds. P.L. Munhall and C. Oiler Boyd), National League for Nursing Press, New York, NY, pp. 180–212.

Kenny, M., and Fourie, R. (2015). Contrasting classic, straussian, and constructivist grounded theory: methodological and philosophical conflicts. *The Qualitative Report,* **20** (8), 1270–1289. Available at https://nsuworks.nova.edu/tqr/vol20/iss8/9.

Johnsson, L. and Nordgren, L. (2019) How general practitioners decide on maxims of action in response to demands from conflicting sets of norms: a grounded theory study. *BMC Medical Ethics,* **20**: 33. doi:10.1186/s12910-019-0360-3.

MacDonald, M. (2001) Finding a critical perspective in grounded theory, in *Using Grounded Theory in Nursing* (eds. R.S. Schreiber and P.N. Stern), Springer, New York, NY, pp. 113–157.

McMillan, L., Booth, J., Currie, K. and Howe, T. (2012) A grounded theory of taking control after fall-induced hip fracture. *Disability and Rehabilitation,* **34** (26), 2234–2241.

Mead, M. (1934) *Mind, Self and Society,* University of Chicago Press, Chicago, IL.

Melia, K. (1987) *Learning and Working: The Occupational Socialisation of Nurses,* Routledge, London.

Mills, J. and Birks, M. (2015) *Grounded Theory: A Practical Guide,* 2nd edn, Sage, London.

Mills, J., Bonner, A. and Francis, K. (2006) The development of constructivist grounded theory *International Journal of Qualitative Methods,* **5** (1), Article 3. Available at http://www.ualberta. ca/<iiqm/backissues/5_1/pdf/mills.pdf.

Morse, J.M., Bowers, B.J. and Charmaz, K. *et al.* (2021) *Developing Grounded Theory: The Second Generation Revisited,* 2nd edn, Routledge, Oxon, Abingdon.

Munhall, P.I. (ed.) (2012) *Nursing Research: A Qualitative Perspective,* 5th edn, Jones & Bartlett Learning, Sudbury, MA.

Mulholland, P. (2020) A grounded theory of interprofessional learning and paramedic care. *Journal of Interprofessional Care,* **34** (1), 66–75.

Newell, C. (2008) Recovery in anorexia nervosa: the struggle to develop a new identity. Unpublished PhD, Bournemouth University.

O'Reilly, M. and Parker, N. (2013) 'Unsatisfactory saturation': a critical exploration of saturated sample size in qualitative research. *Qualitative Research,* **13** (2), 190–219.

Rieger, K.L. (2019) Discriminating among grounded theory approaches. *Nursing Inquiry;* **26,** e12261. doi:10.1111/nin.12261.

Schatzman, L. and Strauss, A.L. (1973) *Field Research: Strategies for a Natural Sociology,* Prentice Hall, Englewood Cliffs, NJ.

Schreiber, R.S. and Stern, P.N. (eds.) (2001) *Using Grounded Theory in Nursing,* Springer, New York, NY.

Sorensen, D. and Christensen, M.E. (2018) Behavioural modes of adherence for inspiratory muscle training in people with chronic pulmonary disease. *Disability and Rehabilitation.* doi: 10.1080/09638288.2017.1422032.

Stern, P.N. and Porr, C.J. (2011) *Essentials of Accessible Grounded Theory*, Left Coast Press, Walnut Creek, CA.

Strauss, A.L. (1987) *Qualitative Analysis for Social Scientists*, Cambridge University Press, New York, NY.

Strauss, A.L. and Corbin, J. (1990) *Basics of Qualitative Research: Grounded Theory Procedures and Techniques*, Sage, Newbury Park, CA.

Strauss, A.L. and Corbin, J. (eds.) (1997) *Grounded Theory in Practice*, Sage, Thousand Oaks, CA.

Strauss, A.L. and Corbin, J. (1998) *Basics of Qualitative Research: Techniques and Procedures for Developing Grounded Theory*, 2nd edn, Sage, Thousand Oaks, CA.

Thomas, W.I. (1928) *The Child in America*, Alfred Knopf, New York, NY.

Thornberg, R. and Dunne, C. (2019). The literature review in grounded theory. *Sage Handbook of Current Developments in Grounded Theory Research*. https://doi.org/10.1080/14780887.2020.1780357.

Watling, C.J. and Lingard, L. (2012) Grounded theory in medical education research: AMEE Guide No. 70. *Medical Teacher*, **34** (10), 350–361.

Wilson, H.S. and Hutchinson, S.A. (1996) Methodologic mistakes in grounded theory. *Nursing Research*, **45** (2), 122–124.

Further Reading

Bryant. A. (2019) *The Varieties of Grounded Theory*, Sage, London.

Bryant, A. and Charmaz, K. (eds.) (2007) *The Sage Handbook of Grounded Theory*, Sage, London.

Bryant, A. and Charmaz, K. (eds) (2019) *The Sage Handbook of Current Developments in Grounded Theory*, Sage, London.

Charmaz, K. (2000) Grounded theory: objectivist and constructivist methods, in *Handbook of Qualitative Research* (eds. N.K. Denzin and Y.S. Lincoln), 2nd edn, Sage, Thousand Oaks, CA, pp. 509–535.

Hoare, K.J., Mills, J. and Francis, K. (2013) New graduate nurses as knowledge brokers in general practice in New Zealand: a constructivist grounded theory. *Health and Care in the Community*, **21** (4), 423–431.

Kuek, J.H.L., Raeburn, T. and Wand, T. (2020) Using constructivist grounded theory to understand mental-health recovery in multi-ethnic environments. *Nurse Researcher*. doi:10/7748/nr.2020.e1691.

Samuriwo, R.K. (2013) The impact of nurses' values on the prevention of pressure ulcers: a Straussian grounded theory study. PhD thesis, University of Glamorgan.

Tarozzi, M. (2020) *What is Grounded Theory?* Bloomsbury Academic, London.

Urquhart, C. (2013) *Grounded Theory for Qualitative Research: A Practical Guide*, Sage, London.

(Some articles have capitals 'Grounded Theory', others use small letters 'grounded theory'. For consistency we employ the terms GT or grounded theory.)

Chapter 12

Narrative Inquiry

The nature of narrative and story

Stories are reflections on people's experience and the meaning that this experience has for them. Narrative research is a useful way of gaining access to new perspectives, thoughts and experiences in order to analyse them in the context of personal story and sense-making. For many decades, health research had focused on the decision-making and thoughts of professionals and their measurement of the treatment outcomes, while the personal experiences and ideas of the patient, the 'insider', tended to be neglected. This changed with the advent of qualitative health research. The perspectives of patients are uncovered through their stories, particularly in narrative research.

Many researchers apply the terms 'narrative' and 'storytelling' interchangeably, although others make a distinction. Frank (1995) uses the concepts of story and narrative differently: He cites the term 'story' when discussing the tales people tell, and narrative when referring to 'general structures' that encompass a number of particular stories. Paley and Eva (2005) claim that story integrates plot and character – both need to be present – while narrative comprises both sequence of events and causal links between them. An interesting MSc by Carmen Tu (2019), discussing character and plot, points 'towards an embodied model of narrative. Bolt (2012: 2) suggests that 'the term narrative is in dispute', and indeed it can be ambiguous.

Thus, the line between story and narrative is blurred, and for purposes of this chapter we shall use these terms interchangeably. Researchers refer to life stories, biographies or narratives; Labov (1972), one of the first sociologists to carry out research through narratives, sees the term narrative as more specific – as events in the past that are being retold. First person narratives provide much material for research. People remember significant events and experiences; they choose from their vast store of memory and select, judge and interpret what happened to them, with insight into their significance and meaning.

Narrating helps people to make sense of their experience. It unveils the intentions and motives of human beings to the researcher. Individuals remember an experience, tell the story sequentially as they perceived it happening and seek explanations for events and actions while interpreting and reflecting on them. However, narrators prioritise; some events and experiences carry more importance than others; according to the specific social context or the people to whom they speak, they emphasise different aspects of the story. They might neglect or fail to mention some issues or events, or they might exaggerate others, depending on their perspective or the audience to whom they speak. Narratives often express and are linked to identity. Price *et al.* (2013) show, for instance, how nursing identities are connected to certain values and images. Identities change: A suffering individual, for instance, might adopt an illness identity.

Narrative research

Narrative research is a broad term and can incorporate other approaches; a narrative study may be an ethnography, take a phenomenological approach or use discourse analysis, but it can also stand as an approach on its own. It refers to 'any study that uses or analyses narrative material' (Lieblich *et al.*, 1998: 2). In this chapter, it is used as an approach which is separate from other qualitative forms of inquiry.

A few narrative researchers believe, as Elliott (2005) does, that narrative inquiry can be quantitative as well as qualitative; however, to have lengthy stories from participants needs a more flexible approach and open questions and for these quantitative methods are inappropriate.

KEY POINT

Narrative research is based in the participants' stories of their experiences.

Narratives in health research

Although the use of narratives for research and other purposes has gone on in an informal way for a long time, as a research approach in health and illness or in education, narrative inquiry is relatively recent, now even sometimes overused. Narratives develop and contribute to professional knowledge, and through the acquisition of this knowledge professionals can improve care. Stories enable professionals to understand their patients and clients more deeply, to gain access to their embedded experience and the meaning they give to this experience. For clinical and professional practice, it means 'the focus of narrative will enable nursing [and other health professions'] knowledge to be grounded in concrete situations' (Frid *et al.*, 2000: 3). However, it is not easy for health researchers to abandon their own assumptions and focus solely on the stories of ill people. Frank (2000) gives examples of this. He also refers to the difficulty professionals have to truly listen to the voice of patients, to really hear what is relevant to those who suffer, because professionals have more skills to respond to patients as 'medical *subjects*' rather than 'ill *persons*' (our italics). It must, however, be noted that narratives do not always focus on suffering and illness, but also on well-being and quality of life. Haydon *et al.* (2017) discuss the value of narrative research in nursing specifically.

Example 12.1 Patient Stories

Patient stories

In Australia, Haydon *et al.* (2021) explored the experience of individuals with a wide age span who had survived a cardiac arrest through narrative research. The long, taped interviews were held in their homes or other localities, or through video and Skype. The personal feelings of the participants were explored. The authors analysed the interviews by the three-dimensional framework of Clandinin and Conelly and identified several threads which identified a transformation from the ordinary to the extraordinary and a transition to a different and new reality.

Student stories

The aim of the research by Koskinen *et al.* (2011) was to explore what it is like to be in a mental health placement. Twenty Finnish students' stories showed that initially they experienced prejudice and negativity towards mental health patients. They were involved in complex care settings and encountered with patients and eventually were able to face their own attitudes and developed coping skills. This happened when they experienced good support from mentors and had active involvement and time for reflection.

Narrative accounts in healthcare can be obtained from a number of different groups:

- Patients or clients
- Caregivers and relatives
- Colleagues and other professionals

Narratives from the point of view of the patient can be seen in several ways. Patients, for instance, might tell their experience of an illness or a chronic medical condition or of care and treatment by professionals. Ill people tell stories that show what it means to be sick. New mothers tell stories about the meaning of childbirth. Older people tell stories about the meaning of older age in the context of this society. Narratives can also be a reaction to care and medical treatment or as a counterperspective to that of health professionals. Through narratives and narrative interpretations, patients, service users and clients may also attempt to justify their own actions and behaviour. It can be understood that as long as people on the receiving end of care tell their stories, they might feel that they have some control over what is happening to them. In addition, they may use these narratives to achieve an attempt at returning to some sense of normality: for instance, they compare their ill selves to their normal social, physical and psychological conditions. Holloway and Freshwater (2007) summarise some of the reasons for storytelling which many authors have discussed, for instance Riessman (2008), and, to give an example of recent health research in a Canadian study, Molzahn *et al.* (2021). Many others have explored this form of research over a number of years.

Through storytelling, people have the possibility to

- Give meaning to experiences, in particular suffering.
- Interpret and verbalise important events and share them with others.
- Present a holistic view of experience and perspective.
- Try to find adjustment when conditions are unalterable.
- Confirm group membership in a shared culture.
- Attribute blame or responsibility to themselves or others.
- Take more control over their own lives.

McCance *et al.* (2001) use narrative methodology to explore caring in nursing practice. They used it as a means to 'tap into the patient experience'. It is not easy to gain access to people's experiences and thoughts but eliciting a narrative may help in this process. Telling stories about specific experiences rather than giving general accounts or thinking in general terms is 'real' for patients; they will often tell the story sequentially along temporal dimensions. Greenhalgh and Hurwitz (1998: 45) in their book on narrative in medical practice, claim that narratives used in healthcare research can

- Set a patient-centred agenda.
- Challenge received wisdom.
- Generate new hypotheses.

Through their stories, patients help health professionals to focus on their perceptions and experiences rather than applying a professional framework 'from the top-down' that may not make sense to the person or not be a good fit to their situation. If professionals truly listen to patients, they might also hear the unexpected and will be able to change their own assumptions, if necessary. Greenhalgh (2013), a general practitioner and academic, advises on the collection and analysis of shared stories of patients with a particular chronic condition, because they can only be meaningfully informed by professionals about its management if there is an understanding how 'their condition affects both their identity and the practicalities of daily life' (p. 60).

Relatives are also narrators of their caregiving experience as it happened and seek explanations for their own behaviour, for the patients' reactions and for professional care and treatment. Through this, they are able to justify their own thoughts and actions to professionals and researchers. Caregivers of patients with

Alzheimer's disease, for instance, tell the sequence of events and discuss the behaviour of their relatives and their own reaction towards them. Essentially, caregivers can attempt to share what caring means to them through this approach.

Researchers and health professionals use patient narrative to locate the person at the centre of his or her illness. They see the narrative as a useful path to the understanding of sick people and the illness experience, as interpreted by patients in a specific cultural framework. Professionals – be they individual professionals in interaction with particular patients or professional groups who define specific conditions or illnesses within a biomedical framework – give different versions from patients. Both versions are valid and together might give the full picture. Sakalys (2000), in particular, addresses the question of culture in a discussion of narratives and claims that the social and cultural interpretation defines the illness experience and the sick role for the individual. Narratives can also demonstrate the conflicts and dilemmas between individual meanings and healthcare ideologies.

In professional education and practice, narrators might tell the story of interaction in specific situations and of learning or teaching experiences. The researcher's aim is the understanding of the essence of that experience in the context of the participants' lives. Josselson (1995) claims that empathy and narrative show the way to people's reality; understanding of this can be achieved through qualitative research. Kleinman (1988) also urges 'empathic listening'. Health professionals need both empathy for and to be sensitised by stories from their clients. Nurse and midwife teachers, in particular, often use narratives to teach students reflection and clinical decision-making as well as to underpin empathic responses in practice. The story of each individual is unique but there are common elements between people's stories as they share their common humanity and sometimes their culture.

Jovchelovitch and Bauer (2000) list the two dimensions of narrative and storytelling: the chronological dimension where narratives are told in sequential form with a beginning, a middle and an end, and the non-chronological, which is a plot constructed as a coherent whole from a number of events – small tales which combine into a big story. According to Paley and Eva (2005), certain conditions need to be fulfilled in the configuration of a plot:

1 The plot contains a central character.
2 This character encounters a problem.
3 A link exists between character and explanation.
4 The plot and its configuration elicit an emotional response in the listener.

The thread of the narrative depends on the storyteller what he or she wishes to communicate to others or what to leave out of the story. People organise their experience through narratives and make sense of them, not least by relating them to time. Indeed, Bruner (2004: 692) states that the only way to account for 'lived time' is in the form of narrative. Narratives allow access to a person's perceived reality in many different ways in their particular context. Richardson (1990) describes many of these types of stories:

1 Everyday stories
2 Autobiographical stories
3 Biographical stories
4 Cultural stories
5 Collective stories

Often, narratives contain a number of overlapping stories. We shall try to illustrate these by examples:

The everyday story

In the everyday story, people relate how they undertake everyday things and carry out their normal tasks: '... And then I went out into the garden and did some work, and then I came inside and sat down'. Most patients import these everyday stories into the history of their condition, care and treatment, thereby offering a natural contextualization.

For instance, when researching people's experience in hospital, one of our students found that participants' narratives always tended to start at a time before they arrived in hospital. 'We were watching television, I had just made a cup of tea when it happened ... and then my wife called the ambulance, I could hardly walk, and then they went through the night with all lights blazing and a lot of noise'. There is often such a 'pre-experience' narrative to add to the sense-making of what happened.

Autobiographical and biographical stories

In an autobiographical story people link the past to the present and future in uniquely personal ways: 'I used to go dancing, but now I can't dance any more, I shall probably never dance again because of my pain'. Through autobiographical stories people also justify and explain their actions: 'Because I had such an awful pain in my back, I could not have regular work'. In autobiographies in which individuals tell for example, their illness history, they demonstrate that they see their own stories as unique and quite separate from those of others. The storyteller can link together various disparate events through narrative (Polkinghorne, 1995): '... And then I went into the garden, and I did some work, and then my back went ... and that's why I am unemployed now'.

Frank (2013) uses his own illness to discuss the journey from patient to person in a narrative. First person perspectives which are usual, can reveal new understandings that are useful for practice, and offer novel contextualised insights.

Biographical stories are narratives which are told of other people. They offer second person perspectives. They might concern the life story or illness trajectory of one person, or of several individuals. Reading and listening to biographical stories enable individuals to share and compare their experiences and link with others who had similar experiences. These narratives, be they on well-being, illness or career, are integrated into the life course of individuals, and they form explicit links between present, past and future. The stories guide beyond the subjective to intersubjective understanding and can contribute to empathic responses by engagement with a shared world. By writing accounts of others' stories, researchers help readers understand the vulnerability of others. An element of the autobiographical or biographical tale could also be a 'victory story' in which individuals demonstrate how they overcame adversity by describing their perspectives and actions (Sandelowsky, 1996). The writing by Sparkes *et al.* (2011) is an example of a biographical story to reveal far-reaching impacts of illness on life, through describing the cancer experience of one individual, an elite athlete. In addition to communicating 'what it has been like', narratives can also be used as a teaching aid; for instance, Maina *et al.* (2013) used various types of narratives to teach nursing students to become aware of the social complexity of HIV/Aids and the social/cultural dimensions that surround these conditions.

Cultural stories

Through the cultural story participants tell, they make visible and demonstrate meanings in a particular cultural context, for instance the meaning of death or the understanding of disease: 'I had epilepsy. In our society people do not understand that, and I was labelled as not quite normal'. Or 'My back pain is invisible, nobody believes that it exists, if I had a broken leg, I would not be labelled lazy or work shy'. Or 'Everybody wants you to have the baby in hospital, in an earlier time, you could have it at home. Luckily times are changing again'. Cultural perspectives can be made visible through narrative.

Collective stories

In narrative research, the collective story is also significant. By retelling a number of stories, for instance of patients, professionals or students, researchers reflect the thoughts and paths of a group or collective of people with similar experiences and give a portrayal of a condition or patterns of experience. Mertova and Webster (2020) state that people tell both personal and social stories.

For instance, a person suffering from pain might mention that others are much worse off (a social comparison story), or that new mothers tell tales that are embedded in the culture of motherhood. Collectivity creates a *Gestalt* or whole picture of the condition or experience. For health professionals, this means that they might recognise the needs of the group members and be able to improve their care by attending to patterns that have emerged from a group perspective.

Illness narratives

The classic book on narrative by Kleinman (1988) *The Illness Narratives* contains probably the best-known examples of narrative in the health and illness arena though not in research. His text was ground-breaking, an early text on this topic by a medic.

Patients use narratives to seek meaning and make sense of their experience, and they want to share this with 'significant' others. The researcher on the other hand, re-tells stories in order to give voice, and to share participants' perspectives, experiences and thoughts. It is questionable, however, that the account is always the authentic voice of the participants because researchers translate and interpret the narrators' tales. Paley and Eva (2005) query the concept of truth as it is sometimes applied to narrative. They believe that 'truth' in the factual sense is irrelevant and that meaning and interpretation are important, not whether the story is factually 'real', Mertova and Webster (2020) prefer the term 'verisimilitude', that is plausibility, credibility and likelihood. Nevertheless, researchers make an attempt to represent the ideas expressed through the stories of the participants. Although the narration may be true in its meaning, it is not always based on fact or objective reality but is a social construction and perception of what has happened to the narrator. At a time when people have little power to act – for instance, when they have experienced an illness, breaking up of a relationship or another trauma in their lives – they attempt to explain this in a different language from that of those in power. To paraphrase Bruner (1991: 11): the patient tells the tale in 'life talk' (that is, in ordinary language) while the professional listens to it and translates it into professional language.

People often tell stories about their illness, particularly when the condition threatens their lives such as in an acute illness, or when it restricts their daily activities and intrudes on normal life. Through illness and suffering, individuals often have an impaired sense of self, and on this they reflect. As it is of such importance to them, they attempt to tell their story to their significant others such as family and friends, employers and work colleagues. They tell it also to the health professionals, doctors and nurses. For each of these groups, ill people adopt different ways of telling.

Illness narratives differ from other stories in that they have an altered temporality while in ordinary tales, the present connects effortlessly to the past and future. The future of those talking about their illness is sometimes uncertain and occasionally non-existent.

Example 12.2 Titles for Narrative Research from the Perspective of Different Health Professions

Cussen, A., Howie, L. and Imms, C. (2012) Looking to the future: adolescents with cerebral palsy talk about their aspirations – a narrative study. *Disability and Rehabilitation*, **34** (24), 2103–2110.

Engblom, M., Alexanderson, K. and Rudebeck, C.E. (2011) Physicians' messages in problematic certification: a narrative analysis of case reports. *BMC Family Practice*, **12** (18), 1–8.

France, E.F., Hunt, K. and Ziebland, S. (2013) What parents say about disclosing the end of their pregnancy due to fetal abnormality. *Midwifery*, **29** (1), 24–32. (secondary analysis of narrative data)

Kurunsari, M., Tyujala, P. and Piiranen, A. (2021) Stories of professional development in physiotherapy education. *Physiotherapy Theory and Practice*. doi:10.1080/09593985.2021. 1888341.

Price, S.L., McGillis Hall, L. and Angus, J.E. (2013) Choosing nursing as a career: a narrative analysis of millennial nurses' career choice of virtue. *Nursing Inquiry*, **20** (4), 305–316.

Soundy, A., Smith, B., Cressey, F. and Webb, L. (2010) The experience of spinal cord injury: using Frank's narrative types to enhance undergraduates understanding. *Physiotherapy*, **96** (1), 52–58.

Frank (1995) proposes three different forms that narratives can take:

1 The *restitution* narrative
2 The *chaos* narrative
3 The *quest* narrative

The different types of the narrative are not always distinct. Frank's justification for differentiating between narratives is to create 'listening devices' – the wish to sort out narrative threads in order to help listeners attend these stories, not to question the uniqueness of an individual's tale nor to give a unifying view of experience. In any case, most stories combine elements of all three forms of narrative. Each of these forms is a reflection of both the culture and the person of the storyteller. Frank also suggests, however, that individuals use different forms of these stories at a different stage in their illness; some use only one and others tell all three forms in one overarching narrative.

The restitution narrative

The restitution narrative permeates the tale of those who have been ill. This includes the wish to get well soon. It can be connected with the concept of sick role of Parsons (1951). Individuals are sick – they receive treatment and care – it is seen as their duty to get better – they will be better in the future. People emphasise not only their desire to get better, but they often claim that they are well and have achieved the state of normality: 'I am OK now'. Most restitution tales reflect Parsons' ideas about the sick role: the person inhabiting the role is not at fault; the patient is exempt from normal role responsibilities; he or she is expected to ask for expert help, comply with the advice and make every attempt to get better.

The restitution narrative reflects the predominant Western culture. Indeed, Frank claims that 'it is the culturally preferred narrative'. It takes the machine as a model: the machine breaks down, one takes it to a repair shop, and it is repaired. It is reconstructed, almost 'as good as new'. It also implies that people have control over their bodies and minds, and that the future is, to some extent, predictable.

The chaos narrative

The chaos narrative suggests that the person will not ever get well again and encompasses his or her suffering in words and silences. This tale is not always tolerated in the predominant culture that focuses on cure (the 'machine' can be fixed or repaired). Perhaps a chaos narrative is easier to listen to for nurses because they focus on care. This narrative has no order and little structure, and it is told by people who have a serious chronic condition, or a life-threatening or terminal illness. This tale is more difficult to understand because it is never linear; it does not have a proper beginning, middle and end nor does it follow the same direction.

For the story to be effective, the storyteller must have some distance from it as the person in the middle of an experience finds it difficult to talk about it. There is iteration with narrators going backwards and forwards much of the time. The chaos narrative implies the narrators' lack of control over their lives. Illness, particularly if it is chronic, generates complete 'biographical disruption', a term used by Bury (1982). Frank claims that health professionals should not hurry patients on when they are telling the tale as this denies the patients the right to their experience. He advises professionals to have tolerance for chaos within a story.

The quest narrative

The quest narrative is told by people who are on a mission, who accept the challenge to learn something from their experience and feel that they are on a journey during which they change their identity. People think they must transmit to others what they have learned. They tell the story chronologically. Disability stories often contain the element of challenge and mission. We have all read of people with a serious illness who tell their story to the newspapers or on television 'to help others'. They often maintain that the illness has transformed them; the narrative has a moral dimension. Even though the condition may not improve, the ill person has control over his or her life.

Thomas-MacLean (2004) demonstrates all three types of narratives and claims that in her research, the quest narrative is rare. She gives examples of the determination to experience life as much as possible by people who realise they have cancer, the different priorities they now have, and how they attempt to assist others in the same position.

The following is an example from health research which contains chaos, restitution and quest.

Example 12.3 An Illustration of Frank's Different Forms of Narrative

An American study on the menopause by Nosek *et al.* (2012) shows, through the analysis of one woman's narrative, how chaos, restitution and quest might be present in one person's story. They demonstrate how a physically fit woman's life is disrupted by physical problems and loss of identity – at work, in her self-image, in her femininity and as a sexual being (chaos narrative). After a variety of attempts to improve her life, she eventually had hormone therapy which alleviated her condition. She shows in her story how she improved physical health and regained a new perspective (restitution narrative). In re-examining her life, she searches for meaning in her previous suffering, tries to make sense of it and sets out on a new journey through her life course (quest narrative).

Losek *et al.* warn the reader that not every person goes through all these stages or forms of narrative.

Narrative interviewing

To obtain a narrative from participants, researchers use narrative interviews in which individuals can tell of their experience. The tale is not the experience itself but a representation of the experience as it is stored in the memory of the individual. Ochs and Capps (2002: 127) suggest 'remembering is a subjective event'; but participants see it as true, although it cannot necessarily be corroborated or verified. Nevertheless, the perception of the 'truth' of the event, treatment or care determines, or at least influences, both perception and action.

Narrative interviewing does not break a story into pieces as other types of qualitative research often do. Rather it aims to hold onto 'the thread that connects', whether this is, for example, temporal, about identity or resolution. Narrative interviewing has a main area of deep interest to participant and researcher. A stimulus or reminder provides the trigger for the story. Riessman does stress that narratives differ distinctly from other types of discourse such as question and answer interviews. Nevertheless, many health researchers use in-depth interviews which contain some key questions to prompt the stories of the participants, and sometimes they analyse naturally occurring shared stories of patients.

Jovchelovitch and Bauer (2000) state that the topic area must be both familiar and also experiential to the participant. The initial question must be broad enough to trigger a long story. For instance, 'Tell us about your time in hospital' might encourage patients into narrating a lengthy tale about what happened to them in the hospital setting. If the interviewer interrupts this story continually, it cannot flow. When the narrative is completed, however, the interviewer might ask some questions to develop the story by including the words of the participant. For instance: 'You said to me that time hung heavily while you were in hospital, can you tell me more about that?' Narrative interviews, like all other forms of interview, are affected by the relationship between the researcher and the participant, perhaps even more so as the researcher does not just ask questions to receive some answers but gives the participants control of the interview and as much time as they need to tell their story. Narrative interviews sometimes contain elements of question-and-answer exchange but mostly sections of narrative. It is not always possible to draw boundaries and discover where the narrative starts and finishes. There is a worrying tendency to carry out semi-structured interviews and call these narrative interviews, but in true narrative interviews, there is little interruption by the researcher. Sools (2013: 95) speaks of 'minimal interviewer interference'.

Narrative interviews often focus on life histories or life stories as they show development of experience and perspective over time. The journey through diagnosis, progress and treatment of a condition, for instance, might be explored. The career of health professionals such as physiotherapists, nurses and doctors could also be examined through their narratives of 'being and becoming'.

KEY POINT

In narrative interviewing it, is important that the participants are able to tell their stories without too much interruption.

Narrative analysis

This whole chapter is about narrative analysis and what it implies. Riessman (2008) does not acknowledge a specific standard set of procedures for analysing the data but offers a choice to researchers. The actual data analysis of narratives is similar to that in other types of qualitative research and depends on the methodological framework. Polkinghorne (1995: 15) defines narrative analysis as 'the procedure through which the researcher organizes the data elements as into a coherent and developmental account', and this cannot be carried out without taking account of the context. The main steps include data transcription and reduction. The first step is the verbatim transcription of the narrative data (see the section on transcribing and sorting, in Chapter 17).

There are different approaches to analysing narrative data, for instance, thematic, structural and dialogic/performance analysis which Riessman (2008) describes, but other ways of analysing narratives are also legitimate.

Thematic and holistic analysis

The researcher analyses a narrative as a whole. In this type of analysis, it is important to identify the main statements – the core of the experience that reflects and truly represents the narrators' accounts, even though they might not have given the story in a sequential and ordered way. It centres on the contents of the participants' story and the meanings inherent in it. The units of text in the transcription are reduced to a series of core sentences or ideas. The core statements of the experience integrate its various elements. This essence of experience is highly auditable in the examples below:

Your life is pain.

It stops you doing … Going out.

Just trying to be a normal person.

I don't feel like doing anything.

All you want to do is to dwell on your own suffering.

Pain becomes an obstacle.

To any type of performance.

(Excerpt from participants' tales in a pain experience study.)

The essence of these statements and the core of the experience is that 'the pain takes over'. Other themes can be linked to this statement. Both Riessman and Elliott advocate this type of analysis in applied research, particularly for novice researchers; Riessman calls it thematic analysis and claims that it is the most straightforward. In this type of analysis, researchers interpret and theorise from the whole story and its meaning, rather than breaking it into categories. The attention focuses on the contents, on 'what' is in the story, rather than 'how' it is told. Unlike analysis in grounded theory, the story is not taken apart but kept together for interpretation. (For further advice, see Riessman (2008: 53–76).)

The term thematic analysis is not unambiguous in narrative inquiry; here it is described the way Riessman uses it in her book.

> **Example 12.4** Thematic Analysis
>
> Swedish research demonstrates narrative thematic analysis. Rejnö *et al.* (2013) explored the next of kin's experiences about their relatives who died unexpectedly of a stroke. The authors analysed the narratives, and found three themes: 'divided feelings about sudden and unexpected death', 'perception of time and directed attention when keeping vigil' and 'contradictions and arbitrary memories when searching for understanding'. The authors do not state in detail how they analysed the narratives, but state that they employed the usual methods of thematic analysis (see Riessman, 2008; Braun and Clarke, 2006).

It is interesting, however, that some researchers use the type of analysis by coding and categorizing the data. This ensures that researchers identify patterns across the data (Braun and Clarke, 2013). However, the downside of this approach is that it 'fractures the data' and can lose the pattern that connects. Riessman (2008: 74) explains that narrative analysts follow the sequence and maintain the story as a whole, unlike grounded theorists, although phenomenological research also takes a holistic stance to data.

> **Example 12.5** Holistic Analysis
>
> The aim of the research by Stenhouse (2013) was to understand what it feels like to be a patient in a psychiatric inpatient ward. The sample of participants consisted of 13 individuals with various diagnoses of mental illness. Their stories were elicited 6 weeks after discharge in two interviews. After the second interview, the data set of each person was examined as a series of small stories set in a big narrative integrating the whole of the experience of what it feels like to be a patient in an acute ward.

Structural analysis

This type of analysis has its origin in the work of Labov and Waletzky (1967). It does not focus on contents but on form, 'how' the story is told, and it is tied to the text of the story. These sociologists developed a structural model of narrative in which they broke down the story and analysed its elements. These six elements are the following (adapted from Riessman (2008: 84) and Elliott (2005: 42). They describe the Labov/Waletzky model):

1 *Abstract:* The summary of the story matter.
2 *Orientation:* The time, place, situation and participants.

3 *The Complicating Action:* The sequence of events, that is the plot with its inherent crisis.

4 *Evaluation:* The appraisal of the story and its meaning for the storyteller.

5 *Resolution:* The outcome of the plot.

6 *Coda:* The return to the present time.

(For a detailed discussion, see Riessman (2008: 77–103).)

Example 12.6 Structural Analysis

Robertson (2014) studied an older woman's perception of her quality of life with dementia. She is in her eighties. Her story shows the narrative process used by this individual to extract meaning and make sense of her identity over the life course. Robertson used Labov's approach to analysis and broke the story into structural units and used the structural constituents to examine the narrative. The woman attempts to make sense of the self and social identity by drawing comparisons with the past. She considers the past and links it with involvement in activities, while the present lacks this immersion, and she keenly feels the loss of important social roles.

    It is interesting that, in spite of structural analysis which breaks down the data, Robertson still manages to grasp the story as a whole and shows the woman's meaning-making within the context of her life course.

The most common types of narrative analysis are thematic, holistic and structural, although many studies use several of these together.

Dialogic/performance analysis

The last of Riessman's approaches to analysis of data is that which she calls dialogic/performance analysis which is a 'broad and varied interpretive approach' (Riessman, 2008: 105) to narrative. Dialogic/performance analysis, according to Riessman, takes certain features from both thematic and structural analyses, but is even more focused on text and context.

It investigates the emergence of interactive talk as well as gestures, mime or other elements of interaction. This seems to be similar to conversation or discourse analysis where the focus is not only on the content and form but also on the people involved and to whom they orient their talk. It focuses on social interaction, relationships and identities co-constructed with others. Riessman calls this a 'hybrid' form of analysis which takes components from other approaches. In any case, many of the previous forms of analysis overlap or are used together in one study.

Visual analysis

The last type of Riessman's narrative analysis focuses on visual images. This is becoming popular and useful in illness narratives, in particular photographs, but sometimes also other images such as painted work, film or theatre. The images can be specifically generated for a topic area or researchers might use existing images from the past or the present (photographs of medical conditions; films of interaction between health professionals and clients; paintings of disfigured people). Lorenz (2007) presented a paper of her work with a survivor of traumatic brain injury. In this, she explored the story of a woman who took photographs of living with her injury over a period of 5 years. The woman showed her pictures to Lorenz and told her what they meant to her. A participant's story can, of course, be told with images, thus having a great visual impact, but the researcher's scholarly work needs analysis and interpretation, and this generally does involve some writing. Riessman (2008: 142) states that 'images become texts to be read interpretively'.

Ongoing debates about narrative

One of the issues in narrative research is that of 'truth'. For the researcher it is difficult to decide on the veracity or falsehood of stories as they are retrospective and also rely on memory. Is the truth being told, or 'the truth as the participants see it'? Hidden motives might underlie the way the narrator tells the story. There are inconsistencies and tensions that lie within it. These problems need reflection and discussion. If the stories fit into the social context and framework, they become more credible, but of course the researcher may never know whether the story was accurate. These issues and the debates about it can become a topic of exploration. People select from their memory banks what they wish to remember or they might forget what 'really' happened. However, the way the story is told, what is withheld or included, what is dramatised or forgotten, is important for the data analysis. Even ostensible 'untruths' might become significant.

The narratives of people and the storytelling by the researcher can be problematic in other ways. On the one hand, Lieblich *et al.* (1998) state that narratives are often seen more as art than as science because they are rooted in intuition and experience. On the other hand, they argue for a structured and coherent approach to storytelling.

Atkinson (1997) highlighted three major issues:

1 Narratives of health and illness play an important part in medical sociology and anthropology (and we would add in nursing and healthcare).
2 Sometimes these narratives are based on inappropriate assumptions and on mistaken methodological and theoretical claims.

3 Narrative analyses must be systematic and should not be seen as single solutions to problems.

Atkinson criticises the unexamined assumptions that underlie these narratives in which researchers take a simplistic view of this form of research; the link between narratives and experiences is complex and they should not be seen as individualistic and romantic constructions of self but located within the context of interaction and social action. They are no more 'authentic' (a favourite word of narrative researchers), he claims, than other forms of research. Readers of narratives need 'thick description' of sociocultural settings in which the narratives are embedded. Atkinson and Delamont (2006) add that overuse and uncritical acceptance is a recurrent problem in narrative inquiry. The research suffers from a lack of analysis and attention to social context and culture. Researchers, they suggest, should approach narrative research with 'a degree of caution and methodological scepticism (p. 18). Narrative research is not merely a re-telling or re-storying of narratives of personal experience that help participants to have their voice heard and represented but also detailed scholarly analysis and evaluation. Atkinson and Atkinson and Silverman started an ongoing debate.

Frank (2000) answers Atkinson by presenting his own ideas on some of the issues important in narrative. He makes five major points:

1 He suggests that, although narrative and story are used interchangeably, people tell stories, they are not telling narratives. Narratives contain structures on which stories are based. Storytellers use these but are not fully aware of them.
2 People share their stories with the listener, and through this sharing of the story the listener becomes part of a relationship in which the story is told.
3 Stories create distance between storytellers and the threats they experience. They do perform the 'recuperative role' that Atkinson attributes to them.
4 Stories are not just the data for analysis to be transformed into text. They affirm the purpose of the story, namely forming relationships.
5 The stories of illness need to be heard. Frank (2000: 355) refutes 'Atkinson's dichotomy' between storytelling and story analysis; he maintains that 'any good story analysis accepts its place in relations of storytelling' and researchers can only listen inside a relationship with ethical and intellectual responsibilities.

Ultimately, Frank sees storytelling in a different way from Atkinson. Frank (2000: 355) states emphatically: 'Storytellers do not call for their narratives to be analysed; they call for other stories in which experiences are shared, commonalities discovered and relationships built'.

The discussion about the purpose of narrative and storytelling is ongoing. Regardless of the stance of individual health researchers, they should be aware of this ongoing debate. Recently, Hammersley and Atkinson (2019) have extended some of the thoughts on narrative and interviewing.

The writer, the participants and the reader together 'create' the final story. The researcher interprets the participants, stories in the research account, and the readers in turn read through the lenses of their own understanding. Researchers interpret and edit the descriptions, thoughts and ideas of the participants. The latter give their individual and personal stories as understood from their own perspective; however, all research reports in narrative research entail collaboration between researcher and participant. The social and cultural world of narrators, whether researcher or participants, is not simple but complex; it always influences the story.

Summary

- Narratives are tales of experience or events and come naturally to human beings.
- Narratives are rarely simple or linear.
- Illness narratives are expressions of illness, suffering and pain.
- Narratives can also be career or education trajectory stories.
- Illness and professional narratives are located in the socio-cultural context as well as in the individual.
- Narrative inquiry is not unproblematic
- There are a number of different ways of analysing narrative data, most of which are legitimate.

References

Atkinson, P.A. (1997) Narrative turn or blind alley? *Qualitative Health Research*, **7** (3), 325–344.

Atkinson, P. and Delamont, S. (2006) Rescuing narrative from qualitative research. *Narrative Inquiry*, **16** (1), 164–172.

Bolt, C. (2012) *Using Narrative in Research*, Sage, London.

Braun, V. and Clarke, V. (2006) Using thematic analysis in psychology. *Qualitative Research in Psychology*, **3** (2), 77–101.

Braun, V. and Clarke, V. (2013) *Successful Qualitative Research: A Practical Guide for Beginners*, Sage, London.

Bruner, J. (1991) The narrative construction of reality. *Critical Inquiry*, **18** (1), 1–21.

Bruner, J. (2004) Life as narrative. *Social Research*, **71** (3), 691–710.

Bury, M. (1982) Chronic illness as biographical disruption. *Sociology of Health and Illness*, **4** (2), 167–182.

Elliott, J. (2005) *Using Narrative in Social Research: Qualitative and Quantitative Approaches*, Sage, London.

Frank, A.W. (1995) *The Wounded Storyteller: Body, Illness, and Ethics*, University of Chicago Press, Chicago, IL.

Frank, A.W. (2000) The standpoint of storyteller. *Qualitative Health Research*, **10** (3), 354–365.

Frank, A.W. (2013) *The Wounded Storyteller: Body, Illness and Ethics*, 2nd edn, University of Chicago Press, Chicago, IL.

Frid, I., Öhlen, J. and Bergbom, I. (2000) On the use of narratives in nursing research. *Journal of Advanced Nursing*, **32** (3), 695–703.

Greenhalgh, T. (2013) Story gathering: collecting and analyzing spontaneously shared stories as research data, in *Understanding and Using Health Experiences: Improving Patient Care* (eds. S. Ziebland, A. Coulter, J.D. Calabrese and L. Lacock), Oxford University Press, Oxford.

Greenhalgh, T. and Hurwitz, B. (1998) Why study narrative? in *Narrative Based Medicine* (eds. T. Greenhalgh and B. Hurwitz), BMJ Books, London, pp. 3–16.

Hammersley, M. and Atkinson, P. (2019) *Principles in Practice*, Routledge, Abingdon, Oxon.

Haydon, G. *et al.* (2017) Narrative inquiry as a research methodology exploring person centred care in nursing. *Collegian.* doi:https://doi.org/10.1016/j.colegn.2017.03.001.

Haydon, G. *et al.* (2021) A narrative inquiry of the time just before and after a cardiac arrest. *Collegian*, **28** (2), 190–196.

Holloway, I. and Freshwater, D. (2007) *Narrative Research in Nursing*, Blackwell, Oxford.

Josselson, R. (1995) Imagining the real: empathy, narrative and the dialogic self, in *Interpreting Experience: The Narrative Study of Lives* (eds. R. Josselson and A. Lieblich), Sage, Thousand Oaks, CA, pp. 27–44.

Jovchelovitch, S. and Bauer, M.W. (2000) Narrative interviewing, in *Qualitative Interviewing with Text, Image and Sound* (eds. M.W. Bauer and G. Gaskell), Sage, London, pp. 57–74.

Kleinman, A. (1988) *The Illness Narratives: Suffering, Healing and the Human Condition*, Basic Books, New York, NY.

Koskinen, L., Mikkonen, I. and Jokinen, P. (2011) Learning from the world of mental health care: nursing students' narratives. *Journal of Psychiatric and Mental Health Nursing*, **18** (7), 622–628.

Labov, W. (1972) *Sociolinguistic Patterns*, University of Pennsylvania Press, Philadelphia, PA.

Labov, W. and Waletzky, J. (1967) Oral versions of personal experience, in *Essays on the Verbal and Visual Arts* (ed. J. Helm), University of Washington Press, Seattle, WA.

Lieblich, A., Tuval-Mashiach, R. and Zilber, T. (eds.) (1998) *Narrative Research: Reading, Analysis and Interpretation*, Sage, Thousand Oaks, CA. (These authors have written a variety of texts about narrative).

Lorenz, L.S. (2007) Living with traumatic brain injury: narrative analysis of a survivor's photographs and interview. Poster Presentation, 26th Annual Conference, Brain Injury Association of Massachusetts, Marlborough, MA, March 22.

Maina, G., Sutankayo, L., Chorney, R. and Caine, V. (2013) Living with and teach about HIV: engaging nursing students through body mapping. *Nurse Education Today*, **34** (4), 643–647.

McCance, T.V., McKenna, H.P. and Boore, J.R.P. (2001) Exploring caring using narrative methodology: an analysis of the approach. *Journal of Advanced Nursing*, **33** (3), 350–356.

Mertova, P. and Webster, L. (2020) *Using Narrative Inquiry as a Research Method*, 2nd edn, Routledge, London.

Molzahn, A.E., Shields, L. Antonio, M. *et al.* (2021) Ten minutes after midnight: a narrative inquiry of people living with COPD and their family members. *International Journal of Health and Wellbeing.* doi:10.1080/17482631.2021.1893146.

Nosek, M., Powell Kennedy, H. and Gudmundsdottir, M. (2012) 'Chaos, restitution and quest': one woman's journey through menopause. *Sociology of Health and Illness*, **4** (7), 994–1009.

Ochs, E. and Capps, L. (2002) Narrative authenticity, in *Qualitative Research Methods* (ed. D. Weinberg), Blackwell, Malden, MA, pp. 127–132.

Paley, J. and Eva, G. (2005) Narrative vigilance: the analysis of stories in health care. *Nursing Philosophy*, **6** (2), 83–97.

Parsons, T. (1951) *The Social System*, Free Press, New York, NY.

Polkinghorne, D.E. (1995) Narrative configuration in qualitative analysis, in *Life History and Narrative* (eds. J.A. Hatch and R. Wisniewski), The Falmer Press, London, pp. 5–23.

Price, L., McGillis, Hall, Angus, J.E. and Peter, E. (2013) Choosing nursing as a career: a narrative analysis of millennial nurses' career choice of virtue. *Nursing Inquiry*, **20** (4), 305–316.

Rejnõ, A., Danielson, E. and Berg, L. (2013) Next of kin's experiences of sudden and unexpected death from stroke. *BMC Nursing*, **12**, 13.

Richardson, L. (1990) Narrative and sociology. *Journal of Contemporary Ethnography*, **19** (1), 116–135.

Riessman, C.K. (2008) *Narrative Methods in the Human Sciences*, Sage, Thousand Oaks, CA. doi:10.1080/17482631.2021.1893146.

Robertson, J.M. (2014) Finding meaning in everyday life with dementia. *Dementia*, **13** (4), 526–543.

Sakalys, J.R. (2000) The political role of illness narratives. *Journal of Advanced Nursing*, **31** (6), 1469–1475.

Sandelowsky, M. (1996) Truth/storytelling in nursing inquiry, in *Truth in Nursing Inquiry* (eds. J.F Kikuchi, H. Simmons and D. Romyn), Sage, Thousand Oaks, pp. 111–124.

Sools, A. (2013) Narrative health research: Exploring big and small stories as analytical tools. *Health*, **17** (1), 93–110. doi:10.1177/1363459312447259.

Sparkes, A.C., Pérez-Smaniego, V. and Smith, B. (2011) Social comparison processes, narrative mapping and their shaping of the cancer experience: a case study of an élite athlete. *Health*, **16** (5), 467–488.

Stenhouse R. (2013) Unfulfilled expectations: individuals' experiences on an acute psychiatric ward. Research output, The University of Edinburgh.

Thomas-MacLean, R. (2004) Understanding breast cancer stories via Frank's narrative types. *Social Science & Medicince*, **58** (9), 1647–1657.

Tu, C. (2019) Unpublished MSc study, McMasters University, Ontario.

Further Reading

Glintborg, C. and Dela Mata, M.I. (2021) *Identity Construction and Illness Narratives in Persons with Disabilities*, Routledge Oxon, Abingdon.

Chapter 13

Phenomenology

Phenomenological research aims to explore and describe phenomena, including everyday experiences of people, and it is sometimes referred to as 'the lived experience' of a situation or condition. Phenomenology is an approach with its roots in philosophy and not specifically a single method of inquiry. It has often been misunderstood. Indeed, Caelli (2001: 275–276) argues: 'Because phenomenology is first and foremost philosophy, the approach employed to pursue a particular study should emerge from the philosophical implications inherent in the question'. To give a basis to phenomenological research, we have traced the complex history of the philosophy of phenomenology and then discussed its adaptation as a qualitative research approach in healthcare. As a method of inquiry, phenomenological research has become popular in health research during the last decades, particularly in postgraduate health studies. Unfortunately, some phenomenological researchers, especially novices, neglect or overlook the philosophical origin of the method. This research is not easy to use and is best employed by more experienced researchers.

KEY POINT

Phenomenology is the study of structures and meanings of experience which includes the study of phenomena.

Various ways of collecting and analysing data, 'doing' phenomenology exist. They all have similar aims however; their data gathering and analytic procedures overlap. The major aim of a descriptive phenomenological research approach is to generate a description of a phenomenon of everyday experience to achieve an understanding of its essential structure, for example the experience of anger or fear, hermeneutic inquiry specifically emphasises understanding more than description which is the method of descriptive phenomenology, and relies on interpretation (see Giorgi, 1992).

Descriptive phenomenologists, such as Giorgi in particular, mainly follow the philosophy of Husserl and his followers. Others incorporate the ideas of

Qualitative Research in Nursing and Healthcare, Fifth Edition.
Immy Holloway and Kathleen Galvin.
© 2024 John Wiley & Sons Ltd. Published 2024 by John Wiley & Sons Ltd.

Heidegger and his colleagues who believe that phenomenology is interpretive, for instance Van Manen (1990, 1998) or Rapport (2005). Either approach can be used; researchers have overlapping though not congruent ideas on the way of doing phenomenological research (see later in this chapter).

Essentially, phenomenological philosophy has developed through three major historical streams: the *descriptive* phenomenology of Edmund Husserl (1859–1938); the *hermeneutic* phenomenology of Martin Heidegger (1889–1976); and the *existentialist* phenomenology of Merleau-Ponty (1908–1961) and Jean-Paul Sartre (1905–1980). There are ongoing philosophical debates about the distinctions and overlaps between these streams, but the differing emphases indicated for the purposes of this chapter generally remain. To read more about the history of phenomenology and its historical context within Continental Philosophy, we recommend Dermot Moran (1999) and to grasp its key philosophical principles, Zahavi (2019).

The term 'phenomenology' derives from the Greek word *phainomenon*, meaning 'appearance' (the concept was first developed by the philosopher Kant). Phenomenological philosophy is partly about the epistemological question – about the theory of knowledge – of 'how we know', the relationship of the person who knows and what can be known (McLeod, 2001). It is also connected to the ontological question: 'what is *being*'. The ontological question is concerned with the nature of reality and our knowledge about it, 'how things really are'. Giorgi and Giorgi (2003) suggest that phenomenology is 'a study of consciousness'.

As philosophy in general, the study of phenomenology is not immediately understandable. It has, however, informed the human sciences and in particular phenomenological psychology where it is used within qualitative research.

It is useful to trace the history of phenomenology. The following section will outline the background of phenomenology from the so-called 'continental philosophy', the subsequent ideas of Edmund Husserl (initially based on Brentano) as well as the later development of the phenomenological movement and schools of phenomenology.

Intentionality and the early stages of phenomenology

Phenomenology begins with Husserl who was the core figure in the development of phenomenology as a modern movement. It is important, however, to trace the earlier history of phenomenology in the influence of Franz Brentano (1838–1917) on the work of Husserl. Brentano was part of the preparatory phase of this movement (Cohen *et al.*, 2000).

One of the main themes of phenomenology is the concept of *intentionality*. Husserl takes this term from Brentano, although he does not use it in the same way. Giorgi (1997: 237) describes the notion of intentionality as Husserl sees it. In Husserl's work, intentionality is 'the essential feature of consciousness', which is directed towards an object. When human beings are conscious, they are always conscious of something. Consciousness in phenomenology relates to the person's consciousness of the world (Langridge, 2007).

This critical statement concerning the notion of intentionality shows the complexity of any attempt to define the act of conscious thought. In the human sciences, according to Giorgi, consciousness overcomes the dilemma of the subject–object debate, the mind–body relationship which is understood holistically and structurally. Philosophers, psychologists and natural scientists, including doctors and psychiatrists, neither agree nor have firmly established what exactly consciousness is, or what is the true relationship between mind and body. The ideas presented in this chapter cannot resolve the mind–body problem. However, it is useful to note that phenomenology is, in fact, one approach that attempts to do this. Priest places phenomenology within mind–body theories arising from the following:

- *Descartes' dualism:* It separates mind and body.
- *The so-called logical behaviourism:* This is a belief that everything concerns behaviour.
- *Notions of idealism:* All that exists can be explained in terms of the mind.
- *Materialism:* Everything in the universe can be explained in terms of matter.
- *Functionalism:* Everything is a kind of cause and effect. The mind is given a stimulus and responds physically or behaviourally.
- *The so-called 'double aspect theory':* The physical and mental are, in fact, merely aspects of something else, another reality, outside notions of the mental and the physical.
- *The phenomenological view:* This is an attempt to describe lived experiences, without making previous assumptions about the objective reality of those experiences.

Whilst these ideas are presented as theories within philosophy, phenomenology is, in fact, also a practice. It is this practice that is so exciting for nursing, health and social care alike, because it offers the possibility of ' … characterizing the contents of experience just as they appear to consciousness with a view to capturing their essential features' (Priest, 1991: 183).

Phases and history of the movement

As has already been stated, phenomenology has philosophical origins. In 1960, the first edition of Spiegelberg's review of the history of the phenomenological movement was published. He described what he termed three phases in the movement, the preparatory, the German and the French phases. Cohen (1987) summarises these in a paper giving her account of the history and importance of phenomenological research for nursing and stated that Brentano influenced this preparatory phase.

The German phase

The German phase involved primarily Husserl and later Heidegger. Cohen *et al.* (2000) discuss Husserl's contribution to the movement and highlight his centrality for phenomenology, his search for rigour, his criticism of positivism (all knowledge is derived from the senses – linked to scientific inquiry of observation and experiment) and his concepts of *Anschauung* (phenomenological intuition) and phenomenological reduction. In the former, a different kind of experience is apparent, closely involved with the imagination. Experience suggests a relationship with something real, such as an event, while *Anschauung* can also occur in imagination or memory. The latter is a process to suspend attitudes, beliefs and suppositions in order to properly examine what is present. Husserl termed this part of phenomenological reduction *epoché* (from the Greek, meaning 'suspension of belief'). Bracketing (a mathematical term) is the name given by Husserl to this process of suspending beliefs and prior assumptions about a phenomenon. Bracketing and phenomenological reduction are important features of the method, the actual 'doing' of phenomenology. The complex approach of various forms of phenomenology and the idea of bracketing in Husserl and Heidegger's work has been debated in many books and articles explaining phenomenology to and for nurses both by well-known and new researchers, for instance, Jasper (1994), Crotty (1996), Berg *et al.* (2006), Streubert Speziale and Rinaldi Carpenter (2010). For the purposes of using phenomenology as qualitative research in health, bracketing can be characterised as a kind of disciplined practice that involves remaining open to what and how the meaning of a phenomenon appears, and to a 'slowing down' so as not to add one's interpretation too readily, but rather to set aside, pre-existing ideas and/or to hold back any leap towards theoretical enflaming or 'going beyond the data'. This is a 'returning to the matters' in themselves and a describing of 'what is there'. Dahlberg *et al.* (2008) have usefully described a process and have coined the term 'bridling'. We think this is a very useful idea particularly for novice researchers who may find the notion of phenomenological reduction or bracketing difficult. The position that bracketing is not possible, is something we do not support, this argument is too simplistic, and particularly in the context of an ongoing controversial debate. See, Halling (2020), as a guiding way through this controversy, ultimately the aim is to be faithful to the phenomenon under study and to show *fidelity* with the phenomenon. Furthermore, there are examples of research in healthcare and nursing that have successfully used bracketing as part of the approach (to explore further see for example, see Dahlberg (2007, 2006) and Dahlberg and Dahlberg (2020)). We now summarise some important elements as identified by the key continental philosophers.

Husserl's major contribution to phenomenology consisted of three elements in particular: intentionality, essences and phenomenological reduction (bracketing).

Several important elements of phenomenology were developed by colleagues and students of Husserl. The major concepts are intersubjectivity and the idea of 'lifeworld' (*Lebenswelt*). Intersubjectivity is about the existence of a number of subjectivities which are shared by a community, that is by individual persons who share a common world. The intersubjective world is accessible because humans have empathy for others. The way of making sense of experience is essentially intersubjective (Schwandt, 2007).

The concept of lifeworld (*Lebenswelt*) is about the lived experience that is central to modern phenomenology. Human beings do not often take into account the commonplace and ordinary; indeed, they do not even notice it. Phenomenological inquiry is the approach needed to help examine and recognise the lived experience that is commonly taken for granted.

The next stage in the German phase of phenomenology involved Heidegger, who was an assistant to Husserl for a while. Due to the upsurge of interest (particularly in North America) in using the phenomenological framework for nursing and midwifery research, Heidegger is often mentioned in the work of a number of health researchers over the years. The phenomenological research of Benner (1984) uncovered excellence and power in clinical nursing practice, and she references, amongst others, Heidegger. Her well-known study had a profound influence, particularly on nursing research. Heidegger's changed direction from Husserlian phenomenology and his break with it occurred in the way he developed the notion of *Dasein*, which is explained fully in his work *Being and Time*, published in 1927 and translated into English in 1962. Heidegger's concern was to ask questions about the nature of being and about temporality (being is temporal). In this sense, he was interested in ontological ideas. Heidegger's notion of *Dasein* is an explanation of the nature of being and existence and, as such a concept of personhood. Leonard (1994) makes five main points concerning a Heideggerian phenomenological view of the person. These are as follows:

1 The person has a world, which comes from culture, history and language. Often this world is so inclusive that it is overlooked and is taken for granted until we reflect and analyse.
2 The person has a being in which things have value and significance. In this sense, persons can only be understood by a study of the context of their lives.
3 The person is self-interpreting. A person has the ability to make interpretations about knowledge. The understanding gained becomes part of the self.
4 The person is embodied. This is a different view from the Cartesian, which is about possessing a body. The notion of embodiment is the view that the body is the way we can potentially experience the action of ourselves in the world.
5 The person 'is' in time. This requires a little more elaboration as outlined below.

Heidegger had a different notion from the one of traditional time, which is perceived to flow in a linear fashion, with an awareness of 'now'. According to Leonard (1994), he used the word 'temporality', which denotes a new way of perceiving time in terms of including the *now*, the *no longer* and the *not yet*.

As well as these ideas, Heidegger developed phenomenology into interpretive philosophy that became the basis for hermeneutical methods of inquiry (in classical Greek mythology Hermes was the transmitter of the messages from the Gods to the mortals). This often involved interpreting the messages for the recipients to aid understanding. Hermeneutics developed as a result of translating literature from different languages, or where direct access to authoritative texts, such as the Bible, was difficult. Hermeneutics became the theory of interpretation and developed into its present form as the theory of the interpretation of meaning. Text means language. Gadamer (1975) suggests that human beings' experience of the world is connected with language.

Linking the ideas of hermeneutics with phenomenology, Koch (1995: 831) states:

> Heidegger (1962) declares nothing can be encountered without reference to the person's background understanding, and every encounter entails an interpretation based on the person's background, in its 'historicality'. The framework of interpretation that we use is the foreconception in which we grasp something in advance.

Heidegger's goes beyond mere description to interpretation. Heideggerian interpretive phenomenology is a popular research approach in nursing. This form of research explores the meaning of being a person in the world. Rather than suspending presuppositions, researchers examine them and make them explicit.

The French phase

Cohen (1987) argues that Heidegger's major contribution to the phenomenological movement was his influence on French philosophy. She points out that the main figures in this phase were Gabriel Marcel (1889–1973), Jean-Paul Sartre (1905–1980) and Maurice Merleau-Ponty (1908–1961). Marcel did not call himself a phenomenologist but viewed phenomenology as an introduction to analysing the notion of *being*.

Jean-Paul Sartre was the most influential figure in the movement but again did not want the label phenomenologist; rather he was termed as an *existentialist*. Phenomenological concepts and terms are difficult to grasp and it is often difficult to find a starting point. Understanding of terminology can be obviously further enhanced in progression from general to specific.

The idea of existence and essence are from Sartre; his famous and often quoted phrase is 'existence precedes essence'. This is Sartre's idea that a person's actual consciousness and behaviour (existence) comes before character (essence) (Cohen, 1987). In this sense, research would focus on real and concrete thoughts and behaviour before imaginary or idealised qualities or essences. The notion of intentionality features also in Sartre's work.

Merleau-Ponty's interest in phenomenology focused on perception and the creation of a science of human beings (for the purpose of this chapter, it is not necessary to develop this further).

Another major figure in French phenomenology is Paul Ricoeur. Spiegelberg (1984) argues that Ricoeur's phenomenology is primarily descriptive and based on a Husserlian eidetic concern with essential structures. Ricoeur, like Gadamer, focuses on the intersubjective and on issues of language and communication.

There are then different approaches within phenomenology. Indeed most researchers acknowledge that phenomenology is not a single and integrated philosophical direction. In the next stage of this chapter, we will examine the schools of phenomenology outlined by Cohen and Omery (1994).

Schools of phenomenology

It has been shown thus far that phenomenology is an approach within continental philosophy. For purposes of qualitative research, however, phenomenology has also been adapted and used as a framework within the so-called interpretive tradition that broadly includes grounded theory and ethnography as Lowenberg (1993) points out. She states: 'Basic to all these approaches is the recognition of the interpretive and constitutive cognitive processes inherent in all social life' (p. 58) and shows that there are many 'quandaries in terminology' which lead to misinterpretations in the nursing and education research literature, and sometimes in social research. She argues that there is a problem with phenomenology, the distinctions between the assumptions that lie behind the theories (e.g. Husserl and Heidegger) and the actual method, the 'doing' of phenomenology. Part of the purpose of this chapter is to try to unravel these perplexities.

A useful outline of phenomenological philosophy, guiding research and describing the development of schools with different approaches, is presented by Cohen and Omery (1994). The broad goal in each school remains the same, that is, to gain knowledge and insight about a phenomenon.

Three major schools can be found, but there is overlap and linkage between them. The first is the *Duquesne* School, guided by Husserl's ideas about eidetic structure (so called because its followers worked at one stage in time at Duquesne University). The second school is about the *interpretation* of phenomena (Heideggerian hermeneutics). The combination of both is found in the *Dutch* School of phenomenology.

The Duquesne School focuses mostly on the notion of description. Giorgi (1985) states that social scientists should describe what presents itself to them without adding or subtracting from it. His advice is to acknowledge the evidence and not go beyond the data, although he believes that description cannot ever be complete. This approach is also known as 'descriptive phenomenology'. The 'interpretation of phenomena' approach concentrates on taken-for-granted practices and common meanings, whilst the Dutch School aims to combine both description and interpretation. More recently, some further innovations in approaches have emerged, which include Reflective Lifeworld Research (Dahlberg *et al.*, 2008) and Dialogical Phenomenology (Halling, 2009). Finlay (2011) has provided an exceptionally helpful analysis of the major kinds and schools of phenomenological research and has also indicated some directions for some of the contested debates within the descriptive and interpretive phenomenological community (Finlay, 2009).

KEY POINT

Phenomenology has developed into several schools. Differences between these are complex and rooted in long-standing philosophical heritage.

The phenomenological research process: doing phenomenology

Giorgi has always recognised the problem in applying a philosophical approach to a practice discipline. This means that new researchers are often uncertain of how to proceed when wishing to use phenomenological research. While developing ideas about complementarities of different phenomenological approaches as a philosophical basis for nursing research, Todres and Wheeler (2001: 2) discuss some philosophical distinctions in the approach to human experience that need to be included when carrying out practical research. They approach three areas in which they show that phenomenology, hermeneutics and existentialism have a contribution to make to health research: *grounding*, *reflexivity* and *humanisation*. Further developments in these applications within practice disciplines are offered by Galvin and Todres (2012).

Grounding

Grounding means taking the lifeworld as a starting point. It includes the everyday world of common experiences. The lifeworld is more complex than that which can be said about it and contains inherent tensions. Lived experience for Husserl is the *ground* of inquiry. There is also a *need* for inquiry. The commonplace, taken for granted, becomes a phenomenon when it becomes questionable. The understanding of the lifeworld demands an open-minded attitude in which prior assumptions are bracketed so that descriptions can clarify meanings and relationships.

Reflexivity and positional knowledge

Hermeneutics has added certain dimensions to phenomenological research. Gadamer (1975) developed Heidegger's ideas about interpretation as integral to human existence. Human beings are self-reflective persons who are based in everyday life. Their personal relationships and experience happen in a temporal and historical context and depend on their position in the world. Preconceptions and provisional knowledge are always revised in the light of experience and reflection. The text is always open to multiple interpretations because researchers or reflective persons are involved in their own relationships with the world and others.

'Humanisation' and the language of experience

Human beings cannot be separated from their relationships in the world. Heidegger's notion of *Dasein*, being-in-the-world, entails a relationship between being human and being-in-the-world. Researchers search for fundamental and general categories of human existence that illuminate experiences that reveal a world. Heidegger (Todres and Wheeler, 2001: 5) reflects on fundamental structures that characterise the essential qualities of being-in-the-world such as

- The way in which the body occurs.
- The way the co-constituting of temporal structures occurs.
- The way the meaningful world of place and things occurs.
- The way the quality of interpersonal relationships occurs.

This is how Heidegger shows that body, time and space reflect the qualities of human presence rather than being notions of quantitative measurement.

From these ideas, Todres and Wheeler (2001) conclude that phenomenology *grounds* research and stays away from theoretical abstraction. They also claim that hermeneutics adds the notion of *reflexivity*, which makes researchers ask questions meaningful and relevant in cultural, temporal and historical contexts. Lastly, these writers state that the ontological existential dimension *humanises* the research so it is not merely technical and utilitarian. A further elaboration of the coherent value base of qualitative research, and lifeworld research in particular, in relation to human dimensions of care (practice) is elaborated by Todres *et al.* (2009).

Phenomenological research focuses on the lifeworld, lived experiences which are described by the participants who reflect on them. These experiences might include 'the experience of diabetes', 'being a first-time father', 'living with epilepsy' and similar phenomena. Thus, phenomenology is an investigation focused on first person perspectives. From the experiences of participants, phenomenologists gain insight and extract common themes – essential structures or essences – which human beings have in common and that go beyond individual cases.

Thus, a phenomenological study presents the essential structure of a phenomenon. Here the concept of bracketing becomes useful for the researcher who, as said before, must exclude (bracket) prior assumptions gained through experience or literature to see the phenomenon with an open mind. It is, however, not sufficient to confirm that bracketing has occurred; the researcher also has to show how and where this took place. This is important for the early stages of the inquiry, while later on, the researcher has a dialogue with the literature about the phenomenon that is being illuminated. Bracketing means that the researchers can experience things as fresh and new as they do not prejudge. Husserl uses the term epoché (from the Greek for cessation) to characterise this suspension of judgement or bracketing. This phenomenological reduction is necessary to gain the essence of a phenomenon. For a further elaboration of these ideas about essences in phenomenology and the development of meaning structures, see Dahlberg (2006).

Van Manen (1990: 5) outlines some of the important features that characterise phenomenological research:

- Phenomenological research is the study of lived experience.
- Phenomenological research is the explication of phenomena as they present themselves to consciousness.
- Phenomenological research is the study of essences or meaning (depending on the specific approach).
- Phenomenological research is the description of the experiential meanings we live as we live them.
- Phenomenological research is the human scientific study of phenomena.
- Phenomenological research is the attentive practice of thoughtfulness.
- Phenomenological research is a search for what it means to be human.
- Phenomenological research is a poetizing activity.

The latter means that reflexive writing and aesthetic presentation is an essential and integral element in phenomenological research. Indeed, it is crucial. Giorgi and Giorgi remind the researcher that phenomenological inquiry should stay as close as possible to the phenomenon to be illuminated. To begin the process of phenomenological inquiry, researchers obviously need an area of interest, puzzlement, concern or a gap in general or specific knowledge about a phenomenon. 'Practising science', as Giorgi (2000, 2009) calls it, is distinctly different from 'doing philosophy'. Indeed, he criticises researchers who write on nursing research, such as Crotty (1996) or Paley (1997) for not distinguishing between the two. Giorgi sees value in the use of phenomenological research in nursing but suggests that this means scientific work rather than doing philosophy. (Giorgi's engagement with the ideas of Crotty and Paley is important but cannot be followed up here.)

In all approaches, the researcher has a responsibility to justify the type of theoretical framework (e.g. symbolic interactionism, phenomenology or any other) and specify and outline the approach to data analysis (e.g. grounded theory for the former, or approaches of Colaizzi (1978) and other writers as regards the latter). Holloway and Todres (2003) argue that there is a need to avoid 'method-slurring' and preserve the integrity of the approach. This is particularly important in phenomenology because of its distinctive underlying philosophy.

In data analysis for phenomenological inquiry, the researcher aims to uncover and produce a description of the lived experience. The procedural steps to achieve this aim vary with the approach taken by the researcher in terms of the three main types of phenomenology previously outlined. Various researchers have developed approaches to data analysis that follow the requirements of bracketing, intuition and reflection. One of these, Colaizzi (1978), outlined a seven-stage process of analysis. Although there has been criticism of pioneering work such as this (Hycner, 1985), this particular process of analysis for the eidetic approach of phenomenology is both logical and credible. Hycner (1985: 279) states, however, that 'there is an appropriate reluctance on the part of phenomenologists to focus too much on specific steps in research methods for fear that they will become verified as they have in the natural sciences'. There are, however, several interpretations of the data analysis process depending on the school of phenomenology chosen. For example, Streubert Speziale and Rinaldi Carpenter (2010) outline the different procedural steps from other earlier authors such as Van Kaam (1959), Paterson and Zderad (1976), Colaizzi (1978), Van Manen (1990) and Giorgi (1985, 2009). Very usefully, Wertz *et al.* (2011) have provided an illustration of phenomenological analysis in the context of the experience of trauma, and further sets this in comparison with, for example, grounded theory and other qualitative data analysis approaches.

Phenomenological analysis ascribes to several specific features: phenomenological reduction (through the phenomenological attitude), description and reflection.

Phenomenology and health research

Streubert Speziale and Rinaldi Carpenter (2010) suggest that professional nursing orientation towards holistic care provides the background for deciding whether to undertake phenomenological research. This should also be so for other health researchers. The holistic perspective, coupled with the study of lived experience, provides the foundation for phenomenological research. These authors like others advise the researcher to ask several questions about the intended topic. For example: Is there some need for clarity concerning a phenomenon? Has there been anything published in relation to this, or is there a need for further inquiry? If there is, the health researcher should question whether inquiry concerning the lived experience is the most appropriate approach to collecting data. As the accounts of those experiencing the phenomenon are the primary data, the researcher needs to consider that this will yield both rich and descriptive data. Streubert Speziale and Rinaldi Carpenter argue that researchers examine their own style, preference and ability to engage with this approach to research. Further considerations for the research process concern completion and presentation of the study to relevant audiences.

Galvin and Holloway (2015) see that this research approach yields very rich data, gives deep insight into the lifeworld of participants and does not stay on the surface. The findings resonate with researchers and readers alike because they concern essential perspectives of human beings. This is one of the reasons why participant observation is problematic as that is seen from the perspective of the researcher, an 'outsider' to the research, while interviews give the ideas of the 'insider'. Researchers need very varied skills, both scientific and communicative; they should be able to do 'good' and rigorous research as well as communicate the findings and meanings in a language that captures the richness of the lifeworld of the participants. It is also stated by Dowling (2007) that phenomenological research is complex and not easy, although it can be successful in exploring the 'human condition' if attempted in a rigorous way and if health researchers place it within its philosophical base. It would be difficult for novice researchers to carry out phenomenological research.

Topics for phenomenological approaches

Wojnar and Swanson (2007) suggest that healing and caring are important phenomena to be illuminated, discussed and understood by health researchers.

Appropriate areas for phenomenological research include topics that are important to life experience such as well-being, suffering, happiness, anger, fear and anxiety or what it means to be a physiotherapist, a doctor or a community midwife. There are other health and illness-related topics such as the experience of having a myocardial infarction, an acute illness or chronic pain. There is also an established literature that draws on phenomenology to explore the meaning of care and practice of caring. Other topics that lend themselves to phenomenological research include, for instance, the meaning of health, suffering, well-being and the experience of growing old, growing up.

KEY POINT

Phenomenological questions in healthcare are generally concerned with describing the structures and meanings of health and illness experiences.

Recently, phenomenological research in healthcare has become very popular. It covers a range of topic areas on meaningful life experiences, including phenomena such as caring, the experience of well-being or its absence, suffering; the meaning of dignity, living with Alzheimer's, the phenomenon of living with breast cancer, fatigue, infertility, first-time motherhood, chronic illness and relationships in healthcare, action learning, addiction, violence and therapeutic touch. The phenomenological approach can also be used in professional education.

There is breadth and depth in phenomenological research and the potential of this method of inquiry. For health professionals, it is a rewarding enterprise but not an easy one because researchers have to understand the underlying philosophies before carrying out a study and decide which type of phenomenological approach to use.

Choice of approach: descriptive or interpretive phenomenology

Researchers usually choose one of these phenomenological approaches. They are similar and many of the ideas overlap as they both have their roots in Husserl's philosophy. Both start with the lifeworld, 'the lived everyday concrete experience' of the participants and focus initially on individual and unique everyday experiences and concrete examples of the phenomenon to be researched. After reflection and analysis, more general ideas about the phenomenon emerge. As stated before, Giorgi and his many students and followers who are descriptive phenomenologists (for instance, Les Todres, Barbro Giorgi and Karin Dahlberg) stay close to Husserl, while hermeneutic phenomenologists, such as Frances Rapport, Kitty Suddick make use of the philosophies of Heidegger, Gadamer and Ricoeur. Van Manen is one of the present-day hermeneutic researchers whose work is particularly known in the field of education. Recently Dahlberg and Dahlberg (2020) have examined 'the fissure' between interpretive and descriptive approaches and pointed to a 'third way'.

Example 13.1 Descriptive Phenomenology Examples

Lundvall *et al.* (2020) described young men's' concerns and challenges about their identity and who they want to be in life, the research focused on descriptions of young men's' experiences of living with existential concerns that they sought support for. The essential description capturing the findings was 'living close to a bottomless darkness, and comprised four constituents – enduring everyday life, striving for a solution, hearing the inner self-critical voice and wearing a hard shell'.

As part of a larger study, Heath *et al.* (2015) reported on research of paediatric outpatient care, underpinned by descriptive phenomenology, from the patients' and parents' perspectives. The description of this phenomenon of care helped the researchers to gain insight into the experience of the participants as lived and a deeper grasp of the meaning of their everyday experience. The research demonstrated that one of the main concerns of those involved meant 'care that fit into their lives'.

> van der Meide *et al.* (2018) provide an excellent illustration of a phenomenological investigation of the embodied experience of living with multiple sclerosis and provide a robust methodological foundation for their phenomenological approach.

These approaches differ in their details. For instance, while descriptive phenomenological researchers find and describe essential and universal structures, researchers who take the hermeneutic approach attempt to interpret the meaning of the phenomenon in context. Bracketing prior assumptions and preconceptions is important for descriptive phenomenologists, but hermeneutic researchers believe that these prior experiences might become sources of knowledge and sensitise the researcher to the meanings that might be presented in the narratives of participants. Interpretive phenomenology uses the term 'fusion of horizons' which has its origin in Gadamer's work on intersubjectivity, one horizon being that of the 'text' and the other that of the interpreter of the text. In the research approach, it indicates the intersection of the researcher's and the participants' ideas. Both have individual perspectives on the phenomenon but they also live in a shared world where they have common perceptions. The term 'hermeneutic circle' also has its origin in the philosophy of Heidegger. In research it means that interpretation of text (participant narratives) looks at parts of the lived experience, then at the whole, and then back again in a spiralling process, the end of which is achieved when the researcher has gained a reasonable understanding and meaning of the text.

Example 13.2 Hermeneutic Phenomenological Analysis in Three Studies

Suddick *et al.* (2019) explored the meaning of space, as lived, in an acute stroke unit. Taking a hermeneutic stance, the meaningful space as lived within by practitioners was illuminated. This also led to a mapping of the spatial context of care as experienced by patients in the stroke unit (2021) drawing on data from patients' everyday experiences and analysing the meaning following a hermeneutic process. Thackery and Eatough (2015) undertook a hermeneutic study exploring the maternal experience of parenting a young adult with developmental disability. An idiographic stance is taken in the analysis of six interviews with mothers aged 48–60. The findings reveal a degree of complexity and are in-depth in communicating the concerns and experiences of mothers.

We also have to mention a branch of phenomenological inquiry which has become very popular, possibly because of an analytic link to grounded theory, namely interpretative phenomenological analysis (IPA), developed by Jonathan Smith and his colleagues (Smith *et al.*, 2009).

Example 13.3 Interpretative Phenomenological Analysis

Fox and Diab (2015) carried out research with six individuals – a homogeneous sample – who were being treated for chronic anorexia nervosa (AN) in two eating disorder units in order to understand how the participants made meaning of their condition. Several broad questions were devised to ask them about living with AN. Their narrative interviews were analysed by IPA by the procedures of IPA through coding, categorising and identifying themes in the data. When themes arose in most of the interview transcripts, they were included in higher order themes presented as findings.

Eatough *et al.* (2008) report a phenomenological study of anger and anger-related regression. Five females were interviewed twice. An interpretive phenomenological analysis showed three aspects of the experience of anger in a way that is highly faithful to the phenomenon.

Example 13.4 Phenomenological Philosophical Analysis

Galvin and Todres (2015) have undertaken a phenomenological analysis of the human experience of dignity using lifeworld theory sensitised reflection. They used phenomenological philosophy as a foundation to reflect on the experience of dignity, its rupture and its restoration. The description of the phenomenon of dignity with its constituents described as 'kinds of dignity' is an example of reflective phenomenological analysis following principles that are rooted in phenomenological philosophy.

Procedures for data collection and analysis

The data collection starts with the specific and proceeds to the general. For instance, in their search for the description of a phenomenon, researchers attempt to ask for a concrete example of their everyday experience of this phenomenon within its context. For instance, a first-time father might be asked: 'What was this experience like for you?' A study of the phenomenon of backpain might start with the researcher's question: 'Describe a situation in which your backpain occurred'. While asking these questions, the researcher brackets prior assumptions and presuppositions. During the rest of the interview the researcher will focus on clarifying the phenomenon. Many such interviews will uncover the essential structure or essence of the phenomenon which is common to all participants.

Phenomenological interviews are distinctive; they are open and not planned as semi-structured, rather the researcher aims to facilitate the participant so that they provide rich descriptions of the phenomenon through examples from everyday life and their own experience. For example, using questions: Can you tell me about your experience of …? And what was that like …? Can you give me an example of when you felt that? What was going on when you felt like that? Can you give me examples of when you do that? Can you give me an example of what happened? What was that like when that happened? Can you describe that for me?

Many phenomenological research studies originate in the Duquesne School and use the approaches from one of the following authors, Colaizzi (1978), Giorgi (1985) or Van Kaam (1966). Although these authors are still popular – especially Giorgi, who made this his life's work – other approaches, in particularly interpretive phenomenology, have also flourished, although analysis is often similar to that of the following authors. Colaizzi advocates seven steps, Giorgi four and Van Kaam six, but many of these steps are similar or overlap, and they are never rigidly applied.

In selecting a school of phenomenology, the researcher will be guided by the approach to the most appropriate procedural steps in data analysis. For the purposes of this chapter, we outline and discuss those developed by Giorgi (1985, 2000) and Colaizzi (1978). It is, however, a decision for student and supervisor (novice or expert researcher) to select the approach best suited for the phenomenon under investigation and to utilise the appropriate literature to guide the research methodology and analysis.

Both Giorgi (1985, 2000, 2008, 2009) and Colaizzi (1978) argue for a descriptive approach and provide a method for data analysis, for instance from transcribed tapes of interviews with participants. These are just examples of qualitative data analyses.

Giorgi's steps for analysis are as follows:

1 The entire description is read to get a sense of the whole. This is important as phenomenology is holistic and focuses initially on the 'Gestalt', that is the whole.
2 Once the Gestalt has been grasped, researchers attempt to constitute the parts of the description, make and differentiate between 'meaning units' – as the parts are labelled (these parts have to be relevant) – and centre on the phenomenon under study. It is important that these units are not theory-laden but the language of everyday life is used.
3 When the meaning units have been illuminated, the researcher actively transforms the original data and expresses the insight that is contained in them and highlights common themes which are illustrated by quotes from participants.
4 Giorgi suggests making the implicit explicit and to go from a concrete situation as an example to demonstrate of what this situation is an example of. The researcher integrates the transformed meaning units into a consistent statement about the participants' experience across individual sources. This is called the *structure* of experience. In other words, it is the essence of the experience.

Although the researchers uncover structures of experience, finding it from the themes generated by individuals, they look at the phenomenon rather than focusing on individual narratives. This does not mean that there is no interest in individuals, but the search is for the overall structure of experience.

Colaizzi's seven-stage process is another approach to data analysis for the researcher but similar to that of Giorgi. The seven-stage process of analysis occurs as follows:

1 Read all of the subject's [*sic*] descriptions (conventionally termed *protocols*) in order to acquire a feeling for them, and to make sense out of them.

2 Return to each description and extract from them phrases or sentences which directly pertain to the investigated phenomenon; this is known as *extracting significant statements*.

3 Try to spell out the meaning of each significant statement; these are known as *formulated meanings*.

4 Repeat the above for each description and organise the aggregate formulated meanings into *clusters of themes*.

   a. Refer these clusters of themes back to the original protocols in order to *validate* them.

   b. At this point, discrepancies may be noted among and/or between the various clusters; some themes may flatly contradict others, or may appear to be totally unrelated to others. (The researcher is advised by Colaizzi to refuse the temptation to ignore data or themes which do not fit.)

5 The results of everything so far are integrated into an *exhaustive description* of the investigated topic.

6 An effort is made to formulate the exhaustive description of the investigated phenomenon in as unequivocal a statement of *identification of its fundamental structure* as possible. This has often been termed as an essential structure of the phenomenon.

7 A final validating step can be achieved by returning to each participant, and, in either a single interview session or a series of interviews, asking the subject about the findings thus far.

These are descriptions of procedural steps adapted from Colaizzi (1978: 59–61).

Colaizzi encourages researchers to be flexible with these stages, and we have found this to be useful. For example, we have encouraged students to take the exhaustive description back to informants, rather than the final, essential structure, because it appears to be more recognisable for them for comment. This ensures rigour. A formal member check is not useful for phenomenologists as they translate the research to a more theoretical level, that of the researcher. It can be seen that many of the steps overlap in the analysis process of different writers on phenomenological research. However, many writers, including van Manen, have a less structured approach and focus on the general insight that phenomenological research offers. In any case, all inquiry goes beyond the formal steps. When Todres (2000: 43) discusses a specific example of phenomenological research, he lists some signposts that go beyond mechanical stages, and they could gain major importance for other researchers.

The presentation of his discoveries involves the following:

- It will go beyond a definition or a series of statements; it will reflect a narrative coherence.
- It will tell us something that connects with universal human qualities so that the reader can relate personally to the themes.
- It will tell a story with which readers can empathise in imaginative ways.
- It contributes to new understanding.
- It will clarify and illuminate the topic to help the reader make sense of it without wholly possessing it.

These signposts are significant for phenomenological studies. They show that the search for the essence of a phenomenon and its meaning within a defined context is not merely a technique or a series of mechanical steps but an exploration of meaning.

The phenomenological approach is holistic, that is the methods are aimed at striving to achieve understanding of the whole phenomenon through a process that delineates the phenomenon 'as a whole', rather than just a focus on a part of a phenomenon, or a partial view.

Summary

- Phenomenology is primarily a philosophy but is applied as a research approach using defined procedures.
- There are three main phases in the phenomenological philosophical movement: preparatory, German and French. There is overlap and interaction of ideas between the phases.
- Writers developed different conceptual formulations (very broadly): descriptive (Husserl), interpretive (Heidegger) and ontological-existential (Sartre), which have been adapted as methods of inquiry by researchers.
- Researchers who use phenomenological methods have formulated various steps of data analysis.
- The approach should not be mechanical but open, insightful and illuminate the phenomenon under study faithfully to capture its essence (essential characteristics that cohere through variations).
- Phenomenology requires a slowing down, engagement with reflective process and offers rich description.

References

Benner, P. (1984) *From Novice to Expert: Excellence and Power in Clinical Nursing,* Addison-Wesley, Menlo Park, CA.

Berg, L., Scott, C. and Danielson, E. (2006) An interpretive phenomenological method for illuminating the meaning of caring relationship. *Scandinavian Journal of Caring Sciences,* **20** (1), 42–50.

Caelli, K. (2001) Engaging with phenomenology: is it more of a challenge than it needs to be? *Qualitative Health Research*, **11** (2), 273–281.

Cohen, M.Z. (1987) A historical overview of the phenomenologic movement. *Image: Journal of Nursing Scholarship*, **19** (1), 31–34.

Cohen, M.Z. and Omery, A. (1994) Schools of phenomenology: implications for research, in *Critical Issues in Qualitative Research Methods* (ed. J.M. Morse), Sage, Thousand Oaks, CA, pp. 136–156.

Cohen, M.Z., Kahn, D.L. and Steeves, R.H. (2000) *Hermeneutic Phenomenological Research: A Practical Guide for Nurse Researchers*, Sage, Thousand Oaks, CA.

Colaizzi, P. (1978) Psychological research as a phenomenologist view it, in *Existential Phenomenological Alternatives for Psychology* (eds. R. Vallé and M. King), Oxford University Press, New York, NY, pp. 48–71.

Crotty, M. (1996) *Phenomenology and Nursing Research*, Churchill Livingstone, Melbourne.

Dahlberg, K. (2006) The essence of essences/the search for meaning structures in phenomenological analysis of lifeworld phenomena. *International Journal of Qualitative Studies on Health and Well-being*, **1** (1), 11–19.

Dahlberg, K. (2007). The enigmatic phenomenon of loneliness. *International Journal of Qualitative Studies on Health and Well-being*, **2** (4), 195–207.

Dahlberg, K. and Dahlberg, H. (2020) Open and reflective lifeworld research: a third way. *Qualitative Inquiry*, 26 (5), 458–464.

Dahlberg, K., Dahlberg, H. and Nyström, M. (2008) *Reflective Lifeworld Research*, 2nd end, Studentlitteratur, Lund.

Dowling, M. (2007) From Husserl to Van Manen: a review of different phenomenological approaches. *International Journal of Nursing Studies*, **44** (1), 131–142.

Eatough, V., Smith, J. and Shaw, R. (2008) Women, anger and aggression: an interpretive phenomenological analysis. *Journal of Interpersonal Violence*, **23** (12), 1767–1799.

Finlay, L. (2009) Debating phenomenological methods. *Phenomenology and Practice*, **3** (1), 6–25.

Finlay, L. (2011) *Phenomenology for Therapists: Researching the Lived World*, Wiley Blackwell.

Fox, J.R.E. and Diab, P. (2015) An exploration of the perceptions and experiences of living with chronic anorexia nervosa while an inpatient on an Eating Disorder Unit: an Interpretative Phenomenological Analysis (IPA) study. *Journal of Health Psychology*, **20** (1), 27–36.

Gadamer, H. (1975), in *Truth and Method* (eds. G. Barden and J. Cumming) (originally published in 1960), 2nd edn, 1989, Seabury Press, New York, NY.

Galvin, K. and Holloway, I. (2015) Phenomenological research, in The *Research Process in Nursing* (eds. K. Gerrish and J. Lathlean), 7th edn. Chapter 16.

Galvin, K. and Todres, L. (2012) *Caring and Wellbeing: A Lifeworld Approach*, Routledge, he University of Brighton, Abingdon, VA.

Galvin, K.T. and Todres, L. (2015) Dignity as honour-wound: an experiential and relational view. *Journal of Evaluation in Clinical Practice*, **21** (3), 410–418.

Giorgi, A. (ed.) (1985) *Phenomenology and Psychological Research*, Duquesne University Press, Pittsburgh, PA.

Giorgi, A. (1992) Description versus interpretation: competing strategies for qualitative research. *Journal of Phenomenological Psychology*, **23** (2), 119–135.

Giorgi, A. (1997) The theory, practice and evaluation of the phenomenological method as a qualitative procedure. *Journal of Phenomenological Psychology*, **28** (2), 235–260.

Giorgi, A. (2000) Concerning the application of phenomenology to caring research. *Scandinavian Journal of Caring Science*, **14** (1), 11–15.

Giorgi, A. (2008) *Workshop on Phenomenology*, Bournemouth University, Poole.

Giorgi, A. (2009). *The Descriptive Phenomenological Method in Psychology*, Duquesne University Press, Pittsburgh, PA.

Giorgi, A. and Giorgi, B. (2003) Phenomenology, in *Qualitative Psychology: A Practical Guide to Research Methods* (ed. J. Smith), Sage, London, pp. 25–50.

Halling, S. (2009) *Intimacy, Transcendence, and Psychology*, Palgrave Macmillan, New York.

Halling, S. (2020) Phenomenology as fidelity to phenomena: moving beyond the van Manen, Smith, and Zahavi Debate. *The Humanistic Psychologist*. doi:10.1037/hum0000195.

Heath, G., Greenfield, S. and Redwood, S. (2015) The meaning of 'place' in families' lived experiences of paediatric outpatient care in different settings. *Health and Place*, **31**, 46–53.

Heidegger, M. (1962) *Being and Time* (eds. J. Maquarrie and E. Robinson) (translated from the original 1927 publication), Harper and Row, New York, NY.

Holloway, I. and Todres, L. (2003) The status of method: flexibility, consistency and coherence. *Qualitative Research*, **3** (3), 345–357.

Hycner, R.H. (1985) Some guidelines for the phenomenological analysis of interview data. *Human Studies*, **8** (3), 279–303.

Jasper, M.A. (1994) Issues in phenomenology for researchers of nursing. *Journal of Advanced Nursing*, **19** (2), 309–314.

Koch, T. (1995) Interpretive approaches in nursing research: the influence of Husserl and Heidegger. *Journal of Advanced Nursing*, **21** (5), 827–836.

Langridge, D. (2007) *Phenomenological Psychology*, Pearson Education, Edinburgh.

Leonard, V.W. (1994) A Heideggerian phenomenological perspective on the concept of person, in *Interpretive Phenomenology: Embodiment, Caring and Ethics in Health and Illness* (ed. P. Benner), Sage, Thousand Oaks, CA, pp. 43–63.

Lowenberg, J.S. (1993) Interpretive research methodology: broadening the dialogue. *Advances in Nursing Science*, **16** (2), 57–69.

Lundvall, M., Horberg, U., Palmer, L. *et al.* (2020) Young men's experiences of living with existential concerns: living close to a bottomless darkness. *International Journal of Qualitative Studies on Health and Well-being*, **15**, 1810947. doi:10.1080/17482631.2020.1810947.

McLeod, J. (2001) *Qualitative Methods in Counselling and Psychotherapy*, Sage, London.

van der Meide, H., Teunissen, T., Collard, P. *et al.* (2018). The mindful body: a phenomenology of the body with multiple sclerosis. *Qualitative Health Research*, **28**, 2239–2249. doi:10.1177/1049732318796831.

Moran, D. (1999) *Introduction to Phenomenology*, Routledge, Oxford.

Paley, J. (1997) Husserl, phenomenology and nursing. *Journal of Advanced Nursing*, **26**, 187–193.

Paterson, J.G. and Zderad, L.T. (1976) *Humanistic Nursing*, John Wiley & Sons, Inc., New York, NY.

Priest, S. (1991) *Theories of Mind*, Penguin Books, London.

Rapport, F. (2005) Hermeneutic phenomenology: the science of interpretation of text, in *Qualitative Research in Health Care* (ed. I. Holloway) Open University Press, Maidenhead, pp. 125–146.

Schwandt, T.A. (2007) *Dictionary of Qualitative Inquiry*, 3rd edn, Sage, Newbury Park, CA.

Smith, J., Flowers, P. and Larkin, M. (2009) *Interpretative Phenomenological Analysis*, Sage, London.

Spiegelberg, H. (1984) *The Phenomenological Movement: A Historical Introduction*, 3rd edn, (1st edn, 1960), Martinus Nijhoff, The Hague, The Netherlands.

Streubert Speziale, H.J. and Rinaldi Carpenter, D.R. (2010) *Qualitative Research in Nursing: Advancing the Human Imperative*, 5th edn, J.B. Lippincott & Co., Philadelphia, PA.

Suddick, K.M., Cross, V., Vuoskoski, P. *et al.* (2019) The acute stroke unit as meaningful space: the lived experience of health care practitioners. *Health and Place*, 57, 12–21.

Suddick, K.M., Cross, V., Vuoskoski, P. *et al.* (2021) Holding space and transitional space: stroke survivors' lived experience of being on an acute stroke unit. A hermeneutic phenomenological study. *Scandinavian Journal of Caring Sciences*, **35**: 104–114

Thackery, C.A. and Eatough, V. (2015) 'Well, the future, that is difficult': a hermeneutic phenomenological analysis of exploring the maternal experience of parenting a young adult with developmental disabilities. *Journal of Applied Research in Intellectual Disabilities*, **28** (4), 265–275.

Todres, L. (2000) Writing phenomenological psychological descriptions: an illustration to balance texture and structure. *Auto-Biography*, **8** (1/2), 41–48.

Todres, L. and Wheeler, S. (2001) The complementarity of phenomenology, hermeneutics and existentialism as a philosophical perspective for nursing research. *International Journal of Nursing Studies*, **38** (1), 1–8.

Todres, L., Galvin, K.T. and Holloway, I. (2009) The humanization of healthcare: a value framework for qualitative research. *International Journal of Qualitative Studies on Health and Well-being*, **4** (2), 68–77.

Van Kaam, A. (1959) A phenomenological analysis exemplified by the feeling of being understood. *Journal of Individual Psychology*, **15** (1), 66–72.

Van Kaam, A. (1966) *Existential Foundations of Psychology*, Dusquesne University Press, Pittsburgh, PA.

Van Manen, M. (1990) *Researching Lived Experience: Human Science for an Action Sensitive Pedagogy*, State University of New York Press, New York, NY.

Van Manen, M. (1998) *Researching Lived Experience: Human Science for an Action Sensitive Pedagogy*, 2nd edn, State University of New York Press, New York, NY.

Wertz, F.J., Charmaz, K., McMullen, L.M. *et al.* (2011) *Five Ways of Doing Qualitative Analysis Phenomenological Psychology, Grounded Theory, Discourse Analysis, Narrative Research, and Intuitive Inquiry*, The Guilford Press, New York, NY.

Wojnar, D.M. and Swanson, K.M. (2007) Phenomenology: an exploration. *Journal of Holistic Nursing*, **25** (3), 172–180.

Zahavi, D. (2019). *Phenomenology: The Basics*, Routledge, New York, NY.

Further Reading

Dahlberg, K., Dahlberg, H. and Nyström, M. (2008) *Reflective Lifeworld Research*, 2nd edn, Studentlitteratur, Lund.

Galvin, K.T. and Holloway, I. (2014) Phenomenology, in *The Research Process in Nursing* (eds. K. Gerrish and A. Lacey), Blackwell, Oxford, pp. 224–238.

Todres, L. (2011) *Embodied Enquiry: Phenomenological Touchstones for Research, Psychotherapy and Spirituality*, 2nd edn, Palgrave Macmillan, Basingstoke.

Chapter 14

Action Research

Action research (AR) or participatory action research (PAR) is generally carried out by practitioners who are, or become, researchers or work in partnership with academic researchers. Action research is a useful approach in working with patients and service users to investigate practice and to explore improvements or develop new approaches. It can also take the form of cooperative inquiry (also known as collaborative inquiry (Heron, 1996; Reason, 1988)) and concerns research 'with people' rather than 'on people'. In the widest sense it is oriented towards social transformation and has its roots in social justice. For example, most recently it has been used to underpin explorations of sustainability (Apgar *et al.*, 2019).

KEY POINT

Action research can only be carried out through meaningful collaboration between researchers and participants.

   AR is carried out through a cyclical process in which each cycle builds on the cycle preceding it. The aim is to solve practical problems in a specific location or context and improve the situation or develop new understandings of it. It is a useful approach to organisational or professional change and improvement; it has been increasingly applied to professional and organisational settings in education since the early 1990s and in nursing and other forms of healthcare in the late 1990s. Seminal work in nursing by Meyer (2000) demonstrates that practitioners can work as both informants and researchers to examine issues and practical problems in their own clinical or educational settings. Community development is another area in which AR is often carried out. Researchers can use both qualitative and quantitative methods and give priority to triangulated sources of data and information about the context of the study. AR is not a 'pure' research approach but a particular style and development, and researchers can use many of the well-known methods and strategies. AR is not distinguished from other types of research by the use of different research procedures, but it

---

differs in some of its aims and processes; any of the conventional approaches may be carried out in its research phase. As the name implies, AR includes both research and action. Other terms often used instead of AR are co-operative inquiry or collaborative research.

Action research is more than mere production of knowledge about a problem, a topic or an area of study and involves situations where change is necessary or desirable, and researchers employ interventions to improve practice. At its most radical level, AR can support transformation in ecological and systemic breakdown (Bradbury and Divecha, 2020).

Action researchers claim that AR differs from other research mainly because:

- It has different aims, two of them being evaluation and reflection.
- Researchers collaborate with practitioners, stakeholders, or are themselves participants in the setting to be studied.
- The process integrates action as an essential element.
- As well as research, it can include intervention and change in the situation under study.
- It is research in the setting where the changes take place.
- The findings can be of immediate benefit as solutions to problems can be implemented and assessed straight away.

Because of its complexity and time consumption, AR is more appropriate for small rather than large studies. Language use also differs from that of other approaches as it must be understood by all the participants and not be full of academic terminology or researcher jargon.

The origins of action research

AR does not have a very long history but it started in the 1940s. It is becoming popular and interdisciplinary, but in education it has been used often and for a long time. Lewin (1946), the social psychologist, was one of the early pioneers to develop AR, although he used it differently from more recent action researchers. The concept of change, however, was already present in this type of research, and he wanted to employ AR to bring about change in behaviour. Lewin adopted a number of stages, which consisted of

- Planning an initial step to change a setting or individuals' behaviour.
- Implementing the change.
- Evaluating the results of the change.
- Modifying the actions in the light of the evaluation.
- Starting the process all over again.

Although modern action researchers still use the stage approach, much has changed; in particular AR has become more democratic and participatory. Action researchers now take account of the power relationships inherent in a setting as a central tenet of the approach.

The Tavistock Institute of Human Relations set up organisational AR from the late 1940s onwards – although at this stage the type of research was not called AR. The members of the Institute, in general psychologists, developed a problem-solving approach. At a later stage, this problem-solving approach was also used to help deprived communities to solve social and educational problems and ameliorate the 'cycle of deprivation'. Since the work of the Tavistock Institute, AR has been carried out in many disciplines including management, sociology, healthcare and other disciplines. Often it is interdisciplinary and interprofessional.

Critical social theory

Many ideas of modern AR have their basis in critical social theory and critical social science. Carr and Kemmis (1986), in an education context have provided an overview of these, and some of their longstanding ideas are summarised here.

Critical theory is critical of positivist and complementary to interpretive research. Critical theorists of the 1950s, such as Horkheimer, Adorno, Marcuse and others, criticised the dominance of positivist social science in the twentieth century, which conformed to rigid rules and stifled critical and creative thinking, although they did agree with the scientific aim of generating rigorous knowledge about social life. While retrieving for social science, those elements that are connected with values and human interests, they also tried to integrate these into a new framework that included ethical and critical thought. Like positivists, however, they still considered rigorous knowledge about social life as a requirement of social science.

Habermas (1974) discusses human behaviour in terms of interests and needs. He argues that knowledge consists of three constitutive interests, which he calls the *technical*, the *practical* and the *emancipatory*. The technical interest helps people to gain knowledge in order to achieve technical control over nature. This instrumental knowledge requires scientific explanations. Habermas suggests that, although this form of knowledge is necessary, not everything can be reduced to scientific explanations, and people need to grasp the social meanings of life to understand others. Generating knowledge through interpretive methods can serve 'practical' interests, but this still does not suffice. Human beings need 'emancipatory' knowledge in order to achieve freedom and autonomy, overcome social problems and change power relationships. This will diminish alienation. The thinking of Habermas (1972, 1974) (developed in his books) is based in Marxist philosophy. (His theories cannot be developed here; this section merely gives a flavour of the thinking behind modern AR. Habermas also discusses the relationship between theory and practice.)

Educationists in the 1970s and 1980s developed ideas for AR, because they pressed for change in educational settings and society within a critical theory framework. The concept of 'conscientization' discussed by Freire (1970), the Marxist educationist, is also connected to critical social science. Freire believed that people become increasingly aware of the social and historical reality that influences their lives and are able to take action in order to change it. McTaggart and Kemmis (1982) developed guidelines in an AR planner, also intended for educational research and several texts on AR planning are available (Kemmis *et al.*, 2014; Sagor and William, 2016; Mills 2017). Although educational and community development studies are not directly connected to AR in nursing and healthcare, the underlying ideas are important and transferable as health researchers too desire the empowerment of patients, users of services, the public who will be able to take control of their own lives and change their situation. AR has, however, lost much of the ideas of its Marxist antecedents, while valuing democracy and equality in action. Indeed, McNiff (2013: 50) contends that 'the aim of critical theory is to critique not to initiate or manage change'.

Action research in healthcare

As AR focused on improving education and society, it was also seen as useful in nursing and other healthcare arenas. In the words of Hart and Bond (1995: 3) who provide clear typologies, 'It represents a counter to positivism and can develop reflexive practice and general theory from this practice'. It is, in their view, a tool for practitioners, as knowledge is vital for improving healthcare practice; only those involved in the setting are fully able to apply this knowledge. AR generates practical knowledge intended to assist in raising standards of care and delivery of service in general. It is not 'blue skies research'. Health workers now use it but do not always go back to its base and develop it merely on a practical level rather than taking into account its added importance in developing theory. Because of its complexity and length of time for development, AR is growing but not as fast as in the 1990s or 2000s.

One of the aims of AR is bridging the theory–practice gap as this gap has been seen as detrimental to professional and clinical work. The main justification for doing health research is improvement in practice. In the health professions, AR is also a useful way of attempting and evaluating change in order to improve settings and care in the clinical arena. Professionals are able, through AR, to undertake research into their own practices. Earlier deeply held assumptions might be questioned. This is linked to the reasons McNiff (2013) gives for engaging in AR, and these can be applied to nursing and health research. She suggests that the aims are political, professional and personal. Through AR, health professionals are able to make sense of the clinical situation and become aware of the impact of policies and practices imposed on them through the system. They will also recognise more clearly that the health services and guidelines for care and treatment should exist initially for the good of the patients and ultimately for the health of society. Meyer and Cooper (2015: 305) give some examples where AR is useful in nursing and healthcare research:

- When evidence is lacking for refuting or confirming current practices.
- When not enough skills or information is available.
- When gaps in knowledge have been identified.
- When service provision is inadequate.

As professionals, health researchers make independent decisions while adopting procedures based on theory and research rather than being controlled by outside forces. AR helps professionals to make decisions in the interest of their clients (Carr and Kemmis, 1986). Rather than accepting unsatisfactory decisions imposed on them, they observe and diagnose problems as well as plan and implement changes that are based on the knowledge gained through the research. In AR, professionals need to adopt a thinking and self-critical stance towards their practice which enables them to justify what they do.

On a personal level, AR not only improves the situation for people and patients, but also enlightens the practitioners themselves and enhances their lives through reflection and engagement in the situation. The clinical setting provides the opportunity for active involvement and personal satisfaction and hence for personal growth.

Example 14.1 Review of Action Research in Mental Health Nursing Care

Sixteen studies, half of which used PAR, were included in a systematic review by Moreno-Poyato *et al.* (2022). Nurses, with other stakeholders, were actively engaged in the action research process. The authors categorized the main areas of inquiry as improving the adoption of a person-centred approach to care and improving decision-making procedures. The authors also observed that the use of action research helped participants identify the meaning they attached to the topic of interest to be improved in the AR studies, and also helped identify needs and strategies for improving care alongside an enhanced sense of empowerment for participants.

The main features of action research

Action research is more than just the generation or production of knowledge about an area of interest in which change is seen as necessary or desirable to improve practice. Researchers carry out interventions in the setting to be investigated. The main features of good AR include the following:

- AR draws data and information from a range of sources.
- AR is cyclical and dynamic.
- AR is collaborative and participatory.

- The aim of AR is to devise solutions to practical problems and to develop theory.
- Researchers and practitioners are critical, self-critical and reflective.

AR draws data from a range of sources and perspectives: for instance, data sources might be interviews and observation, documents or diaries. AR is cyclical in the sense that it represents an action cycle consisting of planning, implementing action, observing and reflecting. Then the process starts again. Lewin (1946) already demanded these four stages, which he developed into a 'spiral'. The difference between his and modern AR is that present-day research is not imposed from outside the organisation or setting but planned and carried out by insiders, namely participants in the setting.

Lewin's (1946) stages still form the basis for AR, and Parahoo (2014) describes the use of the process in nursing where the stages are similar, though the aims and character of AR are different in some ways in clinical and educational nursing from those of earlier AR:

- Researchers identify a problem in practice.
- They carry out research to assess the problem.
- They plan and implement the change.
- They evaluate the outcome.
- After this, the cycle starts again.

AR is collaborative. It involves individuals who choose this approach in the design, data collection and analysis and evaluation of the research as well as in its dissemination. This fulfils the criterion of empowerment and assists emancipation. Because the research influences and intervenes in the participants' working lives, they should be included in decision-making.

Once a problem or an important issue has been highlighted and the need for change and improvement is clearly observed, participants develop the focus for the research as co-researchers. The research centres on the problem or issue in the situation in which they work or learn and on a specific location. Modern-day AR is always collaborative and participatory. The researchers are often themselves involved in the system they study, but even when they are not, they work with practitioners and professionals to carry out the research.

KEY POINT

Action research is based in a specific situation and context with a view to change in practice.

The methodological continuum

There are different types of AR as suggested earlier and many of these are used depending on the intentions of the co-researchers. The most common in nursing were identified early by Hart and Bond (1995) and Holter and Schwartz-Barcott

(1993), but the differences between them are not vast, and they overlap. Because the typology of the latter is inclusive, it will be discussed here.

Holter and Schwartz-Barcott distinguish between three approaches:

1 Technical collaborative
2 Mutual collaborative
3 Enhancement

In the *technical collaborative* approach, the researcher acts as a professional expert who pre-plans the research, carries out the research with practitioners, advises on action and acts as facilitator. It has a pre-specified framework and theory and is rarely qualitative.

The *mutual collaborative* approach entails a more democratic process. The researcher(s) as facilitator and the practitioners collaborate to identify a problem. They plan intervention and change together, and they work as equal partners. Theory is developed rather than predetermined. This mode of AR is more flexible than the technical approach. It is designed to solve immediate and practical problems and needs quick decision-making. There is the danger, however, that the practitioners will not continue when the facilitator leaves the clinical area.

The goals of the *enhancement approach* are, firstly to bridge the theory and practice gap to solve problems and explain them and, secondly, to raise awareness so that practitioners can identify problems and make them explicit. While the mutual collaboration approach fosters mutual understanding, the enhancement approach leads to emancipation of all participants. Some suggest that one of the aims of this approach is the creation of action-oriented policy, which means that this type of AR continues after the facilitator leaves. Berg and Lune (2014) state that groups in particular need a skilled facilitator or moderator.

The link between theory and practice generates empowerment because practitioners gain deeper understanding and are therefore able to apply it in different settings, not just in one location at a particular time.

Although now over 20 years old, Lax and Galvin (2002) describe the differences between AR and PAR, as the two terms remain often used interchangeably; indeed, Koshy *et al.* (2013) state that there are various names for this type of inquiry such as co-operative inquiry, action science and so on. Although often used in community development, PAR has not as often been used in nursing. Kemmis and McTaggart (2000) stress the significance of participation in PAR, which has a stronger element of participation than other types of AR. They state that it usually has three main features of importance:

• *Shared Ownership*: The projects are owned by all who take part in them.
• *Community-Based Analysis*: The collaborators investigate social problems that occur in a community.
• *Orientation Towards Community Action*: The findings will be acted upon among the participating group.

Early developers of PAR include Reason (1988), Heron (1996) and Fals Borda (2001), who claim that it is a way by which participants can take power and control in the research. These ideas have been updated by the later work edited by Reason and Bradbury (2013). Its aim is empowerment, emancipation and the generation of knowledge that benefits them directly. The researchers in this type of AR are much more aware of the elements of power and control.

Example 14.2 Participatory Action Research

In Denmark, Steensgaard *et al.* (2022) undertook a 2-year Action research study investigating nursing initiatives in a spinal cord injury rehabilitation setting. Eight nursing staff participated as co-researchers. Their findings demonstrated that action research processes facilitated the development of four communicative initiatives and they were able to delineate a demonstrable shift in the nursing staff's support of the patient. The process supported an awareness of the patient's perspective which in turn facilitated a caring, attentive and engaged approach from the nursing staff, this promoted rehabilitation tailored to the individual.

Practical steps

We will now describe an example of the practical steps which researcher-practitioners take while going through an AR cycle in clinical or educational practice. Meyer (2006) calls these phases the exploration, intervention and evaluation phase.

1 Researchers and practitioners carefully observe what is happening in the setting. Before starting the AR, all participants should agree on their participation in the project. Usually, they formulate the question together and take decisions. This entails a number of meetings in which procedures will be discussed. These meetings include managers and policymakers who need to give permission for the project to proceed and for access to all the participants. Initially, there is a critical assessment of all the aspects of current practice and a review of its effectiveness, quality and cost-effectiveness. In this early stage, much negotiation between different factions takes place.

2 Researcher–practitioners identify problem areas that they want to improve and thoroughly examine the practices that seem to need change and intervention. They 'explore the nature of the problem' (Meyer, 2006: 282) and then discuss this with their colleagues and others interested in the project, including clients, and ask for their ideas and confirmation of the areas in need of improvement. Observations, interviews and brainstorming and focus group sessions take place to ascertain the problem.

   At this stage, researchers plan changes and interventions and implement them in the practice setting. Planning includes drawing up a budget, suggesting a timescale and giving the details of procedures happening.

3 During the implementation of change or intervention, an evaluation process takes place which carefully monitors all the steps and procedures. This is done through a number of meetings with the people in the setting as well as observation and interviewing.

4 In the light of this careful evaluation, practitioners modify their practices to improve on the intervention or change. Meyer states that there is no tidy end to AR; processes are often ongoing beyond the formal project, or they are sometimes disrupted because of new managers and colleagues that enter the setting.

The action and monitoring process continues until practitioners are satisfied with the level of improvement. Throughout the whole process there will be meetings and discussions. The number of meetings depends on the size and duration of the project. Record keeping is also of major importance and participants write progress reports and give account of their actions to each other and to their managers. One can use both focus groups, individual interviews, meetings and discussions about the research and the outcomes of actions, but groups might also be fruitful as these can give more opportunity to participants to discuss their experiences with others (Stringer, 2014).

Much useful AR can be carried out with patients, users of the services and lay carers. Dowswell *et al.* (1999: 751) advise researchers on the stages of AR while describing their own project. The following are some excerpts from their account and demonstrate what needs to be done by other researchers.

- *Preliminary Stage:* All participants are involved in the proposal and understand the reasons for the project. It is important that they all agree and willingly take part in it.
- *Assessment Phase:* Ethical issues are clarified and anonymity ensured. Aims and limitations are truthfully described.
- *Planning Phase:* Participants find innovative ways of solving problems and carry out agreed tasks and reflect on decision-making.
- *Implementation Phase:* All participants, regardless of ability, must be comfortable with the materials and incorporate both theory and practice.
- *Evaluation Phase:* Interviews, observations and written reviews are used to evaluate the project.

The processes of data collection and analysis are those of other qualitative research.

It is advisable that all collaborators are trained in research skills to carry out observation and interviews as well as acquiring skills to analyse the data. They also learn to reflect on their own beliefs and assumptions and to make them explicit as well as on the situation. This also means identifying the audit trail of the research process, explaining in detail what they have done and thought. The ongoing documentation of what goes on also helps planning and avoids chaos.

Example 14.3 New Approaches to De-colonise Research

Rumsey *et al.* (2022) have developed a novel approach designed to advance qualitative methods in cross-cultural health research. This methodology was developed by synthesising several research methods and involved in-depth stakeholder consultation with participants of a Pacific-based nursing and midwifery health leadership program. They examined the ways in which PAR and local Pacific methods can be synthesised to produce' PARcifi'c – a methodological framework for cross-cultural research in the collectivist cultures. The PARcific methodology, combines PAR, *Talanoa* and *Kakala*, to provide researchers with a framework for guiding their behaviour and interactions with research participants in the Pacific region, with potential application for the wider community. The PARcific framework and methodology is still in early development. This provides a useful example of how wide ranging the use of AR can be in the pursuit of transformative action, which is at the historical heart of the approach.

Trustworthiness in AR

The criteria for validity or its equivalent are often discussed and developed by qualitative researchers. Waterman claims that an unquestioning acceptance of general criteria for qualitative research does not suffice for AR and describes three types of validity:

1 *Dialectical Validity:* tensions and processes
2 *Critical Validity:* moral responsibilities
3 *Reflexive Validity:* valuing ourselves

First, Waterman (1998) points to the importance of examining the inherent tensions of an AR project. It implies attention to and description of details in the ongoing process as well as the conflicts and tensions between practice, theory and research. Second, she describes the moral responsibility of researchers who have to be aware and take account of the problems of people in the setting. Decision-making not only includes action but also knowing when not to take action. Waterman goes on to say that researchers have the responsibility to give reasons for their decisions and argue their cause, as the ultimate aim is 'to improve people's lives'. Third, the reflexive nature of AR is acknowledged. The final report of an AR project should reflect the variety of perspectives that were examined. There is the important dilemma of the multiple roles of researchers who are, in the same study, research participants, change agents and evaluators of change. This position needs a reflexive stance by researchers on their own practices and assumptions. Whilst 'valuing themselves', researchers must also be aware of their own biases and limitations. Another important aspect for judging AR is the existence of more than one cycle. Some researchers who maintain that they have used AR do not go further than a single cycle.

Whatever the criteria for trustworthiness might be, all the collaborators involved in an AR study must agree on the issues. For a project to be truly based on AR, they should reflect together on data collection, analysis and other methodological and procedural issues, because reflection on action is inherent in this approach. In AR, researchers need perhaps more reflection and reflectivity than in other research projects. Evaluation of a programme or action needs careful consideration, particularly when further actions are based on it. Meyer (2006: 284) asks the questions that can identify whether an AR project had 'quality'. This includes questions about the usefulness of the research and whether it led to major improvement, the involvement of all people in the setting, and the appropriateness of research methods. AR depends on active collaboration.

Guidance on assessment of the quality of AR projects and proposals can be found in Waterman *et al.* (2001: 43).

Problems and critique

Of course, AR can be problematic for a number of reasons. First, it is obvious that not everybody may wish to be involved. It takes diplomacy and persuasion to recruit reluctant participants. While undertaking the research, practitioners may be in conflict with each other. Managers, too, may make objections especially if the process takes too much time or is expensive.

AR is not always appropriate, and it can be atheoretical. Morton-Cooper (2000: 25) suggests certain situations in which it should not be used:

- If the policy or service to be implemented is forced on the people in the setting, especially when managers have already made their own decisions about this.
- If the procedures and methodology used have not met the same quality criteria as other clinically based studies.
- If the members of the team giving care, treatment or service do not work well together.
- If the researchers want to enhance their own status and reputation.

We would have to add that AR takes time and is complex because of its cyclical nature.

Meyer (1993) also notes some problems and limitations of AR. She identifies the problem of defining stages in AR when it is difficult to describe them before the start of the research as they develop during its process. This also means that informed consent is problematic because the stages are unknown beforehand. She warns researchers that the members of the participating team – which may consist of practitioners and facilitators as experts in research – should be able to collaborate willingly and with a common aim rather than by edict and selection of management. Power relationships may also have inherent problems: research experts from outside have to negotiate rather than using their expertise as control. Waterman *et al.* (2001) suggest, among other problems, that the familiarity of co-researchers with the setting might result in 'cloud understanding'. Again, this means that they have to become 'professional strangers' or naïve observers of their own situation.

While researchers in other types of inquiry are advised to avoid research in their own setting, AR is carried out in their own location and thus situationally specific and unique. This of course, makes it more difficult and ethically complex. When undertaking research in one's own setting, issues of anonymity and confidentiality might become problematic; because of the different personalities and backgrounds of the people involved, it is not always easy to gain consent. Indeed, often tensions and conflicts between individuals occur which have to be resolved. All must be consulted and agree to the steps that will be undertaken and the decisions that are being made. As in all health research, participation should be voluntary.

Sustaining relationships might also present problems in AR as the research and action cycles can go on over a long stretch of time (Algeo, 2013), and the people in the setting become partners in the research. All the participants should be able to trust each other; the relationships become problematic if the participants feel under threat.

Some health professions still do not see AR as a credible, scientific research because it is not generalisable. It is, however, used in healthcare because it can offer transferable practical solutions to complex problems and also contribute to the enhancement of theory. Morrison and Lilford (2001) describe the dilemma inherent in AR. Action researchers have developed innovative and imaginative ways of developing practice and theory that could be applied in all research approaches. In their enthusiasm, however, they maintain that a major difference from traditional research (or mainstream research) exists. In fact, Morrison and Lilford argue, many of the tenets of AR could be applied to mainstream research. There is only one major difference: AR takes account of its unique social context. However, one might argue that this is true for much of qualitative research which is context-bound, meaning that the specific context in which it takes place has to be taken into account. This does not necessarily indicate that the findings of one specific context cannot be applied in other contexts, or that the theoretical advances are not useful in other settings. The researcher should also be able to apply what is learnt from one situation to another setting. AR is, nevertheless, of most use in a specific context in which a local problem needs a solution or where actions and thinking need improvement. This supports the claim by Waterman *et al.* (2001) about AR as 'real-world research'.

This chapter does not elaborate on how to carry out the data collection procedures in action research, as the research strategies may include many types of qualitative (and indeed, quantitative) methods. Action research offers a framework for research with people drawing on a range of data sources and methods. Data collection and analytic procedures can be found in the other chapters of this book.

Summary

- Inherent in AR is the wish for empowerment, at minimum collaborative working.
- The outcome of AR is improvement in a specific situation or deep understanding of its complexity in partnership with people in the situation.
- AR draws data from a range of data sources.
- Researchers can apply a number of different approaches.
- AR bridges the theory–practice gap and is 'real-world' research.
- AR includes planning, action or intervention and evaluation.
- It is cyclical, reflective and dynamic.
- Highly useful in transformative practice

References

Algeo, C. (2013) The researcher–participant relationship in action research: a case study involving Australian project managers. International Conference of Education, Research and Innovation Proceedings, pp. 6042–6049.

Apgar, M., Ortiz Aragón, A. and Gray, P. (2019). Bridging the territory between me, we, and living earth: six explorations into action research for sustainability. *Action Research*, **17** (3), 279–291. doi:10.1177/1476750319864413.

Berg, B.L. and Lune, H. (2014) *Qualitative Research for the Social Sciences*, 8th edn, Allyn and Bacon, Boston, MA.

Bradbury, H. and Divecha, S. (2020). Action methods for faster transformation: relationality in action. *Action Research*, **18** (3), 273–281. doi:10.1177/1476750320936493.

Carr, W. and Kemmis, S. (1986) *Becoming Critical: Education*, Knowledge and Action Research, The Falmer Press, London.

Dowswell, G., Forster, A., Young, J. *et al.* (1999) The development of a collaborative stroke training programme for nurses. *Journal of Clinical Nursing*, **8**, 743–752.

Fals Borda, O. (2001) Participatory (action) research in social theory, in *Handbook of Action Research: Participatory Inquiry and Practice* (eds. P. Reason and H. Bradbury), Sage, London, pp. 27–37.

Freire, P. (1970) *Cultural Action for Freedom*, Centre for the Study of Change, Cambridge, MA.

Habermas, J. (1972) *Knowledge and Human Interest* (translated by J. Shapiro), Heinemann, London.

Habermas, J. (1974) *Theory and Practice* (translated by J. Viertel), Heinemann, London.

Hart, E. and Bond, M. (1995) *Action Research for Health and Social Care: A Guide to Practice*, Open University Press, Buckingham.

Heron, J. (1996) *Co-operative Inquiry*, Sage, London. (Later edition in 2015).

Holter, I.M. and Schwartz-Barcott, D. (1993) Action research: what is it? How has it been used and how can it be used in nursing? *Journal of Advanced Nursing*, **18** (2), 298–304.

Kemmis, S. and McTaggart, R. (2000) Participatory action research, in *Handbook of Qualitative Research* (eds. N.K. Denzin and Y.S. Lincoln), Sage, Thousand Oaks, CA, pp. 567–605.

Kemmis, S., McTaggart, R. and Nixon, R. (2014) *Action Research Planner: Doing Critical Participatory Action Research*, Springer, Singapore.

Koshy, E., Koshy, V. and Waterman, H. (2013) *Action Research in Healthcare*, Sage, London.

Lax, W. and Galvin, K. (2002) Reflections on a community action research project: interprofessional issues and methodological problems. *Journal of Clinical Nursing*, **11**, 1–11.

Lewin, K. (1946) Action research and minority problems. *Journal of Social Issues*, **2**, 34–46.

McNiff, J. (2013) *Action Research: Principles and Practice*, 3rd edn, Routledge, London.

McTaggart, R. and Kemmis, S. (1982) *The Action Research Planner*, Deakin University Press, Geelong, Victoria.

Meyer, J.E. (1993) New paradigm research in practice: the trials and tribulations of action research. *Journal of Advanced Nursing*, **18** (7), 1066–1072.

Meyer, J.E. (2000) Using qualitative methods in health related action research. *BMJ*, **320** (7228), 178–181.

Meyer, J.E. (2006) Action research, in *The Research Process in Nursing* (eds. K. Gerrish and A. Lacey), 5th edn, Blackwell Science, Oxford, pp. 274–288.

Meyer, J. and Cooper, J. (2015) Action research, in *The Research Process in Nursing* (eds. K. Gerrish and J. Lathlean), pp. 304–317.

Mills, G. (2017) *Action Research: A Guide for the Teacher Researcher*, 6th edn, Pearson, UK.

Moreno-Poyato, A.R., Subias-Miquel, M., Tolosa-Merlos, D. *et al.* (2022) A systematic review on the use of action research methods in mental health nursing care. *Journal of Advanced Nursing*, 1–13. https://doi.org/10.1111/jan.15463.

Morrison, B. and Lilford, R. (2001) How can action research apply to health services? *Qualitative Health Research*, **11** (4), 436–449.

Morton-Cooper, A. (2000) *Action Research in Health Care*, Blackwell Science, Oxford.

Parahoo, K. (2014) *Nursing Research: Principles, Process and Issues*, 3rd edn, Palgrave, Macmillan, Basingstoke.

Reason, P. (ed.) (1988) *Human Inquiry in Action: Developments in New Paradigm Research*, Sage, London.

Reason, P. and Bradbury, H. (eds.) (2013) *Handbook of Action Research: Participatory Inquiry and Practice*, 3rd edn, Sage, London.

Rumsey, M., Stowers, P., Sam, H. *et al.* (2022) Development of PARcific approach: participatory action research methodology for collectivist health research. *Qualitative Health Research*, **32** (8–9), 1297–1314. doi:10.1177/10497323221092350.

Sagor, R.D. and William, S. (2016). *The Action Research Guidebook. A Process for Pursuing Equity and Excellence in Education*, 3rd edn, Sage.

Steensgaard, R., Kolbaek, R. and Angel, S. (2022) Nursing staff facilitate patient participation by championing the patient's perspective: an action research study in spinal cord injury rehabilitation. *Health Expect*, **25** (5), 2525–2533. doi:10.1111/hex.13574.

Stringer, E.T. (2014) *Action Research: A Handbook for Practitioners*, 4th edn, Sage, Thousand Oaks, CA.

Waterman, H. (1998) Embracing ambiguities and valuing ourselves: issues of validity in action research. *Journal of Advanced Nursing*, **28** (1), 101–105.

Waterman, H., Tillen, D., Dickson, R. and de Koning, K. (2001) Action research: a systematic review and guidance for assessment. *Health Technology Assessment*, **5** (23), iii–157.

Further Reading

An issue exclusively dedicated to health is: *Action Research* (2019) **19** (4) Health and healthcare as the context for participatory action research. Sage Journals.

Bradbury, H. (ed.) (2015) *The Sage Handbook of Action Research*, Sage, London.

Brandstorp, H., Kirkengen, A.L., Sterud, B. *et al.* (2015) Leadership practice as interaction in primary care team training. *Action Research*, **13** (1), 84–101.

Davies, J., Lester, C., O'Neill, M. and Williams, G. (2008) Sustainable participation in regular exercise among older people: developing an action research approach. *Health Education Journal*, **67** (1), 45–55.

Friesen-Storms, J., Moser, A., van den Loo, S. *et al.* (2014) Systematic implementation of evidence based practice in a clinical nursing setting: a participatory action research project. *Journal of Clinical Nursing*, **24** (1–2), 57–68.

Kenny, A., Nankervis, K., Kidd, T. and Connell, S. (2012) Models of nursing student employment: an Australian action research study. *Nurse Education Today*, **32** (5), 600–605.

Kjellstrom. S. and Mitchell, A. (2019) Health and healthcare as the context for participatory action research. *Action Research*, **19** (4), 419–609.

Koch, T. and Kralik, D. (2008) *Participatory Action Research in Health and Social Care*, Wiley, Blackwell, Oxford.

McNiff, J. (2017) *Action Research: All you need to know*, Sage, London.

Munn-Giddings, C. and Winter, R. (2013) *A Handbook for Action Research in Health and Social Care*, Routledge, London (kindle edition).

Williamson, G.R., Bellman, L. and Webster, J. (2014) *Action Research in Nursing and Healthcare*, Sage, London.

Delgado-Baena, A., Serrano, L., Vela-Jiménez, R. *et al.* (2022). Epistemic injustice and dissidence: a bibliometric analysis of the literature on Participatory Action Research hosted on the Web of Science. *Action Research*. doi:10.1177/14767503221126531.

Woelder, S. and Abma, T. (2019) Participatory action research to enhance the involvement of residents in elderly care: about power, dialogue and understanding. *Action Research*, **17** (4), 528–548.

Chapter 15
Additional Approaches

There are a number of approaches which are used in qualitative research, but in the last decade, only a few have been developed in health inquiry. The most popular are case study research and performative social science, while the others seem now less prevalent. Researchers use conversation analysis and discourse analysis (DA) mainly in studies about language and interaction through language.

Case study research

Case study research is not specifically a qualitative approach and can be analysed through various means and methods. In this sense, it does not stand alone as a separate approach. The term is used for a research approach with specific boundaries and can be both qualitative and quantitative. Stake (2000, 2005) states that much qualitative research is called case study research but argues that it is very specific, 'a bounded system' and both a process as well as a product of the inquiry. Simons (2009) calls it 'the study of the singular, particular, unique'. Some researchers call anything that has boundedness and specificity a case study, but in this chapter it is referred to more specifically as research in a specific unit in an organization or with a particular individual and unique case. It can be the study of a single individual, although it need not be. A case study is an entity studied as a single unit, and it has clear confines and a specific focus and is bound to context. The boundaries of the case should be clarified in terms of the questions asked, the data sources used and the setting and person(s) involved.

Although it can be conducted as a qualitative, quantitative or mixed method design, Bryman (2016) suggests that it is usually qualitative. We shall here summarise the main features of the qualitative case study, which tends to be more common in health research. It is often combined with a specific approach to research.

Qualitative Research in Nursing and Healthcare, Fifth Edition.
Immy Holloway and Kathleen Galvin.
© 2024 John Wiley & Sons Ltd. Published 2024 by John Wiley & Sons Ltd.

Overview

The case study is used in a number of disciplines such as anthropology, sociology or geography, although not all studies of limited cases are case studies. It has been most popular in business studies, but is also used in social work and nursing.

The best-known writer on this type of research, Robert Yin, has discussed case studies in various editions of his books (the latest edition is Yin (2018)). Although his writing, on the whole, focuses on the quantitative framework, he sees the qualitative approach as valid. Case study research is not to be confused with other types of case work, case history or case study as sometimes used in student education to give examples and flavour of cases in clinical settings or indeed in business studies. Creswell and Poth (2017) suggest that the case study is bounded by both 'time and place'.

Features and purpose of case study research

Generally, researchers who develop case studies are familiar with the case they explore and its context before the start of the research. Health professionals study cases because they may be interested in it for professional reasons or because they need the knowledge about the particular case.

Example 15.1 Case Study Research

The example cited here is an investigation into the bounded phenomenon of care transitions of frail older people in acute hospital wards to community healthcare or community hospital wards. The authors carried out qualitative research study (Baillie et al., 2014). The sample consisted of staff members and frail older people. The data were collected through one-to-one interviews and focus groups. The case was the phenomenon of transition and its problems, a case with clear boundaries but with a large number of participants.

In citing this example, we wish to demonstrate that the case can be complex and multimethod while at the same time having clear boundaries.

As in other types of qualitative research, the case study is a way of exploring a phenomenon or several phenomena in context or studying the ideas or behaviour of a group or a single individual. The researchers therefore use a number of sources in their data collection, such as observation, documentary sources and interviews so that the case can be illuminated from all sides. Observation, interviewing and documentary research are the most common strategies used in case study inquiry. The case study is neither a method nor a methodology as data collection and analysis occur through specific research approaches, but it can make use of a variety of methods (Van Wynsburghe and Khan, 2007). It is something within boundaries that the researcher chooses to study. Travers (2001) gives a range of qualitative approaches which can be applied to case study research which can be used; for instance, ethnography, grounded theory, narrative analysis or other ways of inquiry can be useful in doing case study research.

The case study is determined by the individual case or cases, not by the approach that the researcher uses. The analysis of qualitative case studies involves the same techniques as that of other qualitative methods: the researcher codes and categorises, provides exhaustive descriptions, develops typologies or generates theoretical ideas depending on the approach adopted. Creswell and Poth (2017) describe features of qualitative case study research, some of which we discussed before. One of these is the in-depth understanding of the unique case; another is to give a detailed description of the case. He also differentiates between different types of qualitative case study which are distinguished by their intentions: the single instrumental case study, the multiple case study and the intrinsic case study. The instrumental case study focuses on a specific problem and then focuses on one example of this; the intrinsic case study illustrates a unique case of particular interest, while the multiple or collective case study includes several cases to illustrate the issue under investigation.

In nursing and healthcare, studies focus on individuals such as a patient or a group which might consist of individuals with common experiences or characteristics, a ward or a hospital. Life histories of individuals would also be interesting examples of cases. A process or procedure might also constitute a case. Cronin (2014) suggests that one of the aims of CSR is 'an accurate and complete description of the case', but we would argue that accuracy and completeness is the aim of other qualitative approaches too. Cronin uses an example of workplace learning to demonstrate the rigour of this form of inquiry.

In health research with a psychological emphasis, cases often focus on individuals and an aspect of their behaviour, while the sociologist is more interested in groups. In any health organisation, single or multiple cases can be examined. The local 'case' focuses on both the physical and social elements in the setting.

Example 15.2 Case Study Research

Dodds *et al.* (2020) investigated through an exploratory case study approach the facilitation of end-of-life care on three sites which had a new service for older people – in community settings within the individuals' own homes. Participants consisted of older people themselves and their informal and formal carers. The research was carried out through focus group interviews, non-participant observation and discussion workshops. The researchers concluded that "flexible, responsive, person-centred care in the liminal space between the person's lifeworld and formal health care systems" (p. 350) seemed to be beneficial in many ways.

As in other qualitative research, case studies explore the phenomenon or phenomena under study in their context, and indeed contextualisation is an important feature of all case studies. The lines of division between the phenomenon under study and the context, however, are not always clear (Yin, 2013).

When carrying out case studies, the unit of analysis has to be chosen carefully (Baxter and Jack, 2008). One might pose the question whether to analyse a programme or an individual, an organization. All these can be case studies.

Case studies can be exploratory devices, for instance as a pilot for a larger study or for other, more quantitative research, or they could illustrate the specific elements of a research project. One of our students demonstrated all the ideas she obtained from informants by writing up the case of one single participant. Usually the case study stands on its own and involves intensive observation. The description of specific cases can make a study more lively and interesting.

Case study research is used mainly to investigate cases that are tied to a specific situation and locality, and hence this type of inquiry is even less readily generalisable than other qualitative research (a debate can be found in Gomm *et al.* (2014)). Therefore, researchers are often advised to study 'typical' and multiple cases (Stake, 1995, 2010). Atypical cases, however, may sometimes be interesting because their very difference might illustrate the typical case. It is important, however, that the researcher does not make unwarranted assertions on the basis of a single case. Although there can be no generalisability of the findings from a single case, there might be some transferability of ideas if the researcher has given a detailed audit trail and used 'thick description' so that this case can illuminate other, similar cases.

Conversation analysis

Within the great variety of qualitative methods, some emphasise language and language use. Any professional–client interaction relies on language as a major communication device; body language and movement are part of this communication. Conversation(al) analysis (CA) is a type of DA that examines the use of language and asks the question of how everyday conversation works; in its basic form, it is the study of talk in everyday interaction (Hutchby and Wooffitt, 2008). This type of inquiry focuses on ordinary conversations and on the way in which talk is organised and ordered in speech exchanges. While researchers often examine speech patterns, they also analyse non-verbal behaviour in interaction such as mime, gesture and other body language. As Nofsinger (1991: 2) explains: 'If we are to understand interpersonal communication, we need to learn how this is accomplished so successfully'.

KEY POINT

CA is language-based research and a way of analysing everyday interaction and naturally occurring talk. It examines both verbal and non-verbal behaviour.

The origins of conversation analysis

Harold Garfinkel, Harvey Sacks, Emmanuel Schegloff and others initially developed CA in the 1960s and 1970s in the United States within the ethnomethodological movement. While some other types of DA have their roots in the field of linguistics, CA originates in ethnomethodology, a specialist approach in sociology and phenomenology. Ethnomethodology focuses in particular on the world of social practices, interactions and rules (see Turner, 1974). Garfinkel attempted to uncover the ways in which members of society construct social reality. Ethnomethodologists focus on the 'practical accomplishments' of members of society, seeking to demonstrate that these make sense of their actions on the basis of 'tacit knowledge', their shared understanding of the rules of interaction. This is confirmed by recent texts such as that of Hepburn and Potter (2021).

The use of conversation analysis

CA focuses on what individuals say in their everyday talk, but also on what they do (Nofsinger, 1991). Through conversation, movement and gesture, we learn of people's intentions and ideas. The sequencing and turn taking in conversations demonstrate the meaning individuals give to situations and show how they inhabit a shared world. Body movements too, are the focus of analysis. Conversation analysts do not use interviewing to collect data but analyse ordinary talk, 'naturally occurring' conversations. Most sections of talk analysed are relatively small, and the analysis is detailed. According to Heritage (1988: 130), CA makes the assumptions that talk is structurally organised, and each turn of talk is influenced by the context of what has gone on before and establishes a context towards which the next turn will be oriented. There are two other fundamental tenets of CA according to Heritage: sequential organisation and empirical grounding of analysis. Talk happens in organised patterns; the action of the member who takes part in the conversation is dependent on and makes reference to the context, and researchers should avoid generalities and premature theory building (Silverman, 2014).

CA is more often used in sociological or education studies than in nursing or other disciplines within the healthcare arena. There are a few studies in journals of health research, though not many. It can contribute a valuable research approach in nursing and healthcare and lead to changes in the interaction between health professionals and patients. Researchers generally audio- or videotape these interactions and transcribe the conversations in a particular way (techniques and notation system discussed in the handbook by Sidnell and Stivers (2014)) largely developed by Gail Jefferson who was involved in the formation of CA with Schegloff.

There are examples in health research of doctor–patient or nurse–patient interaction, particularly in consultations which show how talk is generated and organised by the participants and follows an orderly process in which a turn-taking system exists (Sharrock and Anderson, 1987; Bergstrom *et al.*, 1992; Chatwin, 2014). The recent examples we discovered were in the area of health professional and client interaction (see, for instance, Campion and Langdon, 2004). These interactions are usually taped and the tapes show what actually takes place in a setting.

Example 15.3 Conversation Analysis

Wu (2021) conducted research in two Chinese hospitals considering the relationships and interactions between nurses and patients through CA. According to this inquiry, the project described the empathy nurses had, by sequencing and listening to nurses talk during interaction with patients. This explored and illuminated the expression of empathy for nurses and helped to improve the interaction skills of nurses.

CA has been used in different health settings, especially in primary healthcare. Chatwin (2014) gives examples of interaction being videotaped such as helping clients from a chair, giving them food and so on. CA uncovers rules and routines in interaction but also shows how these can affect a situation. The approach has implications for care. The recent scandals in care homes have demonstrated the impact of filming in interaction. Analysing tapes for research purposes could be useful, although, of course, in a less dramatic way.

Jones (2003) investigated the communication and interaction between nurses and patients in healthcare consultations and found that CA was a useful way to undertake this. He regrets that this way of studying talk is not often used in the field. Sequences of talk can be studied, and he suggests that they illuminate processes such as treatment, advice and assessment. The disadvantages of CA he sees as the length of time that is needed for this research approach, and the potential lack of context as the focus on direct interaction and communication might become isolated from the social context.

The analysis of CA includes the discovery of regularities in speech or body movement, the search for deviant cases and the integration with other findings without overgeneralisation (Heritage, 1988). One of the disadvantages is the way in which conversation analysts emphasise the formal characteristics of interaction at the expense of content; however, much can be discerned from the way the communication and interaction proceeds. Ten Have (2014) describes ways of analysing CA data, and researchers might find his book useful. Turn taking is also of particular importance.

Example 15.4 Conversation Analysis

In Switzerland, Schoeb *et al.* (2014) analysed physiotherapist and patient consultations about goal setting, with 37 patients presenting with musculoskeletal problems. Twelve physiotherapists were involved. The emphasis was on the sequences of communication. The first five consultations were videotaped, and the focus was on expectations about treatment. Again, Jefferson's system of notation of talk was used. The study, among other factors, re-affirmed the findings of other research, namely the asymmetry between health professionals' ideas about goal setting and those of patients. This is important knowledge for physiotherapists.

CA is difficult, highly complex and very detailed. Researchers might not find it easy, and we would not recommend it to novices or undergraduate students.

Discourse analysis

DA is a complex concept and confusion exists about this area of research (Cheek, 2004), in other words, it is an umbrella term. It cannot be easily identified, as people use it in different ways; it is more a framework or holistic theoretical stance. Discourse in general is applied to talk and text, such as that in conversations, interviews or documents. Traynor (2006) re-emphasises that it is an analysis of naturally occurring talk, one of the most important sources of data, although talk is not the only discourse that might be analysed.

Example 15.5 Discourse Analysis

McCabe and Sambrook (2013) carried out a DA about the links between psychological contracts and professional and organisational commitment of nurses and nurse managers within a large acute and a small community organisation in the NHS. The researchers interviewed 12 nurses and 11 nurse managers. They considered DA as the appropriate approach to investigate the topic. The discourses examined were those surrounding healthcare delivery 'expressed through competing professional versus basic job discourses and between local and business discourses' (p. 965). The overall findings showed that nurses are controlled by relational psychological contracts based on commitment to the profession. Perceived breaches in contract led to dissatisfaction and turnover as well as to lower organisational commitment and job performance, depending on the type of psychological contract.

DA in psychology is an analysis of text and language drawing on 'accounts' of experiences and thoughts that participants present and their behaviour in interaction. This type of DA has been carried out mainly by psychologists. Accounts consist of forms of ordinary talk and reasoning of people, as well as other sources of text, such as historical documents, diaries, letters or reports and even images such as photographs, drawings or paintings. It can also be used to analyse films or videos of interactions between health professionals and patients. DA is not a method but a specific approach to the social world and research (Potter and Wetherell, 1987; Potter, 1996; Cheek, 2004). It focuses on the construction of talk and text in social action and interaction. In common with other types of qualitative inquiry, discourse analysts initially use an inductionist approach by collecting and reviewing data before arriving at theories and general principles as does other qualitative researchers. The way people use language and text is taken for granted within a culture (Gill, 1996) and this shows that discourse is context-bound. DA as the structural analysis of discourse is often used in media and communication research to analyse data. An example would be an analysis of the speech messages of politicians.

Language itself and reality are socially constructed. The vocabularies which individuals and groups use are located in interpretive 'repertoires' that are coherent and related sets of terms. Crowe (2005: 55) adds to this that discourses show how 'social relations, identities, knowledge and power are constructed in spoken and written text.

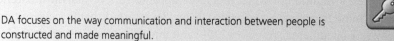

KEY POINT

DA focuses on the way communication and interaction between people is constructed and made meaningful.

It is important to read the documents and transcripts of interviews carefully before interpreting them. The first step in the analysis is a close look at and detailed description of other, less language-based sources. The relevant documents are read and re-read until researchers have become familiar with the data, be they textual or visual. Immersion in the data, after all, is a trait of all qualitative research. Important issues and themes can then be highlighted. The analysis proceeds like other qualitative research: analysts code the data, look for relationships and search for patterns and regularities that generate tentative propositions. Through the process, they always take the context into account and generate analytical notes as in other forms of qualitative inquiry. Analysis of ordinary talk and language proceeds in the same way.

Also, like for other qualitative research, the findings from DA are not instantly generalisable; indeed, researchers are not overly concerned with generalisability, because the analysis is based on language and text in a specific social context. There are a number of similarities between conversation analysis – another way of handling data – and DA: both CA and DA focus on language and text. While DA generally considers the broader context, CA emphasises turn-taking and explains the deeper sense of interaction in which people are engaged, particularly 'naturally occurring' talk, while discourse analysts look at the material more holistically, and they can also use records, newspaper articles or reports of meetings and so on. McMullen discusses DA and gives an example of it in the book by Wertz *et al.* (2011: 205).

Discourse analysts are interested in the ways through which social reality is constructed in interaction and action. DA is based on the belief that language (and presentation of images) does not just mirror the world of social members and cultures but also helps to construct it.

Potter and Wetherell (1987) developed the notion of 'interpretative repertoires', which they saw as a set of related concepts organised around one or several important metaphors. These provide researchers with common sense concepts of a group or a culture. Language is 'action oriented': It is used so people can 'do' and be shaped by the cultural and social context in which it occurs. Social groups possess a variety of repertoires and use them appropriately in different situations. The discourses or narratives of people about various specific areas in their lives generate a text. Discourse analysts must therefore be aware of the context in which action takes place so that the context can be analysed as well. The same text can be interpreted in different ways: different versions of reality exist in different contexts. The DA of psychologists and linguists focuses on language and text. Readers can make judgements about this type of research because they themselves possess knowledge of everyday discourse and its construction. Potter and Wetherell (2007) have since updated their work.

Critical discourse analysis (CDA)

Researchers sometimes distinguish between DA and critical discourse analysis (CDA). The latter is related to the concepts of power and inequality, and analysis shows how these are constructed and maintained. Morgan (2010) also asserts that CDA is political and shows powerful groups create dominant discourses. It is often used in discussing welfare policies, racism and sexism. It is interesting, for instance, how the language about welfare reforms and policy is produced and reproduced in newspapers or journals. Traynor (2006) stresses that people persuade others, present themselves to others and act in particular ways; how this occurs is important and involves power relationships. This can be shown in speech, text or image. For instance, professionals or politicians use particular types of discourse to impose their own or the official version of reality on their audience or readership. DA can be applied to micro-settings but also in a larger context. The following study encompasses both. Laura Funk, a Canadian researcher, for instance, investigated home healthcare and family responsibility through a critical analysis of talk and text in qualitative interviews of homecare decision-makers and opinion leaders in this field. In the larger research project, nine government and agency documents about home healthcare and family responsibility were examined as well as handbooks concerning the latter.

Example 15.6 Critical Discourse Analysis

According to Munro and Beck (2021), the reforms intended in wound care nursing education provision and practice, are not implemented by those at whom they are aimed. The authors explored this area through CDA and provided an insight into the problem. They concluded that policy makers should use an 'active approach' to policy making. This article illuminates the usefulness of CDA but has to be read in full for an understanding of DA.

McHoul and Grace (1995) differentiate between Foucauldian and non-Foucauldian discourse (although these are not completely separate). Michel Foucault, the French historian and philosopher, made the concept of discourse famous while describing the links of language with disciplines and institutions. For him, discourses are bodies of knowledge, by which he means both academic scholarship and institutions, which exist in disciplines. Indeed, he claims that discourse reproduces institutions. In Foucault's work, discourse is focused on power. Social phenomena are constructed through language. Specific language is connected with specialist fields, for instance 'professional discourse', 'scientific discourse' or 'medical discourse'; for instance, Rayner *et al.* (2006) examine the values of the National Health Service Framework for coronary heart disease and identify three different discourses, the managerial, the clinical and the political, all with different messages and overtones. Wilson (2014) carried out a CDA, exploring mental health crisis intervention and examined the language used by people with experience of the service such as service users, their families, professionals and the police. Images or situations can be analysed critically; for instance, the way a health professional approaches a patient or a manager in a hospital talks to the staff might uncover power relationships between people. DA can also be used in healthcare to analyse documents or politicians' speeches to uncover underlying ideologies or hidden messages. CDA discovers the language that operates within the particular discourse under study and which has almost moral connotations.

Morgan (2010) lists a variety of ways in which discourse can be analysed; no orthodox, one way to do this.

Performative social science

In conversation with Patricia Leavy, Kip Jones (Jones and Leavy, 2014) describes performative or performance-based social science (PSS) which Leavy labels arts-based research (ABR). Jones and Leavy (p. 1) call PSS 'the use of tools from the Arts (and Humanities), in carrying out Social Science research and/or disseminating its findings', and it can be used at any point from generating research through communicating the findings and interpreting them. This way of doing research is an innovative and unconventional approach to collecting, presenting or disseminating data through images, poetry and performances such as theatre or dance. Even novels can be based on social science research. It is established in educational and sociological inquiry, and now is becoming increasingly used in qualitative health research. The researcher thus uses tools borrowed from the arts and humanities as is suggested by Jones, and seeks different ways from conventional reports to generate and present research. PSS is being used across a variety of disciplines but is also interdisciplinary and crosses the boundaries between disciplines. It uses a wide range of techniques, media and creative processes. In research, it indicates a change from text to performance and it has become increasingly popular, although text is still the preferred way of presenting qualitative data. Yallop *et al.* (2008) claim that performative data presentation could reach a wider audience as it might be easier to understand than traditional ways of researching and presenting. A lay audience in particular will find it easier to grasp complex issues this way because of its greater accessibility, but it can also have an impact on academic peers and funding agencies. Performance is, however, not suitable in all studies.

The concept of performance in research emerged in the 1970s. It is linked to the enactment of research in various ways. Austin, the philosopher, for instance, uses the term 'performative' in relation to utterances in text or speech which perform and enact (Schwandt, 2007). A text itself might be a performative production. The concept of PSS relates, however, mostly to the visual and audible. In the last two decades, qualitative researchers have often translated their data, findings and presentations into performances. Indeed, Denzin (2001: 26) states that we 'inhabit a performance-based dramaturgical culture'. Film, poetry and video for instance, open up new ways for qualitative inquiry and are often appropriate to evoke emotion and response in the audience; hence, they help listeners and viewers to grasp human concerns more fully.

Drama, dance and music and other tools also are performance-based modes of presenting research; it is not all image-based. Saldaña (2003) speaks of 'dramatizing data' where the participants play roles and are characters in a play. Some of our students, for instance, showed a fictional film about old people in a care home which presented the findings from their research. Rossiter *et al.* (2008) show how and why findings can be usefully communicated, through theatre for instance.

New and innovative technology is often the medium through which performative events can happen and films or dramatic presentations are obvious choices. Jones ties performativity to post-modernity and social constructionism, because of its multi-voiced and interdisciplinary character and for its diversity and lack of linearity. Roberts (2008: 1), however, warns against the collapsing of artistic or social science or activity into mere performance or simply transferring it, as this needs careful examination of 'skills, purpose, tradition and context'.

Gergen and Gergen (2000; 2012) have used performances in their work for decades. They declare that in research, writing is only one way of expression. Films, drama and other modes of presentation can be used to this end, while in the past they were merely complementary to scientific writing. They also believe that in this genre boundaries between data collection and report become blurred in the process of research. Collecting data through images, poems and other means empowers the participants and centres on their perspectives.

The data collected by these techniques have to be analysed in detail to be used by researchers. Indeed, vigorous and rigorous analysis is essential to make performance-based collection and presentation of data acceptable, particularly in academic settings. Nevertheless, through presentation in a storytelling or image-based way, the audience, particularly an audience of patients or users of services, is able to grasp the experience of pain and joy, stigma and other problems which are made more visible and concrete. Jones (2013) produced a professionally made film, 'Rufus Stone', as part of a long research project (*the New Dynamics of Ageing*), a segment of which considered the life of gay men and older lesbian women in the rural area of South West England. Jones (2017) gives an overview in the *Encyclopedia of Communications Research Methods*.

PSS in health research

PSS is useful in health research as it can present vividly the voices of the participants – be it in film, theatre or other media. It is more immediate than reading a report produced by researchers, and assists the audience or readership in understanding the experience of patients or health professionals. The producer of a performance, whether it is in a play, a film or any other form, becomes a recorder of experiences. Their observations evoke a response in audiences who bring their own interpretations to the situation in interaction with the data or their presentation. Kara (2015) re-conceptualises creative methods in the social sciences and points to the extensive the range and scope that has developed over a short time, including arts-based approaches.

KEY POINT

Performative Social Science helps to make research accessible and illuminates issues from another perspective.

Example 15.7 Performative Social Science

Gregory (2014) reported on her PSS project which was developed by four artists and a social scientist (artist). The aim of this work was to explore dementia and the stigma associated with it. The two parts of this research focused on a piece of ongoing qualitative inquiry and an arts exhibition. The latter was created in collaboration with people who had dementia. The exhibition consisted of poems, photographs, songs and collages. The participants were also interviewed about their condition and the stigma attached to it. This study is an example of integration of arts and social sciences.

Example 15.8 PSS

As part of a nation-wide project on ageing, Bournemouth University developed a project into ageing of older lesbian women and gay men in rural areas of the West Country from their own experiences and narratives. These participants recounted their problems and fears. From the findings of this research, Kip Jones (2009–2011), in collaboration with the London filmmaker Appignanesi as director, produced a film 'Rufus Stone' based on the stories of the participants; he labelled this 'research as fiction'. It had its premiere in 2011 and has become an oft-quoted example of PSS.

In the collection of data vignettes, brief stories of issues or problems in health can generate interview data, as one of the examples shows. One of our colleagues used photo elicitation to find how older people perceived 'the meaning of home'.

Keen and Todres (2007) give several examples of dissemination through performance methods and discuss the value of this type of presentation of findings. They show that it can communicate the findings in an insightful way. They give key examples of research which has been disseminated through dramatic presentations such as communication of diagnoses. All the examples they gave were based originally on social science data. Cash (2009) produced a film to demonstrate the findings of her research about the life of older people with dementia.

PSS should not be used as a superficial or merely beguiling and interesting work where the performance becomes more important than the data and ideas on which it is based. Arts-based qualitative research needs to be even more systematic and organized than traditional research to have credibility and quality.

Summary

This chapter is aimed at giving an overview of some qualitative research approaches that are either embedded in other methods, such as case study research and CIT, or those that are more (DA, PSS) or less (CA, CIT) frequently used in health research. Many more exist. Often used feminist research is based on a specific standpoint, and a feminist stance can be adopted in most of the approaches discussed. All qualitative researchers need to have at least some knowledge about the major methods of research. We have focused on mainstream approaches in the preceding sections and not treated additional approaches in depth.

References

Case Study Research

Baillie, L., Gallini, A., Corser, R. *et al.* (2014) Care transitions for frail, older people from acute hospital wards within an integrated hospital system in England: a qualitative case study. *International Journal of Integrated Care*, **14**, e009.

Baxter, P. and Jack, S. (2008) Qualitative case study methodology: implementation for novice researchers. *The Qualitative Report*, **13** 544–559.

Bryman, A. (2016) *Social Research Methods*, 4th edn, Oxford University Press, Oxford.

Cash, M. (2009) Being together. A film produced as part of a PhD thesis at Bournemouth University.

Cheek, J. (2004) At the margins? Discourse analysis and qualitative research. *Qualitative Health Research*, **14** (8), 1140–1150.

Creswell, J.W. and Poth, C.N. (2017) *Qualitative Inquiry and Research Design: Choosing among Five Approaches*, Kindle edn, Sage, Thousand Oaks, CA.

Cronin, C. (2014) Using case study research as a rigorous form of inquiry. *Nurse Researcher*, **21** (5), 16–37.

Crowe, M. (2005) Discourse analysis: towards an understanding of its use in nursing. *Journal of Advanced Nursing*, **51** (1), 55–63.

Denzin, N.K. (2001) The reflexive interview and a performative social science. *Qualitative Research*, **1** (1), 23–46.

Dodds, S., Preston, N., Payne, S. and Walshe, C. (2020) Exploring a new model of end-of-life care for older people. *International Journal of Health Policy and Management*, **9** (8) 344–351.

Gergen, M.M. and Gergen, K.J. (2000) Qualitative inquiry: tensions and transformations, in *Handbook of Qualitative Research* (eds. N.K. Denzin and Y.S. Lincoln), Sage, Thousand Oaks, CA, pp. 1025–1046.

Gill, R. (1996) Discourse analysis: practical implementation, in *Handbook of Qualitative Research in Psychology and the Social Sciences* (ed. J.T.A. Richardson), BPS Books, Leicester, pp. 141–156.

Gomm, R., Hammersley, M. and Foster, P. (2014) *Case Study Method*, Kindle edn, Sage, London.

Jones, K. (2013) Infusing biography with the personal: writing Rufus Stone. *Creative Approaches to Research*, **6** (2), 6–23.

Jones, K. (2017) *Performative Social Science: Draft Entry for the International Encyclopedia of Communications Research Methods*, Wiley Blackwell, Oxford.

Kara, H. (2015) *Creative Research Methods in the Social Sciences: A Practical Guide*, Policy Press, University of Bristol, UK.

Keen, S. and Todres, L. (2007) Strategies for disseminating qualitative research findings: three exemplars. *Qualitative Social Research*, **8** (3), Article 17.

McCabe, T.J. and Sambrook, S. (2013) Psychological contract and commitment amongst nurses and nurse managers: a discourse analysis. *International Journal of Nursing Studies*, **50** (7), 954–967.

McHoul, A. and Grace, W. (1995) *A Foucault Primer: Discourse*, Power and the Subject, University Press, Melbourne.

Morgan, A. (2010) Discourse analysis: an overview for the neophyte researcher. *Journal of Health and Social Care Improvement*, **5** (1), 1–7.

Munro, J.A. and Beck, A.D. (2021) The effect of nursing policy on higher education wound care provision and practice: a critical discourse analysis. *Politics, Policy and Nursing Practice*, **22** (2), 134.

Potter, J. (1996) *Representing Reality: Discourse, Rhetoric, and Social Construction*, Sage, London.

Potter, J. and Wetherell, M. (1987) *Discourse and Social Psychology: Beyond Attitudes and Behaviour*, Sage, London.

Potter, J. and Wetherell, M. (2007) *Discourse and Social Psychology*, 3rd edn, Sage, London.

Rayner, M., Scarborough, P. and Allender, S. (2006) Values underlying the National Service Framework for coronary heart disease. *Journal of Health Services Research and Policy*, **11** (2), 67–73.

Roberts, B. (2008) Performative social science: a consideration of skills, purpose and context. *Qualitative Social Research*, **9** (2), 1.

Rossiter, K., Kontos, P., Colantionio, A. *et al.* (2008) Staging data: theatre as a tool for analysis and knowledge transfer in health research. *Social Science and Medicine*, **66** (1), 130–146.

Saldaña, J. (2003) Dramatizing data: a primer. *Qualitative Inquiry*, **9** (2), 218–236.

Schwandt, T. (2007) *A Dictionary of Qualitative Inquiry*, Sage, Thousand Oaks, CA.

Simons, H. (2009) *Case Study Research in Practice*, Sage, London.

Stake, R.E. (1995) *The Art of Case Study Research*, Sage, Thousand Oaks, CA.

Stake, R.E. (2000) The case study method in social inquiry, in *Case Study Method* (eds. R. Gomm, M. Hammersley and P. Foster), Sage, London, pp. 19–26.

Stake, R.E. (2010) *Qualitative Research: Studying How Things Work*, The Guilford Press, New York.

Travers, M. (2001) *Qualitative Research Through Case Studies*, Sage, London.

Traynor, M. (2006) Discourse analysis: theoretical and historical overview and review of papers in the *Journal of Advanced Nursing*. *Journal of Advanced Nursing*, **54** (1), 62–72.

Traynor, M. (2006) Discourse analysis: theoretical and historical overview and review of papers. *Journal of Advanced Nursing*, **54** (1), 62–72.

Van Wynsburghe, R. and Khan, S. (2007) Redefining case study. *International Journal of Qualitative Methods*, **6** (2), Article 6.

Wertz, P.J., Charmaz, K., McMullen, L.M. and Josselson, R. (2011) *Five Ways of Doing Qualitative Analysis*, The Guilford Press, New York.

Wilson S.C. (2014) Mental Health Crisis Intervention: a discourse analysis involving service users and the police, PhD thesis, Massey University, New Zealand.

Yallop, J.J., Vallejo, I.L. and Wright, P.R. (2008) Overview of Editorial: Overview of the performative social science special issue. *Qualitative Social Research*, **9** (2), Article 64.

Yin, R.K. (2013) *Case Study Research*, 5th edn, Sage, Thousand Oaks, CA.

Yin, R.K. (2018) *Case Study Research and Applications*, 6th edn, Sage, Thousand Oaks, CA.

Conversation Analysis

Bergstrom, L., Roberts, J., Skillman, L. and Seidel, J. (1992) You'll feel me touching you, sweetie: vaginal examination during the second stage of labour. *Birth*, **19**, 11–18.

Campion, P. and Langdon, M. (2004) Achieving multiple topic shifts in primary care medical consultations: a conversation analysis study in UK general practice. *Sociology of Health and Illness*, **26** (1), 81–101.

Cash, M. (2009) Being together. A film produced as part of a PhD thesis at Bournemouth University.

Chatwin, J. (2014) Conversation analysis as a method for investigating interaction in care home environments. *Dementia*, **13** (6), 737–746.

Chatwin, J., Kennedy, A., Firth, A. *et al.* (2014). How potentially serious symptom changes are talked about and managed in COPD clinical review consultations: a micro-analysis. *Social Science & Medicine*, **113**, 120–136.

Cheek, J. (2004) At the margins? Discourse analysis and qualitative research. *Qualitative Health Research*, **14** (8), 1140–1150.

Crowe, M. (2005) Discourse analysis: towards an understanding of its use in nursing. *Journal of Advanced Nursing*, **51** (1), 55–63.

Denzin, N.K. (2001) The reflexive interview and a performative social science. *Qualitative Research*, **1** (1), 23–46.

Gergen, M.M. and Gergen, K.J. (2000) Qualitative inquiry: tensions and transformations, in *Handbook of Qualitative Research* (eds. N.K. Denzin and Y.S. Lincoln), Sage, Thousand Oaks, CA, pp. 1025–1046.

Gill, R. (1996) Discourse analysis: practical implementation, in *Handbook of Qualitative Research in Psychology and the Social Sciences* (ed. J.T.A. Richardson), BPS Books, Leicester, pp. 141–156.

Hepburn, A. and Potter, J. (2021) *Essentials of Conversation Analysis*, American Psychological Association, Washington, DC.

Heritage, J. (1988) Explanations as accounts: a conversation analytic perspective, in *Analysing Everyday Explanation: A Casebook of Methods*, Sage, London, pp. 127–144.

Hutchby, I. and Wooffitt, R. (2008) *Conversation Analysis*, 2nd edn, Polity Press, Cambridge.

Jones, A. (2003) Nurses talking to patients: exploring conversation analysis as a means of researching nurse–patient communication. *International Journal of Nursing Studies*, **40** (6), 609–618.

Jones, K. (2013) Infusing biography with the personal: writing Rufus Stone. *Creative Approaches to Research*, **6** (2), 6–23.

Jones, K. and Leavy, P. (2014) A Conversation Between Kip Jones and Patricia Leavy: Arts-Based Research, Performative Social Science and Working on the Margins. The Qualitative Report 2014 Volume 19, Article 38, 1–7. http://www.nova.edu/ssss/QR/QR19/jones38.pdf

Jones, K. (2017) *Performative Social Science: Draft Entry for the International Encyclopedia of Communications Research Methods*, Wiley Blackwell, Oxford.

Kara, H. (2015) *Creative Research Methods in the Social Sciences: A Practical Guide*, Policy Press, University of Bristol, UK.

Keen, S. and Todres, L. (2007) Strategies for disseminating qualitative research findings: three exemplars. *Qualitative Social Research*, **8** (3), Article 17.

McCabe, T.J. and Sambrook, S. (2013) Psychological contract and commitment amongst nurses and nurse managers: a discourse analysis. *International Journal of Nursing Studies*, **50** (7), 954–967.

McHoul, A. and Grace, W. (1995) *A Foucault Primer: Discourse*, Power and the Subject, University Press, Melbourne.

Morgan, A. (2010) Discourse analysis: an overview for the neophyte researcher. *Journal of Health and Social Care Improvement*, **5** (1), 1–7.

Munro, J.A. and Beck, A.D. (2021) The effect of nursing policy on higher education wound care provision and practice: a critical discourse analysis. *Politics, Policy and Nursing Practice*, **22** (2), 134.

Nofsinger, R.E. (1991) *Everyday Conversation*, Sage, Newbury Park, CA.

Potter, J. (1996) *Representing Reality: Discourse, Rhetoric, and Social Construction*, Sage, London.

Potter, J. and Wetherell, M. (1987) *Discourse and Social Psychology: Beyond Attitudes and Behaviour*, Sage, London.

Potter, J. and Wetherell, M. (2007) *Discourse and Social Psychology*, 3rd edn, Sage, London.

Rayner, M., Scarborough, P. and Allender, S. (2006) Values underlying the National Service Framework for coronary heart disease. *Journal of Health Services Research and Policy*, **11** (2), 67–73.

Roberts, B. (2008) Performative social science: a consideration of skills, purpose and context. *Qualitative Social Research*, **9** (2), 1.

Rossiter, K., Kontos, P., Colantionio, A. *et al.* (2008) Staging data: theatre as a tool for analysis and knowledge transfer in health research. *Social Science and Medicine*, **66** (1), 130–146.

Saldaña, J. (2003) Dramatizing data: a primer. *Qualitative Inquiry*, **9** (2), 218–236.

Schoeb V., Staffoni L. Parry R. and Pilnick A. (2014) "What do you expect from physiotherapy?": a detailed analysis of goal setting in physiotherapy. *Disability and Rehabilitation*, **36** (20), 679–686.

Schwandt, T. (2007) *A Dictionary of Qualitative Inquiry*, Sage, Thousand Oaks, CA.

Sharrock, W. and Anderson, R. (1987) Work flow in a paediatric clinic, in *Talk and Social Organisation* (eds. G. Button and J.R.E. Lee), Multilingual Matters, Clevedon.

Sidnell, J. and Stivers, T. (eds.) (2014) *The Handbook of Conversation Analysis*, Wiley-Blackwell, Oxford.

Silverman, D. (ed.) (2014) *Interpreting Qualitative Data: Methods for Analysing Talk, Text and Interaction*, 4th edn, Sage, London.

Ten Have, P. (2014) *Doing Conversation Analysis*, 2nd edn, Sage, London. (kindle).

Traynor, M. (2006) Discourse analysis: theoretical and historical overview and review of papers in the *Journal of Advanced Nursing*. *Journal of Advanced Nursing*, **54** (1), 62–72.

Traynor, M. (2006) Discourse analysis: theoretical and historical overview and review of papers. *Journal of Advanced Nursing*, **54** (1), 62–72.

Turner, R. (ed.) (1974) *Ethnomethodology*, Penguin Books, Harmondsworth.

Wertz, P.J., Charmaz, K., McMullen, L.M. and Josselson, R. (2011) *Five Ways of Doing Qualitative Analysis*, The Guilford Press, New York.

Wilson S.C. (2014) Mental Health Crisis Intervention: a discourse analysis involving service users and the police, PhD thesis, Massey University, New Zealand.

Wu, Y. (2021) Empathy in nurse-patient interaction. *BMC Nursing*. doi:10.1186/s12912-021-00535-0

Yallop, J.J., Vallejo, I.L. and Wright, P.R. (2008) Overview of Editorial: Overview of the performative social science special issue. *Qualitative Social Research*, **9** (2), Article 64.

Yin, R.K. (2018) *Case Study Research and Applications*, 6th edn, Sage, Thousand Oaks, CA.

Further Reading

Rapley, T. (2018) *Doing Discourse, Conversation and Document Analysis*, 2nd edn, Sage, London.

Discourse Analysis

Cheek, J. (2004) At the margins? Discourse analysis and qualitative research. *Qualitative Health Research*, **14** (8), 1140–1150.

Crowe, M. (2005) Discourse analysis: towards an understanding of its use in nursing. *Journal of Advanced Nursing*, **51** (1), 55–63.

Funk, L.M. (2013) Home healthcare and family responsibility: a critical discourse analysis of text and talk. *Healthcare Policy* (Special Issue), 86–97.

Gee, J.P. (2014) *How to Do Discourse Analysis: A Toolkit*, 2nd edn, Routledge, Abingdon.

Gill, R. (1996) Discourse analysis: practical implementation, in *Handbook of Qualitative Research in Psychology and the Social Sciences* (ed. J.T.A. Richardson), BPS Books, Leicester, pp. 141–156.

Hui, A. and Stickley, T. (2007) Mental health policy and mental health service user perspectives on involvement: a discourse analysis. *Journal of Advanced Nursing*, **59** (4), 416–426.

Lidcoat, A. (2021) *An Introduction to Conversation Analysis*. 3rd edn, Bloomsbury Publishing, London

McCabe, T.J. and Sambrook, S. (2013) Psychological contract and commitment amongst nurses and nurse managers: a discourse analysis. *International Journal of Nursing Studies*, **50** (7), 954–967.

McHoul, A. and Grace, W. (1995) *A Foucault Primer: Discourse, Power and the Subject*, University Press, Melbourne.

Morgan, A. (2010) Discourse analysis: an overview for the neophyte researcher. *Journal of Health and Social Care Improvement*, **5** (1), 1–7.

Munro, J.A. and Beck, A.D. (2021) The effects of UK Nursing Policy on higher education wound care provision and practice: a critical discourse analysis. *Policy, Politics and Nursing Practice*, **22** (2), 134–145.

Potter, J. (1996) *Representing Reality: Discourse, Rhetoric, and Social Construction*, Sage, London.

Potter, J. and Wetherell, M. (1987) *Discourse and Social Psychology: Beyond Attitudes and Behaviour*, Sage, London.

Potter, J. and Wetherell, M. (2007) *Discourse and Social Psychology*, 3rd edn, Sage, London.

Rayner, M., Scarborough, P. and Allender, S. (2006) Values underlying the National Service Framework for coronary heart disease. *Journal of Health Services Research and Policy*, **11** (2), 67–73.

Traynor, M. (2006) Discourse analysis: theoretical and historical overview and review of papers in the *Journal of Advanced Nursing*. *Journal of Advanced Nursing*, **54** (1), 62–72.

Wertz, F.J., Charmaz, K., McMullen, L.M. *et al.* (2011) *Five Ways of Doing Qualitative Analysis*, The Guilford Press, New York, NY.

Wetherell, M., Taylor, S., Yates, S.J. (eds.) (2001) *Discourse as Data: A Guide for Analysis*, The Open University, Milton Keynes.

Wilson, S.C. (2014) Mental health crisis intervention: a discourse analysis involving service users, families, nurses and the police. Unpublished PhD thesis, Massey University, New Zealand.

Further Reading

Bonnin, J.E. (2018) *Discourse and Mental Health: Voice, Inequality and Resistance in Medical Settings*, Routledge. Abingdon Oxon.

Grue, J. (2020) *Disability and Discourse Analysis*, Routledge, Abingdon, Oxon.

Springer, R.A. and Clinton, M.E. (2015) Doing Foucault: inquiring into nursing knowledge with Foucauldian discourse analysis. *Nursing Philosophy*, **16** (2), 87–97.

Wodak, R and Meyer, M. (eds.) (2016) *Methods of Critical Discourse Analysis*, Sage, London.

Performative Social Science

Cash, M. (2009) Being together. A film produced as part of a PhD thesis at Bournemouth University.

Curtin, A. (2008) How dramatic techniques can aid the presentation of qualitative research. *Qualitative Researcher*, **8**, 8–10.

Denzin, N.K. (2001) The reflexive interview and a performative social science. *Qualitative Research*, **1** (1), 23–46.

Gergen, M.M. and Gergen, K.J. (2000) Qualitative inquiry: tensions and transformations, in *Handbook of Qualitative Research* (eds. N.K. Denzin and Y.S. Lincoln), Sage, Thousand Oaks, CA, pp. 1025–1046.

Gergen, M.M. and Gergen, K.J. (2012) *Social Construction: Entering the Dialogue*, Kindle edn.

Gregory, H. (2014) "I Will Tell You Something of My Own": promoting personhood in dementia through performative social science. *Qualitative Social Research*, **15** (3), Article 18.

Guiney Yallop, J.J., Lopez de Vallejo, I. and Wright, P.R. (2008) Editorial: overview of the performative social science special issue. *Qualitative Social Research*, **9** (2), Article 64.

Holloway, I. (2008) *A-Z of Qualitative Research in Healthcare*, Blackwell Science, Oxford.

Jones, K. (2013) Infusing biography with the personal: writing Rufus Stone. *Creative Approaches to Research*, **6** (2), 6–23.

Jones, K. (2017) *Performative Social Science: Draft Entry for the International Encyclopedia of Communications Research Methods*, Wiley Blackwell, Oxford.

Jones, K. and Leavy, P. (2014) A conversation between Kip Jones and Patricia Leavy: arts-based research, performative social science and working on the margins. *The Qualitative Report*, **19** (38), 1–7.

Kara, H. (2015) *Creative Research Methods in the Social Sciences: A Practical Guide*, Policy Press, University of Bristol, Bristol.

Keen, S. and Todres, L. (2007) Strategies for disseminating qualitative research findings: three exemplars. *Qualitative Social Research*, **8** (3), Article 17.

Parsons, J.A. and Boydell, K.M. (2012) Arts-based research and knowledge translation: some concerns for health-care professionals. *Journal of Interprofessional Care*, **26** (3), 170–172.

Roberts, B. (2008) Performative social science: a consideration of skills, purpose and context. *Qualitative Social Research*, **9** (2), 1.

Rossiter, K., Kontos, P., Colantionio, A. *et al.* (2008) Staging data: theatre as a tool for analysis and knowledge transfer in health research. *Social Science and Medicine*, **66** (1), 130–146.

Saldaña, J. (2003) Dramatizing data: a primer. *Qualitative Inquiry*, **9** (2), 218–236.

Schwandt, T. (2015) *The Sage Dictionary of Qualitative Inquiry*, 4th edn, Sage, Thousand Oaks, CA.

Spiers, J.A. (2004) Tech tips: using video management/analysis technology in qualitative research. *International Journal of Qualitative Methods*, **3** (1), Article 5.

Further Reading

Leavy, P. (2019) *Handbook of Arts-Based Research*, 3rd edn, Guilford Press, New York, NY

Leavy, P. (2020) *Method Meets Art: Arts-Based Research Practice*, 4th edn, Guilford Press, New York, NY.

Rose, G. (2016) *Visual Methodologies: An Introduction to the Interpretation of Visual Materials*, 4th edn, Sage, London.

There are also useful articles in the *Handbook for Qualitative Research*, 5th edn. *See above.*

The special issue of *Forum Qualitative Research*, vol. 9, No. 2, a free online journal, contains a number of important and explanatory articles.

Part Four

Data Analysis and Completion

Chapter 16

Data Analysis: Strategies and Procedures

Qualitative data analysis (QDA), an important step in the qualitative research process, is both complex and non-linear. The research project should not be merely a report on the data collected but contain a thorough analysis. Whilst this is a reflective intellectual process, it is also systematic, orderly and structured. However, not all qualitative forms of inquiry take the same approach to analysis; there are distinctions between different analysis methods as can be seen in the chapters on specific approaches. Indeed, grounded theory (GT) and phenomenology in particular, have very distinct ways of analysing data (and also a different approach to data collection). Data reduction or collapsing, description and/or interpretation, however, are common to many types of QDA, although the approach to these procedures is flexible and creative. There is no single rigid prescription as long as the final research account has its roots directly in the data generated by the participants and is coherent with the research method being used. For the purposes of this chapter, we shall only attempt an overview of generic data analysis in qualitative research. For beginners, an examination of relevant chapters in a clearly written text might be useful, such as that of Boeije (2010), Ritchie *et al.* (2014) or Braun and Clarke (2013). We also recommend specialist texts for specific approaches such as GT, ethnography and phenomenology as indicated in earlier chapters.

Data analysis is an iterative activity. Iteration means that researchers move back and forth from collection to analysis and back again, refining the questions they ask from the data. Knowledge of this process means that researchers will be able to allocate and segment their time appropriately. Health researchers often lack time at the end of their study to carry out the appropriate data analysis, because they do not foresee the complexity of the data and the length of time needed for analysing them. These procedures make qualitative research more time-consuming.

> **KEY POINT**
>
> Data analysis in qualitative research is often non-linear and iterative.

Qualitative Research in Nursing and Healthcare, Fifth Edition.
Immy Holloway and Kathleen Galvin.
© 2024 John Wiley & Sons Ltd. Published 2024 by John Wiley & Sons Ltd.

Qualitative researchers usually collect and analyse the data simultaneously (with the exception of some approaches, for instance phenomenology or narrative inquiry), unlike those involved in quantitative inquiry, who complete collection before starting analysis. Indeed, in GT, data collection and analysis interact (see Chapter 11), and in several other approaches researchers often use data collection and analysis in parallel and interactively (for instance, in ethnography). Even when recording and transcribing initial data, researchers reflect upon them and so start the process of analysis at an early stage.

The process of analysis goes through certain stages common to many approaches:
- Transcribing interviews and sorting fieldnotes.
- Organising, ordering and storing the data.
- Listening to and reading or viewing the material collected repeatedly.

All this means immersion in and engagement with the data. Other stages depend on the approach taken by the qualitative researcher:
- Coding and categorising (in GT, thematic analysis (TA) and IPA, also in other generic approaches).
- Building themes.
- Describing a cultural group (in ethnography).
- Describing a phenomenon (in phenomenology).

Usually these steps also involve storing ideas, interpretations and theoretical thought. The process is carried out through memoing and writing fieldnotes (see Chapters 10 and 11 on fieldnotes and memos, respectively).

Silverman (2017) discusses the status of interview data in particular, which must be taken into account before the process of data analysis can start. These data are rarely raw but have already been processed through the mind of the interviewer and can only be seen in context. In observations too, fieldnotes do not always show how the environment might shape the interaction, in particular elements such as the presence or absence of certain people, the work climate and other factors. Boeije (2010) suggests that there are two strategies in data analysis, namely segmenting the data and then reassembling them again into a coherent entity. We would have to add another step, however – the initial and comprehensive reading of a transcript as a whole. In their eagerness to analyse and break down the data, researchers occasionally forget this stage. Whatever the approach to analysis, it is important to continuously reflect on the meaning of the data during the analysis as they as this is a core purpose of qualitative research. Therefore, any approach to analysis that loses sight of meaning by overly focusing on the fragments or parts of the data alone risks losing thick descriptions and depth that are the cornerstone of insightful qualitative findings. It is sometimes helpful to distinguish between (a) ordering and organising the data and (b) analysing and interpreting the data as two distinct but related activities.

Transcribing and sorting

Transcription of interviews is one of the initial steps in preparing the data for analysis. The fullest and richest data can be gained from transcribing verbatim. We advise that, if possible, novice researchers transcribe their own tapes because this way they immerse themselves in the data and become sensitive to the issues of importance. Transcription takes a long time: 1 hour of interviewing takes between 4 and 6 hours to transcribe. For those who are not used to audio-typing, it can be much longer. Transcription is very frustrating and can take time that researchers often lack. A typist using a transcription machine could do it more quickly, but this would be expensive; on the other hand, it would give more time to the researcher to listen and analyse. The decision depends on the researcher. Any outsider who transcribes must, of course, be advised on the confidentiality relating to the data.

Initial interviews and fieldnotes should be fully transcribed so that the researcher becomes aware of the important issues in the data. Novice researchers should transcribe all interviews verbatim, while more experienced individuals can be more selective in their transcriptions and transcribe that which is linked to their developing theoretical ideas. There is danger that researchers who fail to record the interviews will overlook significant issues, which they could uncover on reflection when listening to the tape or considering the transcript. Pages are numbered, and the front sheet (fact sheet) should contain date, location and time of interview as well as the code number or pseudonym for the informant and important biographical data (but no identifier). Many researchers number each line of the interview transcript so that they can retrieve the data quickly when revisiting the transcript. Transcription pages are most useful when put into a column which takes half the sheet, while the other half is left for analysis and comments.

A minimum of three copies (usually more) should be made of the transcripts and a clean copy without comments for locking away in a safe place in case other copies are lost or destroyed.

Occasionally, researchers use formal transcription systems (some invent their own systems); the best known of these is Gail Jefferson's, which uses symbols for non-verbal actions such as coughing, pausing and emphasising. These systems are more often applied to 'naturally occurring data' such as those from conversation or discourse analysis. However, for some approaches the type of transcribing Jefferson developed would be an anathema; Langridge (2007) reminds researchers that phenomenology in particular does not need a micro-level of transcription, and we would suggest the inappropriateness of this for ethnography and GT too. Silverman (2017) gives a list of simplified transcription symbols which could be helpful in conversation analysis and some forms of discourse analysis. Indeed, health researchers could create their own sheet of symbols.

Of course, they transcribe in detail, and as accurately as possible, as they choose sections from the data which answer their research questions. There is however the danger that they select according to their own assumptions about the importance of data rather than focusing on the participants' words, hence careful reading and listening is advised.

Taking notes and writing analytic memos

Some researchers use the video recorder and also take notes during the interview so that participants' facial expression, gestures and interviewers' reactions and comments can be recorded. Making notes might disturb the participant. We would suggest this only when taping is not feasible or if interviewees do not wish to be tape-recorded. Notes can also be taken immediately after the interview.

When participants deny permission for recording or when it seems inappropriate – for instance, in very sensitive situations – interviewers generally take notes throughout the interview, and these notes reflect the words of the participants as accurately as possible. As interviewers can only write down a fraction of the sentences, they select the most important words or phrases and summarise the rest, and this might distort meaning. Patton (2015) advises on conventions in the use of quotation marks while writing notes, (but this is not necessary for lengthy quotes which can be inset into the text in shorter lines). Researchers use them only for full, direct quotations from informants. Patton suggests that researchers adopt a mechanism for differentiating between their own thoughts and the informants' words. When reading transcripts and writing memos, researchers might also collect a series of pithy quotes, which are representative of the thoughts of the participants and the phenomenon or phenomena under study.

Another method of recording is to take notes after the interview is finished. This could be done as soon as possible after the interview to capture the flavour, behaviour and words of the informants and the concomitant thoughts of the researcher. It should not be done in the presence of the participants.

The process of listening to the tapes will sensitise researchers to the data and uncover ambiguities or problems within them. At this time, any theoretical or other ideas that emerge should be written down in the field diary. The process of writing fieldnotes and memos is in itself an analytic process and not just data recording. It helps the researcher to reflect on the data and engage with them.

During the process of analysis, researchers write analytical memos or notes containing ideas and thoughts about the data as well the reasons for grouping them in a particular way. Sometimes researchers draw diagrams to demonstrate this, and these diagrams can be taken directly into the report when they discuss the methods and the decision trail. Researchers might develop concepts in the memos, ask analytic questions of the data or elaborate ideas from the literature that link directly with the data. There are different ways of keeping memos: in field journals or diaries, or on a computer. This all helps 'tacking', that is, going back and forth between the data and theoretical ideas, between codes and themes. This is part of 'iteration' as mentioned before.

Some researchers do not code or categorise because they wish to perceive the essence of the phenomenon as a whole, a *Gestalt*. Breaking the data into codes may lose this holistic view of the phenomenon and fragment the ideas contained in the data.

Memoing goes on throughout the research process but is of particular importance in assisting analysis. (Specific types of analysis are discussed in the chapters on the various approaches.) Bazeley (2020) adds another tool for the analysis, namely codebooks. These are similar to fieldnotes and memos, but give some detail of coding and show how codes have emerged, short and extended definitions of codes. However, the researcher can include this in the memos or field diary. Codebooks might just help to keep the processes of analysis tidy.

Ordering and organising the data

Qualitative researchers generate large amounts of data consisting of narratives from interviews, fieldnotes and documents, as well as a variety of memos about the phenomenon under study (Bryman, 2016). Many use the relevant literature as data (this is sometimes done in GT). Through organisation and management, the researcher brings structure and order to the unwieldy mass of data. This will help eventual retrieval and final analysis. All transcripts, fieldnotes and other data should have details of time, location and specific comments attached. The use of pseudonyms or numbers for participants prevents identification during the long process of analysis when the data might fall into the hands of individuals other than the researcher. Pseudonyms are better than numbers because this is more personal. Everything has to be recorded, cross-checked and labelled. The material has to be stored in the appropriate files for later retrieval.

From the very beginning of the study, nurses and other health professionals will recognise significant ideas and themes in the material they generated because they are sensitized by virtue of prior knowledge in their field. On listening to tapes, reading transcriptions and other documents or looking at visual data common themes and patterns will begin to emerge and become crystallised.

Borkan (1999) discusses the initial process of analysis and describes two strategies from which researchers can choose depending on their approach, namely *horizontal* and *vertical* 'passes' of the data. The horizontal pass involves

• Reading the data and looking at themes, emotions and surprises, taking in the overall picture.
• Reflective and in-depth reading of the data to find supporting evidence for the themes.
• Re-reading for elements that might have been overlooked.

- Searching for possible alternative meanings.
- Attempting to link discrepancies.
  Vertical passes involve
- Concentrating on one section of the data and analysing it before moving on.
- Reflecting on and reviewing the data in the section.
- Looking for insights and feeding them back into the data collection process.

The horizontal is more holistic than the vertical pass. However, researchers not only analyse according to the methods they adopt, but they also have different personal styles, which demand different ways of looking at the data.

Bazeley (2020) sees the beginning of the research as an important stage and suggests '*read, reflect, play and explore* strategies' and to this end advises the following (p. 101): gain familiarity with the scope and content of each new data source;

- Build a contextualized and holistic understanding of the people events and ideas being investigated, and the connections within and between them.
- Understand the perspectives of the participants.
- Review assumptions to further shape data gathering.
- Develop a framework for further analyses.
- Record any ideas and understandings that are generated as you do these things.

Analytical styles

Different approaches to research have different types of data analysis. Even within one approach, researchers might adopt a variety of analytic strategies. They all involve the steps of listening to, viewing and gaining a holistic view of the data as well as dividing them into units or segments of meaning. Dahlberg *et al.* (2008) ask that each part of the transcribed text, analysed for meaning, should be understood in relation to the whole of the text and the whole understood in terms of its parts. This is so not only for phenomenology but also for other approaches.

In *phenomenology*, Moustakas (1994), a hermeneutic phenomenologist, gives a clear, general overview of analysis styles and comes up with overlapping steps in which researchers carry out the following in phenomenology:

- They reflect on each transcript and search for significant statements.
- They record all relevant statements.
- They delete repetitive and overlapping statements, leaving only invariant constituents of the phenomenon, and organise them.
- They link and relate these into themes.
- Including verbatim quotes from the data, they integrate the themes into a description of the texture of the experience as told by the participants.
- They reflect on this and their own experiences.
- They develop a description of the meanings of the experience.

At all times, researchers search for links and relationships between sections of data, categories or themes.

There are more detailed discussions of analytic procedures in the chapters on specific approaches. (Ethnography, Grounded Theory, Phenomenology, narrative research for instance.)

Coding and categorizing

This is a popular way of analysing and examining data in detail. Coding means marking sections of data and assigning labels or names. It is an early stage in analysis and proceeds towards the development of categories, themes or major constructs (the nomenclature depends on the language of the specific approach). It breaks the data into manageable sections.

Line-by-line coding identifies information which both participant and researcher consider important. In their early coding, many researchers single out words or phrases that are used by participants – these are called *in vivo* codes. This type of coding prevents researchers from imposing their own framework and ideas on the data, because the coding starts with the words of the participants. In the sentence 'When I first started out as a physiotherapist, I was floundering. It was sink or swim', the *in vivo* code might be '*sink or swim*'.

In the beginning, type of coding can be useful, but it would be difficult to carry out in all transcriptions of the interviews and sets of fieldnotes. It does, however, help researchers discern important ideas in the data initially until they become used to coding.

Initial coding gives a name to specific pieces of data. The codes may be words, expressions or other chunks of data. Researchers might start with a mass of codes and reduce them so that each of them represents a concept. These concepts are *units of meaning*. Once simple coding has been completed, researchers group together the codes with similar meanings which are linked to the same incident, event or phenomenon. If different terms are applied to the same concept, the best label is used as a name for the concept. Rather than coding line-by-line or sentence-by-sentence, many researchers code paragraph-by-paragraph. Others seek meaningful statements in the text. Importance however has to be given to the participants' understanding of the event or the condition rather than giving primacy to one's own, the researcher's ideas. This means that the collected data have priority, and not the prior assumptions about themes. The dialogue with the literature takes place not only when ideas emerge but also at all other stages, and finally, when the findings have been established. The relevant literature will then be related and integrated into the findings (see Chapter 3).

There are some problems with coding and categorising. One is the loss of the holistic view or *Gestalt* of the phenomenon, which is the aim of *phenomenologists* (see relevant chapter). The other, according to Silverman (2020), is the loss of important information, because it does not 'fit' the code or category, hence the importance of the search for discrepant and alternative ideas (also called 'deviant cases' or 'contrary occurrences').

When analysing data from different data sources – for instance, from observation, interviews and documents – researchers seek similarities and differences. All the material that has conceptual links is grouped together for later categorisation. Some researchers actually cut up the transcribed data and keep them in a file, after pasting them on pages of paper and putting them into a ring binder, others use coloured pencils or pens to identify closely linked material. Researchers need to keep a list of the categories or themes to compare each section of new data with the early-established themes. The new ideas might fit into these, or new themes have to be uncovered. Eventually, a greatly reduced list might be established to form a diagram. Often, researchers generate a hierarchy of themes and codes with more abstract and general themes at the top. They might also establish a typology. Typologies are classification systems. For instance, a researcher might find that there is a distinction between health professionals who rely on book knowledge and experience. They may have different traits or act differently in specific situations.

Many researchers go further than merely arriving at an analytic or a conceptual description. They take into account conditions under which something occurs, variations in findings according to location and time, the context in which things happen, the strategies that participants adopt to cope with their experiences, causes of actions and events as well as their effects and consequences. (See specific approaches such as GT and ethnography.)

Thematic analysis

TA is a generic approach to data analysis and also includes coding and categorizing Braun and Clarke (2006, 2013, 2019) developed this method which is now often used and allows researchers theoretical flexibility. It refers to a search for patterns in a data set and is particularly based in language and meaning (Braun and Clarke, 2013). The steps in this type of analysis resemble those of other approaches, for instance researchers search for themes in the data and focus on their meanings, that is the central ideas in the research. Familiarity with the data is essential for the analysis as in other approaches. As in all qualitative research, a transparent audit trail is of major importance, so that other researchers can follow the decisions of the analyst. Most researchers use the approach developed by Braun and Clarke; however, other versions do exist. TA is not a 'pure' or sophisticated type of analysis, and it has some critics certain features can be found in other approaches – such as coding and categorizing GT and also in IPA– but it is relatively easy to use, and if applied appropriately, can lead to a good research study. A list of articles and books exist on this approach (Clarke and Braun, 2019). As with most approaches, TA has had its critics.

TA is not a single rigid approach to the data, and several versions exist. *Template analysis for instance*, is a type of TA which imposes a degree of structure on the data (Brooks *et al.*, 2015). Its best-known British proponent is Nigel King from the University of Huddersfield (King, 2004). In this 'style' of TA, a coding template is developed (particularly in the analysis of interviews and diaries – textual data). This type of analysis has not been developed lately.

Meaning and Gestalt

As mentioned before, some researchers do not agree with coding, due to the tendency to fragment data, as their primary aim is to convey the 'essence' (essential characteristics) of the phenomenon as a whole, a *Gestalt*. Breaking the data into codes and categories may lose this holistic view of the phenomenon and fragment the ideas contained in the data. Examples of this type of analysis can be found in phenomenology in all its forms as well as in other types of narrative research (more often called 'narrative analysis').

KEY POINT

Data analysis is an essential process in the development of a qualitative research study transparency is a requirement.

Problems of QDA

Because of the complexities of QDA, a number of problems might arise. Li and Seale (2007) list several, and one of these relates to not knowing where to start the process. This might be solved by asking novice researchers to analyse short sections of data. Many find the resulting themes or codes ambiguous, and of course, there is sometimes overlap of meaning. Reporting or recording problems can be overcome more easily. These issues are often connected with forgetting to note down the identifier of the participant, or not being able to retrieve ideas that had previously been discovered. Some new researchers over-interpret – everything has meaning for them – or they report inaccurately and give no evidence where ideas have their roots.

Inferential leaps and 'premature closure'

As part of the process of data analysis, researchers should avoid inferential leaps. In research supervision, it sometimes became apparent that students would infer conclusions from the data too quickly. In their haste to make sense of the data and develop a full picture, students can too readily make inferential leaps. It seems that health researchers in particular remember concepts or frameworks previously learned or discovered as a background to the research, and they try to fit these to the data. The researcher has to return to the data continually, checking and verifying so that inferential leaps are not made. This is closely connected with the warning against 'premature closure' (Glaser, 1978) that is one of the problems of qualitative research. Often novice researchers decide on a theme or category at an early stage of the research process. In GT in particular, the danger exists that once researchers have generated some theoretical ideas, they then sit back and decide that they have arrived at complete explanations for the phenomenon under study. Sometimes there has been no full investigation of the data; sometimes they close their minds to new ideas. Premature closure and inferential leaps might mean that the research is incomplete or inadequate.

Collaboration in the process of analysis and interpretation

In all types of QDA it is important that researchers stay as close to the data as possible and look at everything connected with the phenomenon under study.

A completed study is never a 'mere' description of the participants' experience. It is important to remember that the final product of research depends on the collaborative effort of participants and researcher. While those observed and interviewed are active agents in their world rather than passive participants and construct their social reality, researcher and participant also construct meaning together. The reader of the study too, will eventually be involved in construction of meaning.

Computer-aided analysis of qualitative data

Computers can of course, assist the researcher to carry out the process much more quickly – even when researchers do not use a computer package for the analysis of data. There are, however, arguments both for and against computer use in qualitative research.

Computers have been used in the analysis of qualitative data mainly since the 1980s, although they do not seem as popular as they once were. They are most useful for storing or retrieving data, and all researchers use them this way. Computers can be useful and make the process of qualitative research less cumbersome, as they offer sophisticated data organisation, data ordering and data management solutions, particularly for example, for complex studies that may have different teams working within a collaborative arrangement.

The type of approach influences the program for analysis of qualitative data. Managing a large volume of data by hand is boring and tiring because the search for specific ideas, words, incidents or events takes time. The computer is, however, merely a tool, if a useful one, for a lengthy study with a large number of partici-pants; it shortens routine and mechanical tasks and can be a device to save labour and time, although a novice researcher might spend a lengthy span of time learning to use a particular computer package. In the past, researchers depended for their analysis to a large extent on cutting, sorting and pasting bits of paper. This meant that the researcher was left with a mass of paper cuttings, a great many boxes and envelopes and/or an elaborate card system. Computers have changed these elaborate processes. We do however believe that the researcher is more intimate with the data when the analysis is not computerised. While computers can usefully assist, the use of technology does not replace the intellectual reflective process that is core in qualitative analysis.

Several types of computer-aided QDA software (CAQDAS) exist, of which the best known are NUDIST (Non-numerical Unstructured Data Indexing, Searching and Theorising) NVivo, Ethnograph ATLAS and others. Ethnograph is one of the earliest packages and NUDIST is one of the most widely used (perhaps because of its name!) The packages have slightly different functions.

Since the early 1980s, when the journal *Qualitative Sociology* (1984, **7** (1), 2) published a special edition on the use of computers in qualitative research, new ideas and packages have been developed. Some programs are more sophisticated than others. Each has its own technical traits depending on the choice of the designer. For researchers who wish to use this software, it is essential to become familiar with it.

For further information and details on particular programs, we advise researchers to refer to up-to-date text books such as Jackson and Bazeley (2019), older texts such as those by Fielding and Lee (1998) and the various writings of Richards (2015), who are advocates of CAQDAS. Lewins and Silver (2007) have written a step-by-step guide updated to Silver and Lewins (2014). A specific text on Nvivo is the book by Woolf and Silver (2018). In some of these books, pro-grams and addresses can also be found. Well known are the courses and books generated by the CAQDAS Network of the University of Surrey (see CAQDAS) Networking Project, n.d.). Gibbs' text (2018) contains two chapters on the use of computers in QDA.

The reasons for computer use

Tesch (1993) lists a variety of tasks, formerly done manually, which can now be performed by computers, some of which we list as the most important. This book is now quite old (though it has been re-edited), but these stages are still appropriate tasks for the analyst and also apply to data analysed without com-puter packages.

- Storing, annotating and retrieving texts.
- Locating words, phrases and segments of data.

- Naming or labelling.
- Sorting and organising.
- Identifying data units.
- Preparing diagrams.
- Extracting quotes.

To us this list is useful, because it also applies to qualitative analysis in general as was stated before.

Storing, annotating and retrieving texts

Storing and retrieving texts, such as interview transcripts, fieldnotes or diaries, is the most common use of computer programs in qualitative research. Data are easily accessible – for instance, interview transcripts and fieldnotes can be stored in separate files and memos attached to the category to which they belong – and can be called upon when needed. Researchers must always label and date these files to keep order among them. *NB:* Copies of files should be made on floppy disks and stored safely in different locations.

Locating words, phrases or segments of data

Researchers may want to find particular words or phrases and the context in which they occur as well as their frequency. Sentences, paragraphs and specific keywords can be recalled. These can indicate the importance, which informants and researcher attach to particular words or concepts (although it is dangerous to rely on the number of instances rather than on an in-depth examination of each instance).

Naming or labelling

These labels are keywords that define an idea, or they can be summaries of the content of data. Categorising starts here and is based on this labelling. Categories are concepts attached to a topic emerging from the data and a step in their interpretation. Researchers give the appropriate label to each segment of data or to instances that belong together. Revision of names in the light of further analysis then becomes less difficult. The creation of categories from the data is a step towards theory building. (See the section on coding and categorising.)

Sorting and organising

Sorting and organising the data segments and topic units according to the named categories or keywords attached to them is one of the procedures undertaken during the analysis process. Organising data into segments (bits, chunks or strips as they are sometimes called) means dividing them into discrete units (although these can sometimes overlap with each other). All segments with the same inherent themes or categories can be grouped together.

Identifying data units

Researchers identify data units relevant to several categories and discover relationships between them. They always try to see a structure and links between categories. While working with the data, these links can be found more easily in and across particular files. This helps in the development of working hypotheses, models or typologies. Of course, the computer does none of these processes; they are based on the researcher's theoretical considerations and decision-making but are helped by the machine. Each proposition can be checked out. For instance, a nurse researcher may infer from examining the data that women prefer male to female doctors. This can be checked quickly through viewing the categories and the links between them.

Preparing diagrams

Diagrams illustrate the relationship between themes or categories. The graphic display can enhance the storyline and help to convey its meaning. Many of our students clarify their findings by showing links and connections through diagrams.

Approaches to qualitative computer analysis

Tesch (1991) describes three main approaches to QDA (described below) but acknowledges that these groupings and their subgroups are not neat and discrete; they overlap and do not reflect reality. Both the content of the text and the process of communication are seen as important.

Language-oriented

These types of analysis are used by researchers who are primarily interested in language and its meaning – examples are conversation and discourse analysis as well as ethnography. These approaches focus not only on words and verbal interaction but also on the way in which people make sense of their world.

Descriptive/interpretive approaches

These deal with narratives and give descriptions of feelings and actions. Examples are life histories and certain types of ethnography as descriptions and interpretations of a culture. Researchers tell stories and provide interpretations of meanings that participants in the research attached to their experiences.

Theory building

In theory building, the researcher finds patterns and links between ideas and attempts to build theory. From insights generated by the data, general principles often emerge. This is more explanatory than other approaches. GT represents this type of research. The process of theory building is not routine or mechanical but demands engagement, immersion and reflection from the researcher.

The practicalities of using computer-aided analysis

Most researchers use word processors for entering and storing data. Word processing programs create and revise text and can therefore be helpful to researchers in the transcription of interviews, fieldnotes and in writing the report.

Many researchers would like to learn the use of computers for qualitative analysis, but the practicalities of this must be sorted out before starting a project. The usefulness of computers depends on the researchers' initial knowledge of computers as well as the time span and size of the project. Some of our students started learning to use the computer for data analysis and found it impossible to do so within the allocated time.

We found it difficult to learn the use of computer packages for qualitative analysis from manuals, although some people seem to be able to do so. It is always easier to let expert users teach rather than relying on a manual, but one must be aware that very experienced individuals might be too far advanced to use beginners' terms and explain the skills in a simple way. They take the language and skills needed for computers for granted. It is far better to have a teacher who is just a few steps ahead.

Not only do researchers store and retrieve data, actions that are mechanical and routine, but they also code and categorise. These tasks involve formulating concepts and theory and hence reflection. These two types of activities, procedures and conceptual thinking are always linked to each other and can both be helped by the use of computers.

KEY POINT

In computer analysis as in other types of analysis, it is necessary to stay close to the data.

Advantages of computer use

Researchers use computers as tools for facilitating processes that were done manually in the past; but it is a fallacy to believe that data can be analysed more quickly by computer programs, because it takes time to learn their use. Once learnt however, they can save time and help researchers to be more organised and systematic and facilitate planning. Bazeley (2020) stresses the speed and flexibility which they allow researchers.

Data are more accessible and fewer hours are spent sorting and coding them (However, this implies that all approaches use coding and categorising, and that, of course, is not so.) Cutting and pasting is easy when computers are used, and more time can be given to thinking through the analysis. Researchers should remember to back up their data by storing copies on floppy disks or other computers in several locations and update them regularly. Computers can make the process of qualitative research more manageable especially if a great number of participants are involved. They are, however, merely tools to make the analysis easier. While decisions and judgements are still made by the researcher, searching, cutting and pasting is done by machine. Computers cannot formulate categories or interpret the data, but they might make the analysis more accurate and comprehensive. Health researchers who are not familiar with computer analysis when starting research should not attempt computer analysis unless they are able to extend their project over a lengthy time period. (Salmons (2016) has a chapter on doing analysis in her book (Chapter 10).)

Problems and critique of computer analysis

Certain problems emerge, however, when using computers. Seidel (1991: 107), one of the early, major proponents of computer use in qualitative analysis, warns of 'analytic madness' and states that the use of technology may be a problem that can interfere with appropriate qualitative analysis. He discusses a number of issues. Researchers may be tempted to collect and manage more data than necessary, especially when they have mostly used quantitative methods in the past. The overload of data might prevent them from looking for the most interesting and significant ideas. Instead of searching for deeper meaning in the data, they try to make up for the lack of depth by focusing on the volume of data. There is also the issue of the relationship between researchers and data. This might become mechanistic if analysts do not see the need to examine and evaluate the data carefully. The number of instances of a code or category is often seen as more important than a single significant occurrence just because counting is easy. The lack of scrutiny might prevent the researcher from seeing the real meaning of the phenomenon under study. This also happens occasionally when the data are analysed manually, but the danger becomes greater through the use of computers. Richards and Morse (2013) caution against compulsive activity in computing which can interfere with the process of reflection and engagement with the data. They also maintain that researchers sometimes try to fit the research to the computer program and also homogenise the data, rather than seeing the program as a tool which assists them in the analysis.

Some researchers believe that computing skills are not only unnecessary but also their use could make qualitative research mechanistic and rigid, the very characteristics which might change its lively humanistic nature. Even now, there are some who think this. For instance, more than two decades ago, Becker (1993) already warned the grounded theorist about the use of computers; she felt that computers can prevent sensitivity to the data and the discovery of meanings. Computers might distance researchers from the data. In nursing midwifery and physiotherapy research where emotional engagement and sensitivity is necessary, the use of computers could be problematic.

The distancing of the researcher from the data is another problem in the use of computers. The involvement with a file on a computer or a printed sheet of paper, which is coded by machine, seems less personal than coding and categorising by hand. The researchers have to keep close to the data, immerse in them and engage with them.

In spite of these potential problems, many well-known qualitative researchers use computer programs when conducting a major piece of research. Computers help researchers to identify and retrieve text from documents quickly.

Computers have largely been accepted in qualitative research. In our experience, some funding agencies are impressed by computer packages because their members are used to computers in survey research and often worry about the scientific value of qualitative research. Computer packages do not, of course, confirm or deny the scientific value or quality of qualitative research, as computer-aided analysis is merely an instrument and as good or bad as the thinking and judgement of the researcher who uses it. The greatest help from computers lies in the management of data, especially when there is a large amount. It is important for researchers, however, not to distance themselves from the data.

Depending on their own stance towards the use of computer-aided analysis, or their individual needs and skills, health professionals can, of course, choose whether or not to use computer-aided data analysis.

Summary

There are a number of different ways in which data are analysed depending on the research question and the specific approach adopted.

- QDA is complex, often iterative and time-consuming.
- Many approaches use coding and categorizing, with a constant comparison of data (such as GT) which proceeds from a basic to a more abstract level, while

others apply a more holistic approach, with focus on the description and meaning of a phenomenon and the relation of parts of the data in explaining the whole picture that has emerged (for instance, phenomenology).

- Data analysis is not rigid or prescriptive, although there are certain essential commonalities in most approaches.
- Computers may be a useful tool in the analysis of data, and in some areas of data retrieval, organisation and management, but they should be used within the context of a clearly thought through rationale for their added benefit and with some caution, particularly for novice qualitative researchers.

References

Bazeley, P. (2020) *Qualitative Data Analysis: Practical Strategies*, 2nd edn, Sage, London.

Becker, P.H. (1993) Common pitfalls in grounded theory research. *Qualitative Health Research*, **3** (2), 254–260.

Boeije, H. (2010) *Analysis in Qualitative Research*, Sage, London.

Borkan, J. (1999) Immersion/crystallisation, in *Doing Qualitative Research* (eds. B.F. Crabtree and W.L. Miller), 2nd edn, Sage, Thousand Oaks, CA, pp. 179–194.

Braun, V. and Clarke, V. (2006) Using thematic analysis in psychology. *Qualitative Research in Psychology*, **3** (2), 77–101.

Braun, V. and Clarke, V. (2013) *Successful Qualitative Research: A Practical Guide for Beginners*, Sage, London.

Brooks, J., McCluskey, S., Turley, E. and King, N. (2015) The utility of template analysis in qualitative psychology research. *Qualitative Research in Psychology*, **12** (2), 202–222. doi:https://doi.org/10.1080/14780887.2014.955224.

Bryman, A. (2016) *Social Research Methods*, 5th edn, Oxford University Press, Oxford.

CAQDAS Networking Project (n.d.) University of Surrey. Available at http://caqdas.soc.surrey.ac.uk/index.htm.

Clarke, V. and Braun, V. (2019) Reading list and resources for thematic analysis. Available at https://cdn.auckland.ac.nz/assets/psych/about/our-research/documents/Reading List and Resources for Thematic Analysis April 2019.pdf.

Dahlberg, K., Dahlberg, H. and Nyström, M. (2008) *Reflective Lifeworld Research*, 2nd edn, Studentlitteratur, Lund, Sweden.

Fielding, N. and Lee, R. (1998) *Computer Analysis and Qualitative Research*, Sage, London.

Gibbs, G. (2018) *Analyzing Qualitative Data*, 2nd edn, Sage (from the Sage Qualitative Research Kit), London.

Glaser, B.G. (1978) *Theoretical Sensitivity*, Sociology Press, Mill Valley, CA.

Jackson, K. and Bazeley, P. (2019) *Qualitative Data Analysis with NVivo*, 3rd edn, Sage, Thousand Oaks, CA.

King, N. (2004) Using templates in the thematic analysis of text, in *Essential Guide to Qualitative Methods in Organizational Research* (eds. C. Cassels and G. Symon), Sage, London, pp. 256–270.

Langridge, D. (2007) *Phenomenological Psychology*, Pearson/Prentice Hall, Harlow.

Lewins, A. and Silver, C. (2007) *Using Software in Qualitative Research: A Step-by-Step Guide*, Sage, London.

Li, S. and Seale, C. (2007) Learning to do qualitative data analysis: an observational study of doctoral work. *Qualitative Health Research*, **17** (10), 1442–1452.

Moustakas, C. (1994) *Phenomenological Research Methods*, Sage, Thousand Oaks, CA.

Patton, M. (2015) *Qualitative Evaluation and Research Methods*, 4th edn, Sage, Thousand Oaks, CA.

Richards, L. (2015) *Handling Qualitative Data: A Practical Guide*, 3rd edn, Sage, London.

Richards, M.G. and Morse, J.M. (2013) *Readme First: A User's Guide to Qualitative Methods*, 3rd edn, Sage, Thousand Oaks, CA.

Ritchie, L., Lewis, J., Nicholls, C.M. and Ormston, R. (2014) *Qualitative Research Practice: A Guide for Social Science Students and Researchers*, Sage, London.

Salmons, J. (2016) *Doing Qualitative Research Online*, Sage, London.

Seidel, J. (1991) Method and madness in the application of computer technology qualitative data analysis, in *Using Computers in Qualitative Research* (eds. N.G. Fielding and R.M. Lee), Sage, London, pp. 107–118.

Silver, C. and Lewins, A. (2014) *Using Software in Qualitative Research: A Step by Step Guide*, 2nd edn, Sage, London.

Silverman, D. (2017) *Doing Qualitative Research: A Practical Handbook*, 5th edn, Sage, London.

Silverman, D. (2020) *Interpreting Qualitative Data*, 6th edn, Sage, London.

Tesch, R. (1991) Software for qualitative researchers, in *Using Computers in Qualitative Research* (eds. N.G. Fielding and R.M. Lee), Sage, London, pp. 16–37.

Tesch, R. (1993) Personal computers in qualitative research, in *Ethnography and Qualitative Design in Educational Research* (eds. M.D. LeCompte, J. Preissle and R. Tesch), 2nd edn, Academic Press, Chicago, IL, pp. 279–314.

Woolf, N.H. and Silver, C. (2018) *Qualitative Analysis Using NVivo* (Developing Qualitative Inquiry) Routledge, Abingdon Oxford.

Further Reading

Miles, M.B. (2020) *Qualitative Data Analysis*, 4th edn, Sage, Thousand Oaks, CA.

Vaismoradi, M., Bondas, T. and Turunen, H. (2013). Content analysis and thematic analysis: implications for conducting a qualitative descriptive study. *Journal of Nursing & Health Sciences*, **15**, 398–405. doi:10.1111/nhs.12048.

Vaismoradi, M. and Snelgrove, S. (2019) Theme in qualitative content analysis and in thematic analysis. *Forum Qualitative Sozialforschung/Forum: Qualitative Social Research*, **20** (3), Art. 23. doi:10.17169/fqs-20.3.3376.

Wong, G. and Breheny, M. (2018) Narrative analysis in health psychology: a guide for analysis. *Health Psychology and Behavioral Medicine*, **6** (1), 245–261.

Chapter 17

Establishing Quality: Validity and Trustworthiness

Quality

To demonstrate the quality of their research health, researchers need to demonstrate its credibility and validity. This involves reflection on knowledge claims arising from the research in the context of epistemological issues in qualitative inquiry.

No single or unitary concept of validity exists in qualitative research which is comparable to its meaning in quantitative inquiry, and, as Onwuegbuzie and Leech (2007) state, there is no single definition of validity in qualitative research.

There are several distinct perspectives on the quality of qualitative research (Murphy *et al.*, 1998), some of which are listed below, and though these authors wrote more than 20 years ago, their thoughts are still valid.

- Qualitative and quantitative research should be evaluated by the same criteria.
- Qualitative research should be evaluated by criteria that have been specially developed for it.
- Criteriology (the emphasis on criteria) should be rejected.

Maxwell (2012: 122) argues that the concept of validity has been controversial, that many researchers see it as too closely linked with quantitative inquiry and do not use it. However, Silverman (2017), among many others, argues for the retention of the criteria of reliability and validity while stating, at the same time, that these cannot be directly translated from quantitative to qualitative research because qualitative inquiry has its own criteria by which it can be evaluated. Indeed, validity in qualitative research has different implications and applications. Although qualitative researchers are flexible and open minded, they are also advised to be systematic and well organised and through this, the research gains validity.

Proponents of another group follow the ideas: Guba and Lincoln (1989) developed the concepts of trustworthiness and authenticity as parallel and alternative criteria on which many researchers base their ideas (recently Amin *et al.*, 2020) The researcher will come across both groups of terms during their

Qualitative Research in Nursing and Healthcare, Fifth Edition.
Immy Holloway and Kathleen Galvin.
© 2024 John Wiley & Sons Ltd. Published 2024 by John Wiley & Sons Ltd.

reading and therefore will have to know about them regardless of the terms they themselves apply. However, a simplistic stance is sometimes taken, and concepts developed here are complex. Different qualitative approaches often have a different view of quality, and Sparkes and Smith (2013) demonstrate that there is no shared understanding of validity or trustworthiness in qualitative research. Researchers find difficulty agreeing on how to judge the 'validity' of qualitative research or how to present convincing evidence of its trustworthiness.

Conventional criteria

We will discuss the traditional criteria generally used in quantitative research, their meaning in qualitative inquiry and their alternatives. Trustworthiness and authenticity are more often used than validity and reliability in qualitative healthcare research, and they are discussed in detail later in the chapter.
- Rigour – trustworthiness
- Reliability – dependability
- Validity – credibility
- Generalisability (external validity) – transferability
- Objectivity – confirmability

Rigour

The concept of rigour has its origin in science, and quantitative researchers use it because of its particular connotations with measurement and objectivity; hence it has a more appropriate place in quantitative research. In qualitative research rigour indicates thoroughness and competence. Sandelowski (1986, 1993) wrote two classic articles on rigour in qualitative nursing research. Her latter article recognises that the term rigour could imply inflexibility and rigidity and that researchers should not be too preoccupied with it. Instead, she advises that they should create 'evocative, true-to-life and meaningful portraits, stories and landscapes of human experience ...' (p. 1), and she criticises 'the reduction of validity to a set of procedures' (p. 2). Indeed, excessive rigour may hinder creativity and artistry (Bradbury-Jones, 2007).

Reliability

Reliability in quantitative inquiry refers to the consistency and stability of the research instrument. It is also linked to replicability, that is the extent to which the study is repeatable and produces the same results when the methodology is replicated in similar circumstances and conditions. As the researcher is the main research instrument in qualitative inquiry, the research can never be wholly replicable. Also, reliability refers to particular points in time.

A qualitative study, however, can be accurate, reflect the words and deeds of the participants and might be similar in related settings and contexts as long as it is clear that the researcher cannot wholly replicate the time and context. Other investigators have different emphases and foci, even when they adopt the same methods and select a similar sample and topic area.

Silverman (2020) maintains that the research process needs be transparent to be reliable. He argues for the retention of the term reliability (Chapter 4), while many qualitative researchers avoid this term in their work because it is closely associated with quantitative inquiry.

Validity

Validity in quantitative research is seen as the extent to which an instrument measures what it is supposed to measure. In qualitative research, the concept is more complex. It is always used in quantitative but also more recently in qualitative research. Description and interpretation by researchers and truth telling by participants are all important.

One of the threats to validity is posed when collecting incorrect or incomplete data. The field diary must therefore be detailed and extensive. In interpretation, researchers are in danger of imposing their own ideas or distorting the meaning of the participants' accounts. Therefore, it is important for the researcher to listen to the participants' voices and let them speak before imposing their own interpretations. Researchers hope that the stories of the participants are true; they do occasionally make mistakes or deliberately tell lies, although the latter seems to be rare. This does not mean that there is no truth: the participants describe their world as they see it from their own perspective in the context of their time and culture as well as their own biography. Researchers generally trust their participants even if they cannot prove the 'truth' of their tales. The description by the researcher should not only be plausible but also trustworthy. Researchers set aside their own thoughts and preconceptions about the phenomenon under study at some stage. Alternative and rival explanations to the researchers' own initial interpretation should be taken into account. Although researchers can never be fully certain that all threats to validity have been eliminated, awareness of these threats helps produce a valid piece of research.

To the term validity, Hammersley (1998) adds that of *relevance* as a criterion for evaluating qualitative research. Relevance means that explanatory factors should have significance related to the purpose of the research and in solving the problems of practitioners in the discipline. The research must not only be meaningful but also useful for those who undertake it.

Internal validity is the extent to which the findings of a study are true, and whether they accurately reflect the aim of the research and the social reality of those participating in it. This can be established to an extent by taking the findings back to the participants (see the section on member check later in this chapter). The researchers can compare their own findings with the perception of the people involved and explore whether they are compatible. Bryman (2012) adds that there should be a match between observations and the theoretical concepts which have their roots in them. However, not all approaches in qualitative research use member checking. It is a contentious issue in the context of the researcher being immersed in the whole research process with the participants, and as such is an active part of the research, bringing with them their own values, worldviews and interpretation, in other words, they discover the findings with participants. For a specialist discussion of these issues in relation to validity in qualitative research from an epistemological perspective, see Giorgi (2002). (Member checking is discussed later in this chapter in more detail.)

External validity, also called generalisability, is described in the next section.

Generalisability or external validity

This is the most contentious concept linked to validity. For some authors, generalisability is not an issue to be discussed at length, for they believe it is not relevant as they speak of specific situations and cases. For others, however, this is problematic. Most funding agencies and research committees in the UK National Health Service demand that the proposed research be generalisable, and this is understandable. If large amounts of money are given to researchers, funding bodies wish to know whether the outcomes are of general use in clinical practice and not just the results of 'blue skies' research undertaken for its own sake or only applicable to specific situations.

Generalisability exists when the findings and conclusions of a research study can be applied to other similar settings and populations, that is when they can be generalised across a variety of settings. The term has its origin in quantitative research with its random statistical sampling procedures. Random sampling ensures that the results of the research are representative of the group from which the sample was drawn. It is clear that this type of generalisability cannot be achieved in qualitative research in which sampling is purposeful or, in grounded theory, theoretical.

Generalisability is difficult to achieve in qualitative research, and it is not the aim of this type of inquiry. Positivist and interpretive research differ in the sense that positivists seek law-like generalities, while interpretivists focus on unique cases even though they might want to establish patterns. As much quantitative research – although by no means all – is carried out in the positivist tradition and uses deductive methods, it can be more easily generalised. Many qualitative researchers, however, do not aim to achieve generalisability as they focus on specific instances or cases not necessarily representative of other cases or populations. The case(s) may even be atypical.

For instance, a nurse, physiotherapist or midwife may want to examine a particular phenomenon important for local practice and patients in a particular area rather than of interest to the whole country. However, the study can still be successful, because it highlights specific non-typical features that can be related and compared to those of other, more typical cases.

Many qualitative researchers attempt to achieve some generalisability, however, because they feel that their research should be useful beyond their own studies. Strauss and Corbin (1998) speak of the representativeness of concepts and applicability of theory to other situations. This means that qualitative research can have external validity through 'theory-based generalisation'. Morse (1994) claimed two decades ago that theory contributes to the 'greater body of knowledge' when it is re-contextualised into a variety of settings. She confirms her claims in 2012 (Morse 2012). Theoretical generalisation involves the application of theoretical concepts found in one situation to other settings and conditions. If the theory developed from the original data analysis can be verified in other sites and situations, the theoretical ideas are generalisable. The findings from multi-site studies are, of course, more easily generalisable than those from a few unique cases from one setting. Additionally, in phenomenological research the general purpose is to delineate and describe universal features and characteristics of a phenomenon and to draw out variances as revealed through the findings. These universal features of, for example, the human experience of anger or of crying, are relevant beyond the specific phenomenological study.

Lewis *et al.* (2014: 349) give more specific suggestions for generalisation. They describe three different types that could be potentially applicable qualitative research:

- *Representational Generalisation:* If the findings of a sample can be generalised to a similar 'parent' population.
- *Inferential Generalisation:* When findings of a study can be transferred to other settings and contexts.
- *Theoretical Generalisation:*

When the theoretical ideas have more general application. However, on reflection, transferability would be a more useful and appropriate word in qualitative inquiry. (See later in this chapter.)

Objectivity and subjectivity

Objectivity and subjectivity are terms often used in quantitative research. Objectivity means that the research is free of biases and relatively value neutral. Qualitative researchers do not find this concept very useful. Objectivity and neutrality are difficult to achieve; in fact, the values of researchers and participants become an integral part of the research, and they must openly acknowledge their own subjectivity. They do not conceal it but examine and then set it aside. Critical subjectivity, a term originally coined by Carr and Kemmis (1986) and later developed by other writers, is useful here which means that the researcher is self-reflexive. Although much knowledge is based on subjective experience, it should not be accepted in a simplistic way but rooted in critical consciousness. Researchers do not disregard their subjectivity; they are aware of it and attempt to have self-reflexivity, so no prior assumptions can introduce bias in the study, the researcher strives to be aware of prior assumptions and make them explicit for the reader.

The concept of validity in qualitative research

The concept of validity is used in some qualitative approaches (descriptive phenomenology for instance), but its meaning and the way in which it is ensured is less precise and prescriptive than in other forms of qualitative research. For instance, Research can be valid through intersubjective knowledge. Moustakas (1994) speaks of 'intersubjective truth'. He states (p. 57) that according to Husserl, 'each can experience and know the other, not exactly as one experiences and knows oneself but in the sense of empathy and copresence'. Initially, truth is based in the unique perspective of unique individuals and their self-knowledge. As individuals inhabit the world of self and others, there is also communication with others. This enhances intersubjective understanding. If the research is to have validity, its readers will have learnt something of the human condition as well as recognise and grasp the essence of the phenomenon under study. This form of 'validity' is similar to, although not the same, the concept of 'ontological authenticity' described by Guba and Lincoln (1989) or that of 'thick description' by Geertz (1973).

In phenomenology and a number of other approaches such as grounded theory, internal validity (being faithful to the ideas of the participants) is a complex concept as the researchers always transform the data and take them to a different level from that of the participants when they describe the phenomenon or interpret the ideas of the participants. The researchers' ideas are more abstract and theoretical than those of the participants, and ultimately the researchers' description and interpretation is presented to the readers of the account, although they are grounded in the participants' thoughts and feelings. Lomberg and Kirkevold develop the ideas about validity in grounded theory, namely those of fit, relevance and modifiability (see details in Lomberg and Kirkevold, 2003). Hope and Waterman (2003) discuss the re-conceptualisation of validity in action research, stressing the importance of contextualisation and rigorous application of the chosen approach. (It is not possible to develop ideas on validity in each approach, but we hope that researchers might gain more details from the references.)

An alternative perspective: trustworthiness

It can be seen that the conventional terms used in quantitative research have different meanings in qualitative inquiry. Guba and Lincoln (1989), as stated before, go further than this and develop alternative terms and criteria. We will show how health researchers can attempt to demonstrate trustworthiness in the last section of this chapter. Barusch *et al.* (2011) suggest that this term gives qualitative researchers at least an opportunity to explain the credibility of their research to others.

Trustworthiness in qualitative research means methodological soundness and adequacy. Researchers make judgements of trustworthiness possible through developing dependability, credibility, transferability and confirmability. The most important of these is credibility.

Dependability

Lincoln and Guba (1985; also Guba and Lincoln, 1989) use the term dependability instead of reliability. If the findings of a study are to be dependable, they should be consistent and accurate. This means that readers will be able to evaluate the adequacy of the analysis by following the decision-making processes of the researcher. The context of the research must also be described in detail. To achieve some measure of dependability, an audit trail is necessary. This helps readers follow the path of the researcher and demonstrates how they achieved their conclusions. It also guides other researchers wishing to carry out similar research. Although the study cannot be replicated, in similar circumstances with similar participants, it can be repeated.

Credibility

Credibility corresponds to the notion of internal validity (p. 252). This means that the participants recognise the meaning that they themselves give to a situation or condition and the 'truth' of the findings in their own social context. The researcher's findings are, at least, compatible with the perceptions of the people under study.

Transferability

Lincoln and Guba use transferability instead of generalisability. This means that the findings in one context can be transferred to similar situations or participants. The knowledge acquired in one context will be relevant in another, and those who carry out the same research in another context will be able to apply certain concepts originally developed by other researchers. It seems to us that the concepts of transferability and generalisability are not too different but that transferability is a more appropriate concept.

Confirmability

Confirmability has taken the place of the term objectivity. As the research is judged by the way in which the findings and conclusions achieve their aim and are not the result of the researcher's prior assumptions and preconceptions, Lincoln and Guba demand 'confirmability'. This again needs an audit or decision trail where readers can trace the data to their sources. They follow the path of the researcher and the way he or she arrived at the constructs, themes and their interpretation. For this, details of the research and the background and feelings of the researcher should be open to public scrutiny. When confirmability exists, readers can trace data to their original sources.

Authenticity

Trustworthiness, which relies on the methodological adequacy of the research, does not suffice according to Guba and Lincoln (1989), and therefore they add the concept of authenticity. A study is authentic when the strategies used are appropriate for the true reporting of the participants' ideas. Authenticity consists of the following:

1 *Fairness:* The researcher must be fair to participants and gain their acceptance throughout the study. Continued informed consent must be obtained. The social contexts in which the participants work and live also need to be taken into account.
2 *Ontological Authenticity:* This means that those involved, readers and participants, will have been helped to understand their social world and their human condition through the research.
3 *Educative Authenticity:* Through understanding, participants improve the way in which they understand other people.
4 *Catalytic Authenticity:* Decision-making by participants should be enhanced by the research.
5 *Tactical Authenticity:* The research should empower participants.

A study is authentic when the strategies used are appropriate for the true reporting of the participants' ideas, when the study is fair and when it helps participants and similar groups to understand their world and improve it. It means that there is new insight into the phenomenon under study.

Trustworthiness and authenticity are achieved by following certain strategies. Indeed, Lincoln and Guba developed and systematised these within their writing. The concept of authenticity has not found the same response in qualitative research as the term trustworthiness, which is now popular as an alternative for validity in qualitative research, especially in the United States.

Bryman (2012) suggests that the preceding concepts are an adaptation of the term's validity and reliability for qualitative research.

Strategies to ensure trustworthiness

There are a number of ways in which qualitative researchers can check and demonstrate to the reader whether the research is trustworthy. The most common strategies are the following (although not all of these are accepted by all qualitative researchers and they remain contested):

- Member checking
- Searching for negative cases and alternative explanations
- Peer review (also called peer debriefing)
- Triangulation
- The audit or decision trail
- Thick description
- Prolonged engagement
- Reflexivity

It is more likely that the study is trustworthy if researchers have been involved in the setting for a lengthy period of time as this may eliminate the reactivity of participants, because they learn to trust and are more likely to tell the truth, and also because their own assumptions can be examined in the process of prolonged engagement, persistent observation and immersion in the setting. This does not seem problematic for health professionals who are deeply involved with clinical practice. However, they occasionally bring preconceptions to the research and it is important to be aware of these.

Member checking

Throughout interviews and observations, a check is needed on the understanding of the data with the people who are studied. Researchers do this by summarising, repeating or paraphrasing the participants' words or by talking about their understanding of the participants' words or actions. They then ask whether the participants feel that the interpretation is a true and fair representation of their perspective. This is called a *member check* (Lincoln and Guba, 1985) or *member validation*. The main reasons for member checking are the feedback of participants, their reaction to the data and findings and their response to the researcher's interpretation of the data which are obtained from them as individuals.

The specific purposes of member checking are as follows:

- To find out whether the reality of the participants is presented.
- To provide opportunities for them to change mistakes which they feel they might have made.
- To assess the researcher's understanding and interpretation of the data.
- To give the participants the opportunity to challenge the ideas of the researcher.

Feedback from others ensures the trustworthiness of the research, and a member check is one of the strategies for achieving this. The procedure will help avoid misinterpretation or misunderstanding of the participants' words or actions. If a member check is carried out, it is more likely that the researcher presents the participant's point of view. After all, the aim of the study is to give a true and accurate picture of the participants' different perspectives.

There are a number of ways to carry out member checks:

1 The researcher presents participants with a transcript of their interview or fieldnotes of observations and asks them to comment on the contents. This is a very time-consuming process, and research participants cannot comment on the researcher's interpretations of their perspectives. Although this is an acceptable procedure, we would not advise researchers to do this, because of the time it takes.

2 The interviewer can give the participants a summary of their interview, and his or her own interpretation of their words. This is a more useful way of confirming the ideas and the meaning of the account. The interviewers can discuss their own interpretations and discuss the meaning of the participants' words and actions. It is a check on the understanding of the account. Participants may change meaning and correct errors. The check may also add clarity or trigger and extend ideas that go beyond the original interview. The comments can be included in the final report.

3 The researcher might present the final copy or substantial sections of the report and ask the participants to comment on the contents. Again, this is a lengthy process that demands time commitment and thought from participants, which they may not be able or willing to give. Although all or any of these procedures could be employed, we would suggest the second strategy as the most practical. Member checks do not only help in achieving validity in the study, but they also empower participants and give them control to confirm their words and actions and thus some control in the research itself. Member checking demands a large time commitment from both participant and researcher.

4 Finally, researchers could just give a short overview of the findings of the research and find whether they confirm the participants' ideas.

However rigorous and detailed the member check, some problems are inherent in it:

- The researcher's and participants' perspectives may be different.
- The reactions of participants may be defensive.

- The close relationship with the researcher may prevent the participant from adopting a critical stance.
- Perceptions may change over time.
- The researcher develops second-order concepts and theories.

Sandelowski (1993) sees member checking as problematic and complex. She points to the fact that participants and researchers have a different agenda. Members are more interested in their own unique experiences. Researchers wish to portray 'multiple realities', while still representing the experience of each participant.

Some of the issues related to member checks pose ethical dilemmas for the researcher. Participants might become aware and anxious that they have disclosed ideas that might be judged as unacceptable by the researcher or a reader of the report. They might hesitate to disagree because they have built up a close relationship with the researcher whom they see as a friend. Also, if the member check does not take place at an early stage after collection or analysis of the data, the participants might have changed their perceptions, and the researcher has to start again. Change over time is, of course, one of the reasons, why several interviews are better than one, and why immersion in the setting is useful.

Researchers present the participants' perspectives and the meaning they give to their experiences; however, the data are also transformed so that they become uniquely the researcher's who takes them to a more abstract, theoretical level. Bryman (2012) sums up the problematics of member checking. He claims that researchers write for a readership of scholars and peers. This means that they always take the research to the level of developing concepts, an etic view which includes but goes beyond the participants' perspectives. He also suggests that participants may be defensive of their words or reluctant to be critical and change their minds (p. 391).

Searching for negative cases and alternative explanations

It enhances the validity of the research if the researchers identify data that do not easily fit into the developing theory or their own ideas. There may also be contrary occurrences that do not easily fit into developing patterns. These may provide alternative explanations. In the critical analysis, researchers may find notions and events that do not fit their explanations and challenge the themes and patterns arising from the data. It means thinking about other possibilities. Data that confirm as well as those that challenge and disconfirm have to be examined. Researchers will have to explore whether conclusions gained from them are appropriate. Indeed, even if there is just one case that does not fit or fits a rival explanation, researchers should try to revise their interpretations so they can become confident that the explanations or interpretations derived from the data are the most valid and plausible and can also account for the alternative case.

Negative or deviant case analysis involves addressing and considering alternative explanations or interpretations of the data, especially those which may be contrary to their own view of reality. Working hypotheses or propositions and search for alternative explanations can then be revised. Single or few 'dissenting voices' included in the final report demonstrate the complexity of the research. Negative case analysis always presents challenges: It is not easy to become aware of discrepant data and negative or alternative cases, but at some stage researchers must stop searching when they feel they have exhausted the alternative possibilities and can account for all the cases including those that are 'deviant'.

Peer review

It is also useful to employ the strategy of peer review or 'peer debriefing', as Lincoln and Guba (1985) called it. This means that colleagues who are competent in qualitative research procedures might re-analyse the data, compare their own findings to those of the researcher and listen to the researcher's concerns. Peers can be given the draft copy at the end of the research. They might detect bias or inappropriate subjectivity and try alternative explanations to the researcher's own working propositions and warn them against the attempt to 'fit' interpretations and explanations that cannot be substantiated by the data. Peers can thus challenge the coding decisions, interpretations and assumptions of the researcher. The credibility of the research is then established by more than a single researcher.

Peer review can be a useful tool to confirm some of the main ideas emerging from the research and to ensure coherence and plausibility. Some of our colleagues or doctoral students ask us as relative outsiders to carry out peer debriefing, but they often ask close health professional colleagues because they are insiders in the setting.

Triangulation

Another important strategy to establish validity is to adopt triangulation procedures. Triangulation is the process by which the phenomenon or topic under study is examined from different perspectives. Triangulation in research means that the findings of one type of method (or data, researcher and theory) can be checked out by reference to another. This will provide a way of establishing whether there is generalisability in the research, although researchers do not necessarily aim for this. Denzin (1989), decades ago, differentiates between several types of triangulation as listed below.

- *Data Triangulation*, where researchers use multiple data sources and obtain their data from different groups, settings or at different times (multiple sources of data). Data triangulation is the most common way of triangulating.
- *Investigator Triangulation*, when more than one expert researcher is involved in the study. This is common in larger studies but rarely happens in student projects or theses.
- *Theoretical Triangulation*, when the researcher employs several possible theoretical interpretations in the study. Competing explanations or interpretations are developed and tested against each other to find the one which is most likely to describe or explain the phenomenon.
- *Methodological Triangulation*, when researchers use two or more methods in one study to answer a similar question (observations, interviews, documents, questionnaires). These are either between-method or within-method triangulation (see below).

The last method in the list is most often used in a small-scale dissertation. Researchers might consider confirming findings using one method with the findings of another. It is not always necessary, although occasionally desirable, to use quantitative methods to confirm qualitative findings, that is using 'between-method' triangulation. Morse (2001: 210) gives a number of possibilities for triangulation, each of which has different emphases. Studies using quantitative and qualitative methods can be used simultaneously or sequentially depending on the main direction of the research and its underlying assumptions. Morse claims (p. 209) that they may generate 'a more complete understanding.

However, it is more common to check observations with answers from qualitative interviews or documents and thus stay within the same methodology; this is called 'within-method' triangulation. It can include interviews and observations, diaries or other data sources. Indeed, some researchers might argue that this has better 'fit' with the research view of qualitative researchers.

Triangulation takes place when the same phenomenon has been examined in different ways or from different perspectives. Triangulation does not, of course, automatically demonstrate the trustworthiness of the study. It is used to give more depth to the analysis and enhance its validity, although it cannot guarantee it.

The audit or decision trail

All research should have an audit trail by which others are able to judge, to some extent at least, its validity. Halpern (1983) initially discussed the inquiry audit in qualitative research, and Lincoln and Guba (1985) developed the concept of the audit trail. The audit trail is the detailed record of the decisions made before and during the research and a description of the research process. Rodgers and Cowles (1993) suggest four types of documentation:

1 Contextual
2 Methodological
3 Analytic
4 Personal response

The *contextual* documents should contain excerpts from fieldnotes of observation and interviewing, the description of the setting, people and location. The political and social context must also be described. Rodgers and Cowles suggest that *methodological* documents include methodological decision-making and the rationale for these decisions. *Analytic* documents consist of reflections on the analysis of data and the theoretical insights gained. *Personal response* documents describe the thought processes and demonstrate the self-awareness of the researcher. This self-examination is part of 'reflexivity' discussed later in this chapter. An account of the decisions that were made throughout should be incorporated into the research account to point.

Thick description

Thick description too, helps to establish the truth value of the research and is linked to the audit trail. The term was coined originally by the philosopher Ryle but developed by Geertz (1973); it means a detailed description of the process, context and people in the research, inclusive of the meaning and intentions of the participants and the researcher's conceptual developments. Thick description provides a basis for the reader's evaluation of quality.

Thick description is an account of the complex processes in a specific context and a rich and 'holistic' and even 'artistic' portrayal of the phenomenon under study. Readers of the research report should be able to follow the research trail, empathise with the participants and draw similar conclusions to the researcher. There is a chance, however, that the research is not seen as useful if the reader cannot transfer the insight gained from the research to other settings, particularly in the healthcare arena. If the contextual description is rich and the analytical language comprehensive enough to enable readers to understand the processes and interactions involved in the context, it might be possible to generalise to the extent of stating that people in other settings have a similar way of understanding. Thick description necessitates immersion and prolonged engagement in the setting (see also Chapters 7 and 10).

Prolonged engagement

Immersion in the setting, or 'persistent observation' which helps to deepen the research and 'prolonged engagement' which extends its scope (Lincoln and Guba, 1985: 304), is not only useful but also often necessary in qualitative research to discover how people behave, interact and whether their actions confirm what they have told the researcher. Through this immersion in the situation, researchers become aware of the context of the research, and they are able to gain insight into the setting. For some, this is not always possible because of time constraints but the study always improves and gains trustworthiness when these strategies are carried out. It means spending time in the setting.

Reflexivity

Reflexivity means that researchers critically reflect on their own preconceptions and monitor their relationships with the participants and their own reactions to participants' accounts and actions. As the main tool of the research, researchers are part of the phenomenon to be studied and must reflect on their own actions, feelings and conflicts experienced during the research. If they adopt a self-critical stance to the research and their own role, relationships and assumptions, the study will become more credible and dependable. A self-critical stance throughout the inquiry process and location in political and social context enhances the quality of the research. Reflexivity is ongoing through data collection, analysis, interpretation and writing up (see also Chapter 1).

Quality and creativity

There is an essential tension between the focus on method and creativity, which is sometimes neglected by those who endlessly grapple with validity and its equivalents. Thus, there is no complete consensus about the quality of qualitative research and the criteria adopted.

The obsession of qualitative researchers with validity and related issues is due to a defensive stance in relation to the critics of qualitative research by positivist writers. Sparkes (2001) claims that the topic of validity will remain unresolved and different perspectives on it can coexist because of the variety of epistemological and ontological stances. However, we suggest that as long as qualitative inquiry is seen as 'not really' valid by quantitative researchers, those who undertake qualitative studies will have to explain why their work is credible, and that the quality criteria by which to judge it are useful devices to demonstrate this.

Cho and Trent (2006) maintain, however, that just because certain techniques and strategies have been used to establish validity or trustworthiness, there are still no guarantees that the knowledge obtained is valid, especially as the researcher has transformed the data and interpreted the findings.

> **KEY POINT**
>
> Whatever labels health professionals apply, they have to demonstrate that their research has truth value, and they should be consistent in the language, concepts and methods.

Summary

There are several distinct schools of thought about criteria for judging qualitative inquiry.

- Qualitative researchers use either the conventional criteria of validity and reliability or alternatives such as trustworthiness and authenticity. There is some shared understanding of the concepts and the strategies to achieve credibility.
- Strategies to ensure the quality of the research include member checking, the search for alternative cases, peer debriefing, in-method triangulation, disclosing an audit trail, thick description, prolonged engagement and reflexivity.
- It is important for researchers to spend time in the setting and immerse themselves in this.

References

Amin, M.E.K., Norgaard, L.S., Cavaco A.M. *et al.* (2020) Establishing the trustworthiness and authenticity in qualitative pharmacy research. *Research in Social and Administrative Pharmacy*, **16** (10), 1472–1482.

Barusch, A., Gringeri, C. and George, M. (2011) Rigor in qualitative social work research: a review of strategies used in published articles. *Social Work Research*, **35** (1), 11–19.

Bradbury-Jones, C. (2007) Enhancing rigour in qualitative research: exploring subjectivity through Peshkin's I's. *Journal of Advanced Nursing*, **59** (3), 290–298.

Bryman, A. (2012) *Social Research Methods*, 4th edn, Oxford University Press, Oxford.

Carr, W. and Kemmis, S. (1986) *Becoming Critical: Education, Knowledge and Action Research*, The Falmer Press, London.

Cho, J. and Trent, A. (2006) Validity in qualitative research revisited. *Qualitative Research*, **6** (3), 319–340.

Denzin, N.K. (1989) *The Research Act: A Theoretical Introduction to Sociological Methods*, 3rd edn, Prentice-Hall, Englewood Cliffs, NJ.

Geertz, C. (1973) *The Interpretation of Cultures*, Basic Books, New York, NY.

Giorgi, A. (2002) The question of validity in qualitative research. *Journal of Phenomenological Psychology*, **33** (1), 1–18.

Guba, E.G. and Lincoln, Y.S. (1989) *Fourth Generation Evaluation*, Sage, New York, NY.

Halpern, E.S. (1983) Auditing naturalistic inquiries: the development and application of a model. Unpublished doctoral dissertation, Indiana University (cited by Rodgers and Cowles (1993) qv).

Hammersley, M. (1998) *Reading Ethnographic Research: A Critical Guide*, 2nd edn, Longman, London.

Hope, K.W. and Waterman, H.A. (2003) Praiseworthy pragmatism? Validity and action research. *Journal of Advanced Nursing*, **44** (2), 120–127.

Lewis, J., Ritchie, J. Ormiston, R. and Morrell, G. (2014) Generalising from qualitative research, in *Qualitative Research Practice* (ed. J. Ritchie, J. Lewis, C. Nicholls and R. Ormston), Sage, London, pp. 347–362.

Lincoln, Y.S. and Guba, E.G. (1985) *Naturalistic Inquiry*, Sage, Beverly Hills, CA.

Lomberg, K. and Kirkevold, M. (2003) Truth and validity in grounded theory: a reconsidered realist interpretation of the criteria: fit, relevance and modifiability. *Nursing Philosophy*, **4** (3), 169–200.

Maxwell, J.A. (2012) *Qualitative Research Design: An Interactive Approach*, 3rd edn, Sage, Thousand Oaks, CA, Chapter 6.

Morse, J.M. (1994) Designing funded qualitative research, in *Handbook of Qualitative Research* (eds. N.K. Denzin and Y.S. Lincoln), Sage, Thousand Oaks, CA, pp. 220–235.

Morse, J.M. (2001) Qualitative verification: building evidence by extending basic findings, in *The Nature of Qualitative Evidence* (eds. J.M. Morse, J.M. Swanson and A.J. Kuzel), Sage, Thousand Oaks, CA, pp. 203–220.

Morse, J.M. (2012) *Qualitative Health Research: Creating a New Discipline*, LeftCoast Press, Walnut Creek, CA.

Moustakas, C. (1994) *Phenomenological Research Methods*, Sage, Thousand Oaks, CA.

Murphy, E., Dingwall, R., Greatbatch, D. *et al.* (1998) Qualitative research method in health technology assessment. *Health Technology Assessment*, **2** (16), 1–274.

Onwuegbuzie, A.J. and Leech, N.L. (2007) Validity and qualitative research: an oxymoron? *Quality and Quantity*, **41** (2), 233–245.

Rodgers, B.L. and Cowles, V. (1993) The qualitative audit trail: a complex collection of documentation. *Research in Nursing and Health*, **16** (3), 219–226.

Sandelowski, M. (1986) The problem of rigour in qualitative research. *Advances in Nursing Science*, **8** (3), 27–37.

Sandelowski, M. (1993) Rigor or rigor mortis: the problem of rigour in qualitative research revisited. *Advances in Nursing Science*, **16** (2), 1–8.

Silverman, D. (2017) *Doing Qualitative Research*, 5th edn, Sage, London.

Silverman, D. (2020) *Interpreting Qualitative Data*, 6th edn, Sage, London.

Sparkes, A. (2001) Myth 94: qualitative health researchers will agree about validity. *Qualitative Health Research*, **11** (1), 538–552.

Sparkes, A.C. and Smith, B. (2013) *Qualitative Research in Sports, Exercise and Health*, Routledge, Abingdon.

Strauss, A. and Corbin, J. (1998) *Basics of Qualitative Research: Techniques and Procedures for Developing Grounded Theory*, 2nd edn, Sage, Thousand Oaks, CA.

(The older references are often the foundational articles for the discussion in this chapter)

Further Reading

Bryman, A., Bell, E., Reck, J. and Fields, J. (2022) *Social Research Methods*, Oxford University Press, Oxford.

Luciani, M., Campbell, K.A., Whitmore, C. *et al.* (2020) How to critically appraise a qualitative research study. *BMJ Evidence-Based Medicine*. Available at www.profinf.net/pro3/index.php/IN/article/view/700.

(This is a comprehensive overview of the appraisal of quality in qualitative research with references to checklists)

Johnson, J.L., Adkins, D. and Chauvin, S. (2020) Qualitative research in pharmacy education. *American Journal of Pharmacy Education*, **84** (1), article 7120.

Chapter 18

Writing up and Publishing Qualitative Research

The research account

Writing the report of the research is an important task for the researcher; the presentation is in the public domain and it is essential that the researcher's stance, study processes, analysis and findings can be reviewed by others. Even the background and former involvement of the researcher in the setting might be important. Researchers submit the results of their work to external examiners, commissioning or funding agencies or to a journal for peer review either in the academic or professional arena. If the study is a thesis or dissertation, the candidate will have guidelines for presentation and these should be followed. Although conventions for writing up exist, the format may vary from one institution to another. It is of note that the communication of robust and in-depth qualitative research to audiences is quite complex and we suggest readers also seek guidance from specialist texts in writing up qualitative research, especially if a thesis is being produced.

KEY POINT

Researchers should become acquainted with the regulations of their organisation for the production of a research report/dissertation.

The research report mirrors the proposal, although the latter is more detailed and, of course, includes the findings and discussion. There are various forms of presenting findings, some of which have been discussed by Reay *et al.* (2019).

Writers must take into account the potential readership; there is a clear difference between reports that are written for practitioners in the clinical setting, those for funding bodies and a research dissertation or thesis. Employers and practitioners may be more interested in the results and implications of the

---

research for practice and less concerned with philosophical and theoretical issues, while academics see the latter as important and value the process of learning how to research. Occasionally, health professionals or academic writers feel it is more appropriate to write two separate reports on the research, one for the university in which they are taking their degree and the other for the practice setting. In all these reports, anonymity and confidentiality of the research participants are essential elements.

The format should match the research design; in a qualitative thesis, the rationale and the methodology section set a frame for the research. Readers and reviewers must be able to follow all the procedures and processes of the study, thus ensuring that the methods and logic of the study are explicit and open to public scrutiny (see chapter on validity). Background and prior assumptions of the researcher must also be divulged to others. On a practical level it is useful to have a style sheet, similar to the sheet that journal editors present to article writers, where the researcher notes down all the consistent elements, such as certain spellings, the type of referencing both in the chapters and at the end of the dissertation or report, the format for headings and other aspects, so this can be used throughout the report (advice from Wolcott, 2009). Many students lack consistency in style and spelling.

Supervisors will generally ask their students to write an outline for the research well before they attempt to write a full draft so that they have a tentative structure.

Use of the first person

When writing up introduction and methodology, it is our view that it is better that researchers write in the first person to show that they are accountable for their actions, and to implicitly and explicitly acknowledge their role as an active participant in the research. It can sound pompous and dull when they state 'the researcher has found ... the author does ... the writer considers ...' and so on, and Webb (2002), in a now long-standing editorial for the *Journal of Advanced Nursing*, claims that first person writing is more reader-friendly. Writing up qualitative research – and increasingly quantitative research – does not proceed in an objectified and neutral way. Gilgun (2010) too, advocates the use of the first person because researcher roles become integrated into the study. Researchers can use the first person when they describe what they themselves chose to do. For instance, researchers would not say when speaking about their own actions 'the author chose a sample, or the researcher used the methods ...' and so on. They might write 'I chose a purposive sample of ... I collected the data through ...'. It is equally important, however, that the first person is not overused, and the use of 'I think, I feel, I believe' throughout is not appropriate. Those who do not wish to use the first person might choose the passive form (although this is not considered good

English); for instance, 'a purposive sample was chosen ...' and so on. Wolcott (2009) confirms that writing in the first person acknowledges the presence and the crucial role of the researcher who comes to the inquiry with certain subjective assumptions which need be uncovered. Writing this more personal way would also involve the reader of the research account. (We attach a warning here: some universities and many journals wish the research to be written in the third person.)

Geertz (1988) warned two decades ago against the 'author evacuated text'; Charmaz and Mitchell (1996) speak of the 'myth of silent authorship' and encourage the inclusion and presence of the writer in the text. This means writing sometimes in the first person. Occasionally researchers also write in the first-person plural, 'we' to involve the reader, but this is unusual and not advisable as nobody knows to whom 'we' refers.

KEY POINT

Researchers write in the first person to show ownership of their own actions but should not overuse the first-person perspective.

The format of the report

The structure of a qualitative report is often organised in the following sequence, although this may differ between studies depending on the setting, type of method and other factors:

- *Title*
- *Abstract*
- *Table of contents* (in some guidelines this appears after acknowledgements)
- *Acknowledgement and dedication*
- *Introduction*
  - Background and rationale (justification) for the study, including its aim
  - Initial literature review (or overview of the literature)
- *Entry issues and ethical considerations* (sometimes placed in or after the methodology section)
- *Methodology and research design*
  - The philosophical basis
  - Description and justification of methods (including type of theoretical framework)
  - The sample and the setting
  - Specific techniques and procedures (such as interviewing and/or observation)
  - Data analysis
  - Trustworthiness and authenticity (or validity and reliability, depending on the terms used)

- *Findings/results and discussion* (separate or integrated, including a dialogue with the literature)
- *Conclusion*
  - What has been learnt through the research in relation to the aim and research questions
  - Limitations of the research
  - Implications for practice
  - Where the researcher or reader might go on from here
- *Reflections on the research* (this could be in the conclusion section)
- *References*
- *Appendices*

Qualitative writing may differ substantially from a quantitative report, although commonalities exist. The main distinction lies in the flexibility of the qualitative report. The findings and discussion are the most important elements of the final write-up (see Ponterotto and Grieger (2007) for advice on communicating qualitative research).

A list of abbreviations, acronyms and/or a glossary of terms employed and written in alphabetical order is useful before the first chapter or at the end of the study. The first time the terms are mentioned in the writing, they have to be written in full, with the abbreviations in brackets. From then on, abbreviations can be used.

Title

The title of a study is important, especially if it is presented as a student project, dissertation or thesis because it is the first and most immediate contact the reader has with the research, and its impact on judging the work can be considerable. We would argue for a concise but informative title which sounds interesting but not facetious. It must be remembered that it is initially a working title and may change when some of the research has been done, so it can encompass emergent ideas.

Example 18.1 Titles

A psychological structure pertaining to the meaning of recreational programmes in the natural environment for those living with and beyond cancer (Thurlow, 2020)
   Investigation into gendered aspects of older person care with delineation of care service and well-being impacts. (Tauzer, 2023)
   Becoming a Transformational Learning Facilitator (Robinson, 2023).

Writers often use explanatory subtitles; Silverman (2017) prefers two-part titles. The title gives a clear and succinct picture of the study's content. Punch (2016) advises that the title should not be long but contain all essential information. Novice researchers sometimes include redundancies in the title such as 'A Study of ...', 'Aspects of ...' or 'Inquiry', 'Analysis', 'Investigation'. These words clutter up the title and are obvious. Although the title should reflect the aim of the research, it would be clumsy to give the whole aim in the title. Questions usually do not make good titles, although there may be some exceptions.

The title page in a dissertation or thesis contains the title, the name of the researcher, the year and the name of the educational institution at which the student was enrolled. There is generally a pro forma for the title page at most universities. They also specify other details for the finished dissertation such as word allowance or size of margins. Obviously, this differs for other types of research.

Abstract

The abstract is a summary of the study and is written when the research is completed. In a dissertation or thesis, it appears on the page behind the title but before the table of contents and the full report. The abstract provides the reader with a brief overview of the research question and aim, methods adopted, sample and the main findings of the study. It might include the implications of the study in one or two succinct sentences.

Depending on the size and type of study, the abstract should contain between 200 and 500 words, usually contained in one sheet of A4 paper in single spacing and often written in the past tense. Writers should keep to the word limit specified for them by the university or commissioning agency and be selective about the content. Journal editors too, specify the form of the abstract which may be structured.

The abstract for a thesis or dissertation is generally a little longer than that for an article and provides a summary of the research. There is no need for a long rationale or introduction. All important information is included. Sometimes writers forget to include the size of the sample, the method or the results (in short and in clear language).

The abstract is the 'public face' of the study as it appears on databases, websites and in abstract books, so it is of major importance in the research. Alexandrov and Hennerici (2007) maintain that the abstract determines whether the work is chosen for inclusion and has to be presented and communicated in a readable and appropriate way.

Simkhada *et al.* (2013: 1) advise researchers to write the abstract after completion (they speak of academic papers but we suggest this also for other research reports, dissertations and theses). This means the researcher will not forget to include the most important points. They state that the abstract needs to be 'informative and accurate but also interesting'.

Example 18.2 Abstract from a PhD Thesis

This study explores and explains how people make sense of their long-term, potentially life-threatening, health condition. Thrombophilia offers an example of a little-researched condition which may not affect people significantly on a day-to-day basis, but can lead to acute illness. The second condition under consideration, asthma, was selected due to its similarity in this regard. The literature indicates that information about long-term conditions is acquired from various sources and influenced by experience. Such conditions are frequently perceived as being problematic. However, some are accepted, and affected individuals can achieve well-being. The literature does not yet offer insights into how knowledge may support this process of achieving well-being.

A constructivist grounded theory approach was adopted, and interviews used to collect data from 10 individuals affected by thrombophilia. Constant comparison of the data was carried out. Theoretical sampling suggested the inclusion of six people with a second long-term condition, and the process continued until saturation was reached.

Findings indicated a two-stage process. *Gaining knowledge* comprises of phases occurring pre-diagnosis and during diagnosis, and this assists participants in making sense of their condition. *Living with a long-term condition* consists of the phases making informed decisions, accepting the condition and living with it. Previous research has not elucidated this entire process or the importance of the pre-diagnosis phase.

Based on these findings, a theory is offered. This proposes that individuals diagnosed with a long-term condition create constructs about it, based on information and experiences, which are used as the foundation for decision-making.

Some people are able to accept their condition and its nuances. Those who understand their conditions, make informed decisions and accept it are able to live with it. Those who are unable to do so will live alongside their condition and do not integrate it into their lives (Roddis, 2015). (Abstracts from a Master's dissertation might be slightly shorter.)

Example 18.3 Abstract from an Article by Norton *et al.* (2014)

Aims and Objectives. To generate a grounded theory about female adolescent behaviour in the sun.

Background. Nurses have key roles in health promotion and skin cancer prevention. Adolescents' resistance to sun safety messages and their vulnerability to sunburn are of concern internationally. Understanding why young women do as they do in the sun may enhance skin cancer prevention, but their behaviour has not been explained before in the United Kingdom.

Design. The study incorporated a qualitative grounded-theory design using the approach of Glaser.

Methods. Qualitative data were gleaned from group and one-to-one, semi-structured interviews with 20 female participants aged 14–17, research memos and literature. Sampling was purposive and theoretical. Data collection, analysis and theory generation occurred concurrently. Data were analysed using the constant comparative method. Data collection ended when a substantive theory had been generated.

Results. Data analysis revealed five categories of findings: *fitting in*, *being myself*, *being physically comfortable*, *slipping up* and *being comfortable* (the core category). The theory generated around the core explains how young women direct their sun-related activities towards meeting their physical and psychosocial comfort needs.

Conclusions. A contribution of this research is the grounded theory explaining the behaviour of young women in the sun. Furthermore, the theory challenges assumptions that female adolescents necessarily take risks; it explains their sun-related activities in terms of comfort. The theory extends findings from other researchers' descriptive qualitative studies and also appears to apply to young people in countries other than the United Kingdom.

Relevance to Clinical Practice. Understanding the sun-related activity of young women in terms of physical and psychosocial comfort may help nurses to develop new approaches to skin cancer prevention. These could complement existing messages and humanise health promotion.

Acknowledgement and dedication

Traditionally, all researchers, especially PhD or MPhil candidates, give credit to those who supported, advised or supervised the research, and they also acknowledge the input of the participants. Often the writing is dedicated to particular individuals such as parents or spouses. Sometimes writers overwork and exaggerate 'thank you notes' or dedications, but of course, acknowledgement of others' help and support is important.

Contents

Academic research reports have a table of contents before the main chapters begin. It cannot be finished before the whole project is finalised and written. The content is sectioned into chapter headings and subheadings with page numbers. In an undergraduate student project, the table of contents should be concise and need not be too long and detailed. If there are too many short sections, the report could look cluttered with numbers.

Introduction

Background and rationale

In the introduction, the writer informs the audience about the research question or topic. The introduction consists of the background and context of the research as well as the aim – the overall purpose of the project. Writers explain why they have become interested in the question, how their project relates to the general topic area and what gap in health knowledge or education might be filled by the new research through linking the question to the potential implications for practice. In the introduction, the researcher explains the significance of the study for the clinical setting and how it could improve clinical practice or policy. Researchers need to justify the chosen topic, and why it is relevant for the profession and for themselves at this time. The background section sets the scene for the study. It is useful for the researcher to ask the 'so what?' question to keep the background section relevant.

Initial literature review (or overview of the literature)

This section can stand on its own, or it can become an integral part of the introduction. The literature in qualitative studies has a different place from that in quantitative research. Of course, it must show some of the relevant research that has been done in the field. The researchers summarise the main ideas from these studies, their problems and contradictions, and they show how these papers relate to the project in hand. It is important in qualitative reports to strike a balance between justifying a gap in knowledge that can be met by the qualitative study and to present an initial review that offers a comprehensive evaluation of the current state of the research knowledge in the field. This does not necessarily mean exploration of every piece of research in the field at the start of the study, nor to give a critical review of *all* the literature but the main foundational studies, those which are specifically relevant and up-to-date recent research. There will be differences in the kind of initial literature reviews that are written that reflect nuances and distinctions within the field or topic being studied. Gaps in knowledge become apparent at this point. At this stage, the research question is linked to the literature (see Chapter 3 for more details on literature review). By the end of the introductory section, the reader should be in no doubt that qualitative research, in the form suggested by the researcher, is most appropriate to meet the research aim which could be stated at the very beginning or at the end of the initial literature section. It needs to show the gap which needs to be closed by the present project.

Entry issues and ethical considerations

Health researchers describe entry and ethical issues (see Chapters 3 and 4). It must be stated how the participants were first approached and initial recruitment strategy, for instance, whether researchers advertised on a notice board or approached the potential participants personally. How did researchers gain permission from gatekeepers, those in the position of power to grant access to the setting (managers at various levels and local research ethics committees)? If patients are involved, their consultants or GPs might have to be asked for their permission if they are still under treatment.

Last, but most importantly, researchers should make explicit how the ethical principles were followed in the study, and how the participants' rights were protected. It is important that individual participants cannot be recognised in the report. To have permission from ethics committees might be essential, but it does not necessarily ensure that the researcher behaves ethically! The ethical principles and strategies to ensure the reader should form part of the written account.

Methodology and research design

The methodology chapter includes several subsections: the research design and methodology; the methods, including data collection, sampling, detailed interviewing or observation procedures, etc. and a description of the data analysis. In qualitative research, the methodology is of particular interest because the researcher is the main research tool and has to make explicit the path of the research, so that the reader knows about the details of design, biases or pre-understandings, relationships and limitations and is able to follow the decision trail. Hence, the methodology section is often longer than its equivalent in a quantitative study. Methodology and methods should have 'fit'.

Description and justification
The research design usually includes the main methods and the theoretical framework. Researchers briefly describe the methods they will adopt and the reasons and justification for it. They also explain the fit between the research question and the methodology.

The sample and setting
The sample is described in detail. Not all purposive sampling is fixed from the beginning (for instance, not in grounded theory (GT)). This is a feature of much qualitative research which sometimes confuses ethics committees or funding bodies. The writer describes the participants, who they were, how many were chosen and the reasons for the choice. Researchers tell the reader how they obtained their sample and portray the setting in which the study took place. If there is theoretical sampling, this must also be explained (see Chapter 11).

Specific techniques and procedures
The method section gives information about the data collection. The researcher describes the procedures such as interviewing, observation or other strategies that were used and any problems encountered. The outline should not be a general essay on procedures but a step-by-step description of the work in hand so that the reader can follow how the methods were applied. It is necessary that researchers give the reasons for using a particular methodology and research strategies and describe the procedures of collecting data. The reader should also know how the data were collected and stored.

Data analysis

The data analysis needs to be explained in detail and includes the ways in which, for example, data were coded and categorized, or how data were transformed to meaning units, and how theoretical constructs were generated from the data. It is useful, and essential in dissertations or theses, to give examples from the study. A detailed account of the chosen type of analysis is required. The readership is entitled to know whether a computer analysis was used. In a dissertation or thesis, some detail and examples of each step should be presented, so that the audit trail is clearly demonstrated.

Trustworthiness

This section will demonstrate how the researcher ensured the validity (or trustworthiness) of the research (see the relevant chapter for a discussion of this topic).

Findings/results and discussion

There are several ways to present qualitative findings and discussion. The first is written in the traditional format in which findings and discussion are separated and follow one another. Findings without discussion and comments do not always make a good storyline; therefore, the findings and discussion are more often integrated. This gives meaning to the report and shows the storyline more clearly (but again, no rigid rule exists about this). Some writers present a brief summary of the results in a diagram, and then discuss each major category (or construct, or theme) in a few sentences before starting the findings and discussion chapter. In each chapter, the data the researcher collected are discussed first. The relevant literature is integrated into the discussion where it fits best and serves as additional evidence for the particular category or as a challenge to the findings of the researcher. A dialogue with the literature needs to be ongoing throughout the research. There are a range of ways this later literature can be organized, the researcher reads throughout the process, and the literature is integrated with findings, or drawn into the discussion of findings, but this decision depends on preference and also the context and nature of the material in the study.

Telling the tale

In a qualitative report, writers tell a story which should be vivid and interesting as well as credible to the reader. The qualitative findings should communicate a 'sense of aliveness' so that the depth of the findings can resonate with the reader. In addition, a thesis should present an 'arc' with a beginning, middle and end, so as to facilitate 'a coherent sense of the whole' for the reader (as opposed to a fragmentation of many disconnected parts). This sometimes means writing and rewriting drafts until a storyline can be discerned clearly. Although there may be similarities with journalism or fiction, writers have to keep in mind that research accounts have a different purpose, namely to give an accurate and systematic analysis of the data and a discussion of the results. A good qualitative study need not be dry and mechanistic but reflects the researcher's involvement. The events, the people and their words and actions are made explicit, so that readers can experience the situation in a similar way to the researcher, albeit with the researcher's interpretations or more abstract descriptions of the phenomenon under study. The communicative element is of special importance in the presentation of qualitative research so it can make an impact on its readers and remind them that the participants are 'real' people. Holloway (2005: 282) reminds researchers that scientific writing need not be incomprehensible but should capture the audience's attention, have immediacy and present a good story.

The use of quotes from participants

Direct and verbatim quotes from interviews or excerpts from the fieldnotes are inserted at an appropriate place to show some of the data from which the results emerged. Sandelowski (1994) lists some of the uses of quotes in qualitative studies and argues that they give insight into people's experiences and their meanings and interpretations of the situation and illustrate the arguments of the researcher. The content of the quotes helps the reader to judge how the findings were derived from the data, to help establish the credibility of the emerging categories or themes and provide the reader with a means of auditing these. The writers, of course, must take care that the quotes convey the meanings and feelings of the participant and are directly connected with the themes the research seeks to illustrate. Sandelowski gives importance to both content and style of quote. A direct quote of the participants' words in a study makes the discussion lively and dynamic. Long rows of quotes or continuous duplication are not needed, and frequent very short quotes might make the study look fragmented. The choice of quotes should demonstrate that the data come from a wide range of participants rather than just one or two, except when the researcher explores deviant or negative cases. The quotes, according to Green and Thorogood (2018), are indeed examples of particular concepts to demonstrate to the reader that the ideas discussed are based on the data and used to illustrate the analysis. Quotes also confirm the credibility of the data in these authors' view. Corden and Sainsbury (2006: 98) point out that quotes help to 'clarify the links between data, interpretation and conclusions. They report that participants valued the inclusion of their own words as they felt their voices were heard and represented. Corden and Sainsbury advise researchers to consider carefully the ethical issues involved with using quotes such as, for instance, protection of identity and anonymity. Green and Thorogood state that consent for using the quotes must be obtained from participants.

The use of quotations from the literature

Trying to give substance to their own arguments, inexperienced health researchers often quote the words of experts. This can interrupt the storyline of the research. Sometimes it is better to avoid a quotation when it can be paraphrased or summarised, but of course, the idea should still be credited to the originator.

When a specific phrase is critical and written by a well-known expert or author of a classic text on the field of study, a quotation can be used. Occasionally, it does enhance a piece of writing and is appropriate. When using substantial quotes from books or articles, page numbers should be given.

We must warn researchers of two common mistakes. First, researchers often write in a very complex way and use incomprehensible terminology. In their fear of sounding simplistic and not academic, researchers in the field of healthcare often complicate and obscure simple and clear issues. It is important to express ideas in clear and unambiguous terms, although they should not, of course be simplistic. The second flaw is linked to a lack of analysis. It is not enough to simply give a collection of lengthy quotes and summarise their content. This is not analysis. Researchers have to develop their theoretical ideas and interpretations, build them into the study and then illustrate them with the relevant quotes from the participants.

The use of diagrams and flow charts

Diagrams and flowcharts throughout the report could make a research study clearer or demonstrate the pathway of the researcher. Patterns and processes can also be illustrated this way, as mentioned earlier. Pictures can enhance a study but should only be used when appropriate and necessary, their rationale and purpose should be clear. Verdinelli and Scagnoli (2013) provide examples of diagrams and charts.

Conclusion and implications

Generally, studies end with a conclusion. The conclusion is a summary of the findings in context. It must be directly related to the results of the specific study, and no new elements (or references) should be introduced here unless they are necessary. The conclusion reviews what has been learnt in relation to the aim, the theoretical ideas and propositions that emerged from the study. Dramatic and overly assertive conclusions can be dangerous and pretentious in a small project. Novice researchers seldom generate 'formal theory' or come to significant conclusions; their research is small in scope – although extensive in depth; however, the modest scope does not mean that the piece of research has no importance or implications for the clinical area.

Woods (2005) has a list of considerations for the conclusion. He asks researchers whether their writing has answered the questions asked, whether there are weaknesses and limitations, and how these can be addressed. Of course, it is important to demonstrate that the study has contributed to knowledge in the field or that the conclusion provides a new light on the topic. The conclusion should be placed in the context of conclusions of other studies, the more general framework of the area under study and how it fits within the global picture of the topic. The full discussion of relevant related literature has been given however in previous chapters as is usual in qualitative research.

In health research and other projects for clinical and professional settings, the conclusion contains the implications and, if appropriate, the recommendations that could be made on the basis of the results. The implications can be integrated into the conclusion, they can be discussed towards its end or they can form a separate section following on from the conclusion. The implications must be based *directly* on the findings of the study which has just been completed; all too often they are not linked sufficiently to the findings and based on the work of other researchers. Any significant policy implications can also be addressed here.

Some researchers tend to overestimate the importance of their research, and this can be avoided as readers are sceptical about exaggerated claims.

To check the quality of their conclusion, researchers might ask the following questions:

- Why have I included this here? (on reflection about a statement)
- What are the main issues arising from the data?
- Is my argument clear?
- How has the study achieved its aims?
- What were the answers to the research questions?
- What is new and different in my research?
- What new insights have been achieved?
- What has it contributed to knowledge in the area of study?
- How does this fit into the wider context of knowledge in this field?
- What are the limits/limitations of my study?
- What are the implications for my profession (or for policy) that derive from my research?

Reflections and reflexivity

Many academic researchers reflect on their project and adopt a critical stance to it, usually towards the end of their dissertation or thesis. They demonstrate how the research could be improved, extended or illuminated from another angle. At this point, they might point to its limitations and their own biases, which they might not have made explicit in the main body of the study and describe some of the problems they encountered. Not all studies contain this reflective section; sometimes they are part of the conclusion at other times they are built into the study. Nurses and other health professionals who take a reflective stance could discuss at this point how they have professionally and personally developed and changed through the research. The description of their own location in the research is called reflexivity (see Chapter 18).

A statement about validation of a qualitative study by a survey or other quantitative methods might suggest a lack of awareness that a qualitative study can stand on its own, has its own validation procedures and cannot be judged from the quantitative researcher's point of view, but occasionally a direction for a different type of research might have to be indicated.

Referencing

For academic studies the Harvard system of referencing is generally used, but other formal systems of referencing, such as Vancouver style, may be acceptable to the students' supervisors, or required by journals or funding bodies. It is best to find out about this before the start of the study from supervisors, course leaders or handbooks and journals. Sometimes slight variations in advice are given in libraries, reflecting institutional preferences, but the reference information must be current, accurate and detailed in a research report. Sloppy references are the cause of criticism and might well generate 'a negative halo effect'.

The writer should compare the references in the text with the selected bibliography and make sure that every reference is included. We often find that student referencing is incomplete, incorrect or insufficient. Page (the singular) is shortened to p.; pages – the plural – to pp. but for journals the pp. or p. is usually left out. The title of the book or the name of the journal should be underlined or written in italics. Page numbers are stated in the references when an article in a journal is given, or a chapter in an edited book is referenced. Direct quotations from books or articles need page numbers after name and date (for instance: Smith 2021: 7 or Smith 2019, p. 7; Smith 2020, pp. 7–11).

Educational institutions, within certain parameters, may have their own rules about referencing. Publishers of books and articles, too, use different ways of referencing. In this book for instance, we follow the guidelines of our publisher.

Appendices

A table of informants (with pseudonyms), their ages, experience or length of service is sometimes included by writers (making sure, however, that anonymity is preserved, particularly when the participants or informants might easily be recognised). An interview guide and a sample interview transcript (in a study that uses interviews) could be attached as an example for the reader to help in understanding the development of the data collection. Some fieldnotes from observations might be given to demonstrate their use. Appendices depend on the advice given to researchers and on their own common sense, but there should not be too many sections. Sometimes researchers attach the formal initial letter to participants or an example of the letter of permission. A copy of the letter of approval from the ethical committee should be attached, and where appropriate, the researcher blocks out the address and location of the research. The words in appendices do not generally count as part of the dissertation or thesis.

The appendices (plural of appendix) are usually placed at the very end of the study after the bibliography in the order in which they appear in the chronology of the study. For instance, the example of the initial letter to participants would be placed before the exemplar of an interview transcript. Universities might have their own rules about the use of appendices or footnotes.

Particularly detailed advice is given in Panda (2014) which is useful for PhD students. *The origin of this article is not completely clear.*

Critical assessment and evaluation

Researchers must be aware that the readers of a research study or report evaluate and judge the quality and credibility of the research and look for particular components and details. For these reasons, a short guide to evaluating qualitative inquiry follows, which is based on a number of writings by others, such as Horsburgh (2003), Ryan *et al.* (2007) and Green and Thorogood (2018). It is clear that many, although not all, criteria and issues for appraisal are different and distinct in qualitative research. The following checklist contains important factors to consider when evaluating a qualitative research study. It would be useful for researchers to examine their own study in the light of these elements.

Guide to research evaluation

The Research Question and Method
Is the research problem or question suitable and feasible for qualitative research?
Is there a clear rationale for the study and the methodological approach?
Does the study show that the data of the researcher have priority?

The Abstract
Does it state the aim and describe the methodology and methods (including sampling)?
Does it summarise results, conclusions and implications?

The Literature
Is there an initial overview that demonstrates the gap in knowledge?
Are there connections to existing and relevant theories?
Has the appropriate literature related to the findings been integrated into the study?
Are the references comprehensive, relevant and up-to-date, and do they include some foundational texts?

The Sample

Does the researcher use purposive sampling (including theoretical sampling if appropriate)?

Are the criteria for sampling made explicit?

Is the sampling explained adequately?

Is the type and size of sample justified?

Entry and Ethical Issues

Does the researcher state how they gained access to the participants?

Were the rights of participants safeguarded (including their right to withdraw from the study)?

Are issues of anonymity and confidentiality discussed in relation to the study?

Are issues of power taken into account?

If vulnerable people, for example children, are included in the sample, is this inclusion justified?

Are major ethical issues discussed?

Has the study been approved by ethics committees and review boards?

Data Collection and Analysis

What are the data sources, and are they appropriate for the study?

How are the data collected, transcribed and stored?

Is the method of analysis identified and described (with examples)?

Is the data analysis systematic and detailed?

(In GT: Do data collection and analysis interact?)

The Findings and Discussion

Is the presentation of the findings appropriate for a qualitative approach?

How have these findings been discussed in relation to the literature?

Do the findings communicate sufficient depth (avoid superficial analysis)?

Does the researcher explain the trustworthiness (validity) of the study?

Is the 'audit trail' traced in detail?

How have validity issues been managed?

Is there an element of reflexivity?

Conclusions and Implications

Has the study met its aim?

Does the conclusion clearly state what was learned from the research?

Do the conclusions come directly from the data?

Are the implications for clinical practice discussed?

Do they emerge directly from the findings of the study?

Publishing and presenting the research

If the findings are significant, the researcher has the responsibility to disseminate them to a wider group such as colleagues and other health professionals or, if acknowledged as appropriate by experts, to lay people.

Books

Sometimes health professionals produce a book based on their thesis or a chapter in an edited book. Most publishers have guidelines for writing book proposals. The proposal then goes to their editorial board to decide whether the book is worth publishing in their view, and commercially viable. If their proposal is not accepted, the study might be too esoteric or not interesting for a larger market. Commercial considerations are the main concern of publishers, and these depend on the general appeal of the piece of research. Editors are, of course, also concerned about the quality of the content and the ability of the researcher to write clearly and in an accessible style.

Articles

More often, students who have carried out research publish an article in a professional or academic journal, often with their supervisor. The length and style of the article will depend on the type of journal; for instance, articles in the *International Journal of Nursing Studies* and *Journal of Advanced Nursing* are more academic and generally longer than those in professional journals such as the *Nursing Times* (their purpose and readership differ). There are professional journals for most health professions, for instance in pharmacy, physiotherapy, medicine, medical or nursing education, counselling, etc. Articles have higher standing in research circles than chapters in books because articles in international academic journals are refereed by experts in the field, are more likely to be cited (used) by others and therefore are used as an indicator of research quality in, for example, the UK Research Excellence Framework.

The detailed guidelines for manuscripts are laid out at the front or the back of the hard copy journal or available on journal websites labelled 'Guidance for Authors'. Some journal editors want a very detailed description of the methods adopted (for instance, the journal *Midwifery*), others claim that a well-known and widely published methodology, such as GT, can be summarised rather than discussed in great detail (*Sociology of Health and Illness*). Writers must take into account the different styles and guidelines of these journals. As a long research study cannot be fully discussed in article format, researchers choose what to include or exclude. For example, just one chapter, one category or a methodological issue might form the basis of the article. Journal editors or academics sometimes speak of 'salami slicing' the research; this practice is appropriate for lengthy and in-depth studies which cannot be reported in a single article. The European Association of Science Editors (EASE, 2016) offer detailed advice and a toolkit that is available on the World Wide Web.

It is important to write in a lively manner in an article or a book based on qualitative research. This can be achieved through a good storyline and enhanced through vignettes or excerpts from interviews or fieldnotes, taking into account, of course, that individuals should not be recognised in the descriptions. Good diagrams might clarify some of the aspects of the work. Different journals address different audiences.

In an introduction, the researcher gives a short overview of the work, including the research question and aim of the research and a brief justification for both (Anderson, 2010). The method(ology) should be described, and the rest consists of the findings and discussion sections just as in a dissertation or thesis but in very much shorter form. The conclusion summarises what has been learnt with the implications directly drawn from this.

Types of article

The book by Corbin and Strauss (2008) states that three types of paper are published in journals, intended for different readership:
1 For academic colleagues
2 For practitioners
3 For lay readers

Articles for academic colleagues

There are those colleagues who have a particular interest in the theoretical and methodological framework as well as in the research topic and implications of the findings for practice. The *Journal of Advanced Nursing, Physiotherapy: Theory and Practice, Midwifery* and *Qualitative Health Research,* for instance, are examples of journals publishing this type of articles and having high-impact ratings within these disciplines. Even the *British Medical Journal* has recently published articles on qualitative research. The journals *Qualitative Research* and *Qualitative Inquiry* deal mainly with methodological issues but are not professional nursing or healthcare publications (*Qualitative Inquiry* and *Qualitative Health Research* are journals published in the United States while *Qualitative Research* is published in Britain). *International Journal of Qualitative Studies on Health and Well-being* publishes a range of research methods exploring diverse contexts. *Nurse Education Today* covers educational issues and research in nurse and midwifery education. The *International Journal of Nursing Studies* and the *Journal of Clinical Nursing* are also high-ranking journals from the United Kingdom, but there are many others as well. The academic standard and quality of most journals is high, and their editors and reviewers demand high standards in their articles. *Social Science and Medicine* is a particularly prestigious journal but a novice might find it difficult to publish in it.

Articles for practitioners

Examples of journals intended to assist practitioners are *Nursing Times, Journal of Nursing Management,* the *British Journal of Midwifery, Medical Education.* Their purpose it to make potential research impacts more accessible for busy professionals. In these journals, one can find articles which describe findings and address the implications of these findings for clinical practice. Often the writers of these articles develop ideas that assist in the understanding of patients or the work of nurses, midwives and professions allied to medicine.

Articles for the lay reader

Some articles are meant for lay readers and the public. Although health researchers do not always write for this readership, it is good practice as an article in a specialist magazine could actually help members of a group or the general population. For instance, an article on research into hormone replacement therapy in a women's journal might give information to women, although it would have to be short, clear and accessible. It is necessary that researchers write with integrity and factual accuracy; however, the writing should be clear to lay people and not written in an academic style.

Student articles

All students carrying out PhD or MPhil and even MA/MSc research should attempt writing articles; some universities encourage this during the process of the research, others suggest writing after completion of the research degree. There is an academic tradition that candidates publish with their supervisors who, of course, have had a major input in the research and will help in refining the article, critiquing it and possibly writing sections for it. Nevertheless, the student's, not the supervisor's, name should be first on the list of authors. In early articles, it is useful to seek the help and advice of supervisors who know the different journals and their editors' styles and preferences.

It is very useful for all students to publish, if their work is acknowledged as valuable by their supervisors or managers, as they not only get used to disseminating their research but it will also eventually enhance their status within the profession. The research is finally completed when the findings have been written up and published, and Evans (2008: 1) even adds that 'research that is not written up is wasted'.

Alternative forms of presenting or disseminating the research

There are a variety of ways to present or disseminate qualitative research. Keen and Todres (2007) describe some of these non-traditional forms which might include theatrical performances, dance, poetry or others. A doctoral student for instance wrote a play based on her research with old people, others have presented films which are rooted in the research with patients, or included photographs. Some of alternative forms of presenting the data or findings evoke strong feelings in the audience (see chapter on performative social science, in particular the work by Kip Jones).

Summary

The following are the main points to remember when writing up qualitative research:

- There is flexibility in writing research accounts.
- The structure of a qualitative research account often differs from that of a quantitative study.
- Ethical issues and access must be addressed as in all research.
- The findings and discussion are the major part of the study.
- There is a dialogue with the literature, generally in the discussion.
- Reports in qualitative health research need a strong conclusion with new insights drawn out, and implications for the profession and/or clinical practice directly based on the findings.
- The research should have a good storyline which communicates with the reader.
- To be of use in practical terms, the research needs to be disseminated.

References

Alexandrov, A.V. and Hennerici, M.G. (2007) Writing good abstracts. *Cerebrovascular Diseases*, **23** (4), 256–259.

Anderson, C. (2010) Presenting and evaluating qualitative research. *American Journal of Pharmaceutical Education*, **74** (8), 141–152.

Charmaz, K. and Mitchell, R.G. (1996) The myth of silent authorship: self, substance and style in ethnographic writing. *Symbolic Interaction*, **9** (4), 285–302.

Corbin, J. and Strauss, A. (2008) *Basics of Qualitative Research: Techniques and Procedures for Developing Grounded Theory*, 3rd edn, Sage, Los Angeles, CA.

Corden, A. and Sainsbury, R. (2006) Exploring 'quality': research participants' perspectives on using quotes. *International Journal of Social Research Methodology*, **9** (2), 97–110.

EASE (The European Association of Science Editors) (2016). Available at http://www.ease.org.uk/publications/ease-toolkit-authors/how-write-good-qualitative-paper.

Evans, R. (2008) Getting the message across. *Qualitative Researcher*, **8**, 1.

Geertz, C. (1988) *Works and Lives: The Anthropologist as Author*, Stanford University Press, Palo Alto, CA.

Gilgun, J.F. (2010) Grab and good science: writing up the results of qualitative research. *Qualitative Health Research*, **15** (2), 256–262.

Green, J. and Thorogood, N. (2018) *Qualitative Methods for Health Research*, 4th edn, Sage, London.

Holloway, I. (ed.) (2005) Qualitative writing, in *Qualitative Research in Health Care*, Open University Press, Maidenhead, pp. 270–286.

Horsburgh, D. (2003) Evaluation of qualitative research. *Journal of Clinical Nursing*, **12** (2), 307–312.

Keen, S. and Todres, L. (2007) Communicating qualitative research findings: an annotated bibliographic review of non-traditional dissemination strategies. Bournemouth University.

Norton, L., Holloway, I. and Galvin, K. (2014) Comfort versus risk: a grounded theory about female adolescent behaviour in the sun. *Journal of Clinical Nursing*, **23** (13–14), 1889–1899.

Panda, S. and Assistant Librarian Chandigarh (2014). *Writing up a PhD (Qualitative Research)*. Part of this first found in Lynch, T. (2014). Writing up your PhD (Qualitative Research) Independent Study Version. University of Edinburgh. English Language Teaching Centre.

Ponterotto, J.G. and Grieger, I. (2007) Effectively communicating qualitative research. *Counseling Psychologist*, **35** (3), 404–430.

Punch, K.F. (2016) *Developing Effective Research Proposals*, 3rd edn, Sage, London.

Reay, T., Mondeiro, P., Zafar, A. and Glaser, V. (2019) Presenting findings from qualitative research: one size does not fit all!. *The Production of Managerial Knowledge and Organizational Theory: New Approaches to Writing, Producing and Consuming Theory*, 201–216. doi:10.1108/S0733-558X201000009011.

Robinson, P. (2023) Participatory, PhD thesis, Bournemouth University.

Roddis, J. (2015) Living with a long-term condition: a grounded theory. Unpublished PhD thesis, Bournemouth University.

Ryan, F., Coughlan, M. and Cronin, P. (2007) A step by step guide to critiquing research. Part 2: qualitative research. *British Journal of Nursing*, **16** (12), 738–744.

Sandelowski, M. (1994) The use of quotes in qualitative research. *Research in Nursing and Health*, **17** (6), 479–483.

Silverman, D. (2017) *Doing Qualitative Research: A Practical Handbook*, 5th edn, Sage, London.

Simkhada, P.P., van Teijlingen, E. and Hundley, V. (2013) Writing an academic paper for publication. *Health Renaissance*, **11** (1), 1–5.

Tauzer, J. (2023) Ethnography, PhD thesis, Birmingham City University.

Thurlow, O. (2020) Phenomenology, PhD thesis, University of Brighton.

Verdinelli, S. and Scagnoli, N.I. (2013) Data display in qualitative research. *International Journal of Qualitative Methods*, **12**, 350–381.

Webb, C. (2002) Editorial: how to make your article more readable. *Journal of Advanced Nursing*, **38** (1), 1.

Wolcott, H.F. (2009) *Writing up Qualitative Research*, 3rd edn, Sage, Thousand Oaks, CA.

Woods, P. (2005) *Successful Writing for Qualitative Researchers*, 2nd edn, Routledge, London.

Further Reading

Heinrich, K. (2008) *A Nurse's Guide to Presenting and Publishing: Dare to Share*, Jones & Bartlett, Cambridge, MA.

Holloway, I. and Brown, L. (2012) *Essentials of a Qualitative Doctorate*, LeftCoast Press, Walnut Creek, CA.

Murray, R. (2013) *Writing for Academic Journals (Study Skills)*, 3rd edn, Open University Press, Maidenhead.

Lynch, T. (2014) *Writing up your PhD (Qualitative Research)* Independent Study Version. University of Edinburgh. English Language Teaching Centre.

Ramani, S. and Mann, K. (2015) Introducing medical educators to qualitative study design: twelve steps from inception to completion. *Medical Teacher*, **38** (5), 456–463.

Sandelowski, M. and Leeman, J. (2012) Writing usable qualitative health research findings. *Qualitative Health Research*, **22** (10), 1404–1414.

van Teitlingen, E., Simkhala, B., Regmi, P. *et al.* (2022) Reflections and variations in PhD viva regulations; "And the options are…" *Journal of Education and Research*, **12**, 61–74.

Final Note

Researchers need to be aware that qualitative research operates with different tenets and principles from quantitative research as was explained earlier. The exploratory nature of this form of inquiry sometimes generates critical comments, by those who do not wish to use it, even from insiders who know its hazards and difficulties. There are some problems and pitfalls, some of which have been discussed in previous chapters.

Many novice health researchers, particularly students, see a research report and a good story line in an academic journal and think that using this type of inquiry is easy, and that they might do it more quickly than quantitative research. Problems arise from this misapprehension and lack of knowledge about the issues involved and their complexity. The data collection is *relatively* straightforward if ethical guidelines, moral principles and methodological tenets are adhered to, but analysis can often be difficult and complex, especially as researchers do not know whether the participants are 'telling the truth', and even if they do, they tell it as they perceive it. However this is true of all research that relies on self-reports, whether qualitative or not. Research with human beings in their context is difficult.

The most serious claim against qualitative research states that it is not scientific. This statement is based on a 'naïve model of science'. The claim rests on a misunderstanding about the nature of social science methods which are fundamentally different from those based on natural science (discussed in Chapter 2). The researcher's aim in the social and human sciences is a search for meaning and understanding of human experiences and social phenomena. Indeed, there was an open letter to the editors of the *British Medical Journal* (Greenhalgh *et al.*, 2016) when 76 senior academics from 11 countries who are mainly medical professionals challenged the journal editors and asked them 'to consider their policy of rejecting qualitative research on the ground of low priority'. These contributors to research recognise the importance of qualitative inquiry.

It must however be stressed that qualitative research, just like quantitative inquiry, needs a systematic, robust and transparent approach, especially because it can be ambiguous, and participants' thoughts and feelings might not always

---

Qualitative Research in Nursing and Healthcare, Fifth Edition.
Immy Holloway and Kathleen Galvin.
© 2024 John Wiley & Sons Ltd. Published 2024 by John Wiley & Sons Ltd.

be coherent nor well ordered. An advantage of this research is that it represents and illustrates the complexity and diversity of human beings, their behaviour and actions, even though it cannot always fully do so. According to Hammersley (2008: 9), '. . . any idea that it is possible to produce a stable, genuine, complete representation of the social world can only be an illusion . . .'

It is essential to demonstrate validity (trustworthiness), credibility and consistency; outsiders should be able to evaluate it by following the researcher's decision trail (see Chapter 18). The necessary evidence in qualitative research, however, comes from the participants and hence is not wholly predictable or always factual but based on perceptions of participants, researchers and readers (different in degree from that in quantitative research). Of course, it must be taken into account that participants, researchers and readers speak from a particular perspective which is influenced by location and culture.

Another assertion is that qualitative research can be anecdotal and trivial. Anecdotal evidence may be based on personal perceptions and feelings which are important in health research, *Good* qualitative research, however, is never trivial because it searches for in-depth answers to important questions such as the reasons for participants' actions and feelings. One of the strengths of qualitative research is its open-endedness and flexibility; it explores 'underlying values, beliefs and assumptions' (Choy, 2014). Researchers often find new questions and answers which have not been considered before.

Packer (2011: 3) claims that qualitative research is not just a set of techniques and procedures but 'a reconceptualization of the social sciences as forms of inquiry in which we work to transform our forms of life'. This is particularly so in the arena of health and care. Good qualitative research is transformative and should reflect the human condition through exploring perspectives, actions and experiences of the participants.

References

Choy, L.T. (2014) The strengths and weaknesses of research methodology: comparison and complementarity between qualitative and quantitative approaches. *Journal of Humanities and Social Science*, **19** (4), 99–104.

Greenhalgh, T., Annandale, E., Ashcroft, R. *et al.* (2016) An open letter to The *BMJ* editors on qualitative research. *BMJ*, **352**, Pi563.

Hammersley, M. (2008) *Questioning Qualitative Inquiry*, Sage, London.

Packer, M. (2011) *The Science of Qualitative Research*, CUP, New York.

Glossary

Abstract: A short summary of the research including research topic, methods aim, procedures such as sampling, data sources, data collection and analysis and findings and implications.

Aide mémoire (or aide memoir): Words or phrases to remind researchers of the focus or the agenda of the research during in-depth interviewing.

Assumption: A belief, conjecture or preconception of the researcher based on a hunch or experience which has not been verified by evidence.

Audit trail: A detailed description of all the steps taken by the researcher in the research

Authenticity: A term used to show that the findings of a research project are authentic and represent the participants' perspectives.

Autoethnography: An ethnographic approach where writers or researchers explore their own experiences which then become the focus of the research.

Axial coding: Axial coding in GT refers to the process of relating codes, categories and concepts to each other, through an inductive and interpretive process (term used in Straussian GT).

Bias: A predisposition, inclination or even distortion in the processing of research (a problematic concept rooted in quantitative research).

Bracketing (in phenomenology): A process by which researchers set aside their assumptions about the phenomenon under study.

CADQAS: Computer-aided/assisted qualitative analysis software.

Case study: Research on a unit of study (an individual, a group, an event) with clear boundaries.

Category: A group of concepts – a unit of analysis – which shares traits and is given a label by the researcher.

Causality: A link between cause and effect – where the cause generates the effect.

Coding (in qualitative analysis): Examining and breaking down the data into pieces of text and naming them.

Concept: An abstract idea produced by specific instances.

Qualitative Research in Nursing and Healthcare, Fifth Edition.
Immy Holloway and Kathleen Galvin.
© 2024 John Wiley & Sons Ltd. Published 2024 by John Wiley & Sons Ltd.

Confidentiality: A principle in ethics where the communication between the researcher and participants is kept private and not disclosed under the name of the participant (but see confidentiality in research)

Constant comparison (in grounded theory): A technique in data collection and analysis where incoming data are compared with those previously collected.

Construct: A construct is built on concepts or categories and has a high level of abstraction and theory.

Constructionism (social constructionism): A belief or supposition that human beings are creating their own social reality, and that the social world cannot exist independent of human beings.

Context sensitivity: An awareness of context.

Contextualisation: Researchers locate people, data and processes in their specific social context.

Core category (in grounded theory): A central phenomenon which links or integrates all other categories in the research.

Criterion (plural criteria): A standard by which something is judged.

Critical theory: The view that people can critically evaluate social phenomena and change society in order to become emancipated and which has its origin in Marxism.

Data (plural but also in use as singular): The information collected by researchers which they analyse to draw their findings and conclusions.

Data analysis: Organisation, reduction and transformation of the gathered data.

Deductive reasoning: Reasoning that proceeds from general principles to explain specific cases.

Delimitations: The boundaries of the research showing what is included or excluded.

Description: A detailed account of the features of a phenomenon, setting or situation.

Design (research design): The plan of the research, including strategies and procedures for sampling, data collection and analysis.

Deviant case: An occurrence or instance that is contrary to what has been found in the rest of the data; an example where some elements of the data do not fit into the working propositions or initial explanations of the researcher.

Emic perspective: The 'insider's' point of view which is culture-bound (see also etic perspective), a term used specifically in anthropology.

Epistemology: The theory of knowledge, an area of philosophy concerned with the nature of human knowledge.

Ethnography: Anthropological (or sociological) research concerned with a description of a culture or group and its members' experiences and interpretations. An ethnography is the completed product of ethnographic research.

Etic perspective: The outsider's point of view, the perspective of the observer or researcher (see also emic perspective).

Exclusion criteria (singular: criterion): Conditions/factors/people that are excluded on the selection of sample.

Exhaustive description (in phenomenology): Writing that is comprehensive and captures the participants' experience in-depth and exhaustively.

External validity: Generalisability (see generalisability).

Field: The general area and/or the setting of the research.

Fieldnotes: Notes and records made by the researcher from observations in the field.

Fieldwork (initially a term from anthropology): The collection of data 'in the field' by observation, interviewing and so on, outside the laboratory or library.

Focus group: A group of individuals with experience of a particular phenomenon who provide information about it.

Gatekeepers: People who have the power to allow or restrict access to an organisation, a setting, or participants for research.

Generalisability: The extent to which the findings of a qualitative study can be generalised, that is, applied to other settings or situations.

Grounded theory: A research approach which generates theory from the data through constant comparison, initially developed by Strauss and Glaser.

Hermeneutics: A phenomenological research approach which focuses on the interpretation and meaning of text rather than the description of a phenomenon.

Hypothesis: An assumption, theory or tentative statement based on limited evidence of a relationship between variables which can be tested, verified or falsified.

Idiographic methods: An approach to knowledge where methods focus on the unique rather than the general. These differ from *nomothetic methods* (qv) that seek law-like generalities subsuming individual cases.

Immersion: The process whereby researchers are engaged and involved in the field.

In vivo code: A verbatim term from participants (see grounded theory).

Inclusion criteria (singular 'criterion'): Factors or conditions that are taken into account or will be met in the choice of sample (see also exclusion criteria).

Induction: A reasoning process in which researchers move from specific instances to the general.

Informant: An individual who, as a member of the group under study, participates in the research and helps the researcher to interpret the culture of the group (see also key informant).

Informed consent: A voluntary agreement of participants to take part in a study after they have been informed of and understand the nature and aim of its nature.

Interview guide: An array of questions which might be used flexibly in in-depth interviews. (Not interview schedule as in quantitative research.)

Interviewer effect (also observer effect): The effect of the researcher's (interviewer's or observer's) presence on the research.

Iteration: Repetitive movement between parts of the research text and the whole, between raw data and analysed data.

Key informant (in ethnography): A member of a culture or group who is an expert on its customs and rules.

Limitations: Restrictions in the scope of the research.

Member check: Feedback from participants and verification of their perspectives.

Memoing: Records and notes from the field of varying degrees of abstraction.

Method: Strategy for collecting, analysing and interpreting data.

Methodology: The framework of theories and principles on which methods and research strategies are based.

Narrative: The account of experiences and related events.

Nomothetic: Having law-like generalities, tendency to generalise (see also idiographic methods).

Objectivity: A neutral and unbiased stance, not distorted by feelings or personal assumptions, and free from individual perceptions.

Ontology: A branch of philosophy concerning the nature of being, related to assumptions about reality and existence.

Paradigm: A theoretical framework (pattern, model) to reality recognised by a community of scholars. A position that provides the researcher with a set of principles to guide the research.

Participant: A person who takes part in qualitative research.

Participant observation: Observation in which researchers/observers participate in the setting they study.

Phenomenology: A philosophical movement which explores the study of consciousness. In research it explores the meaning of individuals' lived experience through their own description.

Phenomenon: The central occurrence, event or experience to be researched (see phenomenology)

Pilot study: A small-scale trial run or feasibility study of research (not usual in qualitative research).

Positivism: A philosophical approach to scientific methods which aims to find general laws and regularities (oriented towards cause and effect) based on the methods of the natural sciences.

Premature closure: Arriving too early at an explanation before the research is fully analysed.

Progressive focusing: Starting with broad questions which become gradually more specific in the research.

Pseudonym: Fictitious name given to participants to protect their anonymity.

Purposive (or purposeful) sampling: A sample chosen by certain criteria relevant to the research question.

QAQDAS: Computer-assisted data analysis.

Raw data: Unanalysed data.

Reflective lifeworld research: A research method that builds on phenomenological philosophy and has at its core reflection, human intentionality and capacity for finding meanings.

Reflexivity: Reflecting on and critically examining one's own position and influence in the research.

Reliability: Consistency of a research tool.

Research account: A written record or report of a research study.

Research aim: The statement by researchers of what they want to achieve, related to the research question.

Research question: A statement which identifies the problem or question that guides a study.

Rigour: Accuracy and truthfulness.

Saturation: A state where no new data linked to the specific study and developing theory emerge.

Serendipity: An unexpected discovery and a pleasant surprise.

Storyline: The plot of a narrative.

Subjectivity: A personal and individual perspective influenced by one's own background and assumptions based on experience.

Symbolic interactionism: An interpretive approach in sociology that focuses on meaning in interaction, particularly language and signals.

Tacit knowledge: Informal or implicit knowledge often unrecognised and not articulated.

Theoretical sampling: A sampling technique which proceeds on the basis of emerging concepts and is guided by developing theory (see grounded theory).

Theoretical sensitivity: Sensitivity and awareness of meaning in the data.

Theory: A set of concepts, principles and propositions that explains phenomena.

Thick description: Dense detailed and conceptual description which depicts events and actions within a social context.

Triangulation: A way of validating the research by using different methods (the most common way), data collection approaches, investigators or theoretical perspectives in the study of one phenomenon (e.g. qualitative and quantitative methods, interviews and observation).

Validity: The extent to which the research does what it intends to do, the extent to which researchers' findings are accurate, reflect the purpose of the study and represent reality (validity in qualitative research differs from that in quantitative research).

(This glossary has been developed from a variety of sources but mainly from previous editions of this book.)

Index

Qualitative Research in Nursing and Healthcare, Fifth Edition.
Immy Holloway and Kathleen Galvin.
© 2024 John Wiley & Sons Ltd. Published 2024 by John Wiley & Sons Ltd.